Neuroradiology Emergencies

Guest Editor

ALISA D. GEAN, MD

NEUROIMAGING CLINICS
OF NORTH AMERICA

www.neuroimaging.theclinics.com

Consulting Editor
SURESH K. MUKHERJI, MD

November 2010 • Volume 20 • Number 4

SAUNDERS an imprint of ELSEVIER, Inc.

W.B. SAUNDERS COMPANY
A Division of Elsevier Inc.

1600 John F. Kennedy Boulevard • Suite 1800 • Philadelphia, Pennsylvania 19103-2899

http://www.theclinics.com

NEUROIMAGING CLINICS OF NORTH AMERICA Volume 20, Number 4
November 2010 ISSN 1052-5149, ISBN 13: 978-1-4557-0529-0

Editor: Joanne Husovski
Developmental Editor: Natalie Whitted

Neuroimaging Clinics of North America (ISSN 1052-5149) is published quarterly by Elsevier Inc., 360 Park Avenue South, New York, NY 10010-1710. Months of issue are February, May, August, and November. Business and editorial offices: 1600 John F. Kennedy Blvd., Suite 1800, Philadelphia, PA 19103-2899. Business and editorial offices: 6277 Sea Harbor Drive, Orlando, FL 32887-4800. Periodicals postage paid at New York, NY, and additional mailing offices. Subscription prices are USD 314 per year for US individuals, USD 436 per year for US institutions, USD 158 per year for US students and residents, USD 363 per year for Canadian individuals, USD 546 per year for Canadian institutions, USD 461 per year for international individuals, USD 546 per year for international institutions and USD 226 per year for Canadian and foreign students and residents. To receive student/resident rate, orders must be accompanied by name of affiliated institution, date of term, and the *signature* of program/residency coordinator on institution letterhead. Orders will be billed at individual rate until proof of status is received. Foreign air speed delivery is included in all *Clinics* subscription prices. All prices are subject to change without notice. POSTMASTER: Send address changes to *Neuroimaging Clinics of North America*, Elsevier Health Sciences Division, Subscription Customer Service, 3251 Riverport Lane, Maryland Heights, MO 63043. Telephone: 1-800-654-2452 (U.S. and Canada); 314-447-8871 (outside U.S. and Canada). Fax: 314-447-8029. E-mail: journalscustomerservice-usa@elsevier.com (for print support); journalsonlinesupport-usa@elsevier.com (for online support).

Reprints. For copies of 100 or more of articles in this publication, please contact the Commercial Reprints Department, Elsevier Inc., 360 Park Avenue South, New York, NY 10010-1710. Tel.: 212-633-3812; Fax: 212-462-1935; E-mail: reprints@elsevier.com.

Neuroimaging Clinics of North America is covered by *Excerpta Medical/EMBASE,* the RSNA Index of Imaging Literature, *MEDLINE/PubMed (Index Medicus),* MEDLINE/MEDLARS, SciSearch, Research Alert, and Neuroscience Citation Index.

GOAL STATEMENT

The goal of *Neuroimaging Clinics of North America* is to keep practicing radiologists and radiology residents up to date with current clinical practice in radiology by providing timely articles reviewing the state of the art in patient care.

ACCREDITATION

The *Neuroimaging Clinics of North America* is planned and implemented in accordance with the Essential Areas and Policies of the Accreditation Council for Continuing Medical Education (ACCME) through the joint sponsorship of the University of Virginia School of Medicine and Elsevier. The University of Virginia School of Medicine is accredited by the ACCME to provide continuing medical education for physicians.

The University of Virginia School of Medicine designates this educational activity for a maximum of 15 *AMA PRA Category 1 Credits*™ for each issue, 60 credits per year. Physicians should only claim credit commensurate with the extent of their participation in the activity.

The American Medical Association has determined that physicians not licensed in the US who participate in this CME activity are eligible for a maximum of 15 *AMA PRA Category 1 Credits*™ for each issue, 60 credits per year.

Credit can be earned by reading the text material, taking the CME examination online at http://www.theclinics.com/home/cme, and completing the evaluation. After taking the test, you will be required to review any and all incorrect answers. Following completion of the test and evaluation, your credit will be awarded and you may print your certificate.

FACULTY DISCLOSURE/CONFLICT OF INTEREST

The University of Virginia School of Medicine, as an ACCME accredited provider, endorses and strives to comply with the Accreditation Council for Continuing Medical Education (ACCME) Standards of Commercial Support, Commonwealth of Virginia statutes, University of Virginia policies and procedures, and associated federal and private regulations and guidelines on the need for disclosure and monitoring of proprietary and financial interests that may affect the scientific integrity and balance of content delivered in continuing medical education activities under our auspices.

The University of Virginia School of Medicine requires that all CME activities accredited through this institution be developed independently and be scientifically rigorous, balanced and objective in the presentation/discussion of its content, theories and practices.

All authors/editors participating in an accredited CME activity are expected to disclose to the readers relevant financial relationships with commercial entities occurring within the past 12 months (such as grants or research support, employee, consultant, stock holder, member of speakers bureau, etc.). The University of Virginia School of Medicine will employ appropriate mechanisms to resolve potential conflicts of interest to maintain the standards of fair and balanced education to the reader. Questions about specific strategies can be directed to the Office of Continuing Medical Education, University of Virginia School of Medicine, Charlottesville, Virginia.

The faculty and staff of the University of Virginia Office of Continuing Medical Education have no financial affiliations to disclose.

The authors/editors listed below have identified no professional/financial affiliations for themselves or their spouse/partner:
Ashley H. Aiken, MD; A. James Barkovich, MD; Wessam Bou-Assaly, MD; Cynthia Chin, MD; William P. Dillon, MD; Joey D. English, MD, PhD; Nancy J. Fischbein, MD; Christopher P. Hess, MD, PhD; Steven W. Hetts, MD;Joseph M. Hoxworth, MD; Kevin Huoh, MD; Joanne Husovski, (Acquisitions Editor); Jane J. Kim, MD; Carlos Leiva-Salinas, MD; Jason A. McKellop, MD; Sanjay P. Prabhu, MBBS, FRCR; Vincent Y. Wang, MD, PhD; Christine A. C. Wijman, MD PhD; and Tina Young-Poussaint, MD.

The authors listed below have identified the following professional/financial affiliations for themselves or their spouse/partner:
Dean Chou, MD is on the Speakers' Bureau for Stryker Spine.
Alisa D. Gean, MD (Guest Editor) is on the Advisory Committee/Board for Neurologica, Inc.
Christine M. Glastonbury, MBBS is a consultant and owns stock with Amirsys Inc.
Suresh K. Mukherji, MD (Consulting Editor) is a consultant for Philips.
Lubdha M. Shah, MD (Test Author) is a consultant for Amirsys.
Max Wintermark, MD is an industry funded research/investigator for GE Healthcare and Philips Healthcare.
Esther L. Yuh, MD, PhD receives royalties from General Electric.

Disclosure of Discussion of Non-FDA Approved Uses for Pharmaceutical Products and/or Medical Devices.

The University of Virginia School of Medicine, as an ACCME provider, requires that all faculty presenters identify and disclose any off-label uses for pharmaceutical and medical device products. The University of Virginia School of Medicine recommends that each physician fully review all the available data on new products or procedures prior to clinical use.

TO ENROLL

To enroll in the Neuroimaging Clinics of North America Continuing Medical Education program, call customer service at 1-800-654-2452 or sign up online at *http://www.theclinics.com/home/cme*. The CME program is available to subscribers for an additional annual fee of USD 196.

Neuroimaging Clinics of North America

THE CLINICS ARE NOW AVAILABLE ONLINE!

Access your subscription at:
www.theclinics.com

Contributors

CONSULTING EDITOR

SURESH K. MUKHERJI, MD
Professor and Chief of Neuroradiology and Head and Neck Radiology
Professor of Radiology, Otolaryngology Head and Neck Surgery and Radiation Oncology
University of Michigan Health System
Ann Arbor, Michigan

GUEST EDITOR

ALISA D. GEAN, MD
Professor of Radiology and Biomedical Imaging
Adjunct Professor of Neurology and Neurological Surgery
University of California, San Francisco
Brain and Spinal Injury Center (BASIC)
San Francisco General Hospital
San Francisco, California

AUTHORS

ASHLEY H. AIKEN, MD
Assistant Professor of Radiology
Division of Neuroradiology
Emory University Hospital
Atlanta, Georgia

A. JAMES BARKOVICH, MD
Professor of Radiology, Neurosurgery and Pediatrics
Chief of Pediatric Neuroradiology
Department of Radiology and Biomedical Imaging
University of California, San Francisco
San Francisco, California

WESSAM BOU-ASSALY, MD
Department of Radiology at the University of Michigan Health System
Neuroradiology and Nuclear Medicine Division, Department of Radiology
Ann Arbor Veterans Affairs Health System
Ann Arbor, Michigan

CYNTHIA CHIN, MD
Section of Neuroradiology
Department of Radiology
University of California,
San Francisco, California

DEAN CHOU, MD
Associate Professor of Neurological Surgery
Associate Director of Spinal Tumor Surgery
Department of Neurological Surgery
University of California
San Francisco, California

WILLIAM P. DILLON, MD
Elizabeth Guillaumin Professor of Radiology, Neurology, and Neurosurgery
Chief of Neuroradiology
Department of Radiology
University of California, San Francisco
San Francisco, California

JOEY D. ENGLISH, MD, PhD
Assistant Professor of Neurology and Radiology
Co-Chief of Interventional Neuroradiology San Francisco Veterans Administration Medical Center
Interventional Neuroradiologist San Francisco General Hospital
Neurointensivist University of California, San Francisco Medical Center
San Francisco, California

NANCY J. FISCHBEIN, MD
Associate Professor of Radiology and, by courtesy, Neurology, Neurological Surgery
and Otolaryngology-Head and Neck Surgery
Stanford University Medical Center
Stanford, California

ALISA D. GEAN, MD
Professor of Radiology and Biomedical Imaging
Adjunct Professor of Neurology and Neurological Surgery
University of California, San Francisco
Brain and Spinal Injury Center (BASIC)
San Francisco General Hospital
San Francisco, California

CHRISTINE M. GLASTONBURY, MBBS
Associate Professor
Departments of Radiology and Biomedical Imaging
Otolaryngology–Head and Neck Surgery, Radiation Oncology
University of California
San Francisco, California

CHRISTOPHER P. HESS, MD, PhD
Assistant Professor of Radiology
Chief of Neuroradiology San Francisco Veterans Administration Medical Center
Department of Radiology and Biomedical Imaging
University of California, San Francisco
San Francisco, California

STEVEN W. HETTS, MD
Assistant Professor of Radiology
Chief of Neuroradiology at San Francisco General Hospital
Co-Chief of Interventional Neuroradiology
San Francisco Veterans Administration Medical Center Interventional Neuroradiologist
University of California, San Francisco Medical Center
San Francisco, California

JOSEPH M. HOXWORTH, MD
Assistant Professor
Department of Radiology
Mayo Clinic
Phoenix and Scottsdale, Arizona

KEVIN HUOH, MD
Resident,
Department of Otolaryngology–Head and Neck Surgery
University of California, San Francisco
San Francisco, California

JANE J. KIM, MD
Assistant Professor of Clinical Radiology
Departments of Radiology and Radiology and Biomedical Imaging
University of California, San Francisco, San Francisco General Hospital
San Francisco, California

CARLOS LEIVA-SALINAS, MD
Division of Neuroradiology
Department of Radiology
University of Virginia
Charlottesville, Virginia

JASON A. MCKELLOP, MD
Department of Radiology
University of Michigan Health System
Ann Arbor, Michigan
Radiology Resident
New York University Langone Medical Center/Bellevue Hospital Center
New York, New York

SURESH K. MUKHERJI, MD
Professor and Chief of Neuroradiology and Head and Neck Radiology
Professor of Radiology, Otolaryngology Head and Neck Surgery and Radiation Oncology
University of Michigan Health System
Ann Arbor, Michigan

TINA YOUNG-POUSSAINT, MD
Associate Professor of Radiology
Harvard Medical School
Staff Neuroradiologist
Boston Children's Hospital
Boston, Massachusetts

SANJAY P. PRABHU, MBBS, FRCR
Instructor in Radiology
Harvard Medical School
Staff Neuroradiologist
Department of Radiology
Children's Hospital Boston
Boston, Massachusetts

VINCENT Y. WANG, MD, PhD
Department of Neurological Surgery
University of California, San Francisco
San Francisco, California

CHRISTINE A.C. WIJMAN, MD, PhD
Associate Professor
Department of Neurology and Neurological Sciences
Director Stanford Neurocritical Care Program
Stanford University School of Medicine
Stanford, California

MAX WINTERMARK, MD
Associate Professor of Radiology, Neurology, Neurosurgery and Biomedical Engineering
Chief of Neuroradiology, Division of Neuroradiology
Department of Radiology
University of Virginia
Charlottesville, Virginia

ESTHER L. YUH, MD, PhD
Assistant Professor
Department of Radiology
University of California, San Francisco
San Francisco, California

Contents

disability in the world by the year 2020. This article outlines the classification of TBI, details the types of lesions encountered, and discusses the various imaging modalities available for the evaluation of TBI.

This article outlines a practical imaging approach to CNS infection and reviews 5 basic imaging patterns commonly seen: (1) extra-axial lesion, (2) ring-enhancing lesion, (3) temporal lobe lesion, (4) basal ganglia lesion, and (5) white matter abnormality. Opportunistic infections in the setting of HIV are also discussed within the context of these 5 basic imaging patterns. Characteristic imaging features in conjunction with clinical history are also highlighted in order to narrow the differential diagnosis or suggest a specific diagnosis in some cases.

Recognizing typical midface fracture injuries and describing the imaging findings that are relevant to the maxillofacial surgeon are important. Particular attention should be paid to findings that potentially result in significant cosmetic or functional complications. Radiologists should evaluate facial fractures in multiple planes with coronal and sagittal reformats, which are especially helpful for horizontally oriented facial fractures, such as injuries to the orbital floor and the hard palate. 3-D images can also facilitate a broader understanding of the fracture impact on facial width, height, and projection and are useful for an overview of more complex fracture patterns that involve multiple facial bones.

Intracranial pressure (ICP) is the pressure within the intracranial space. Intracranial hypotension is a clinical syndrome in which low cerebrospinal fluid volume (CSF) results in orthostatic headache. Severe cases can result in nausea, vomiting, photophobia, and, rarely, decreased level of consciousness and coma. CSF opening pressure can be within the normal range in spontaneous intracranial hypotension. Imaging tests therefore play a key and decisive role in the diagnosis, as well as treatment, of intracranial hypotension. Intracranial hypertension occurs in a chronic form known as idiopathic intracranial hypertension, as well as in a large variety of neurologic and systemic disorders. Symptoms include headache, nausea and vomiting, blurred vision, and in severe cases, altered level of consciousness that can progress to coma and death. Direct measurements of CSF pressure through lumbar puncture (in idiopathic intracranial hypotension) or invasive ICP monitoring (in acute intracranial hypertension) are the key diagnostic tests. Imaging is used primarily to determine treatable causes of increased ICP, to assess for impending brain herniation, and to evaluate ventricular size.

The various findings observed on computed tomography (CT) and magnetic resonance (MR) imaging examinations in patients with seizures reflect the variety of different causes that give rise to this common neurologic symptom. In the emergency setting, CT is most valuable in its ability to accurately identify acute abnormalities that require emergent medical or surgical treatment. MR imaging, by contrast, is usually reserved for patients with recurrent or refractory seizures. The accurate interpretation of either modality requires familiarity with how seizures are classified clinically, the most common presenting features of different causes for seizures, the relevant neuroanatomy, and the imaging manifestations of both common and uncommon causes of seizures and epilepsy. Of particular practical importance to the radiologist is the ability to recognize (1) the most common findings in patients with recurrent seizures and (2) potentially reversible causes for seizures that require prompt intervention to avoid or minimize permanent brain injury. This article surveys a variety of different causes for seizures and epilepsy, focusing on specific clinical features that can help to refine differential diagnosis, and on imaging findings characteristic of different disorders.

This content presents infectious and vascular spinal emergencies, including epidural abscess, nontraumatic epidural hematoma, vascular malformations, and spinal cord infarction. The spine is subjected to multiple potential insults, such as trauma, infection, ischemia, hemorrhage, tumor, inflammation, and degeneration. All of these processes can lead to the sudden onset of neurologic symptoms, such as motor weaknesses, bowel and bladder incontinence, and sensory changes. Therefore, prompt recognition of these entities is important to reverse or minimize potential neurologic injury. The authors discuss several infectious and vascular spinal emergencies, including epidural abscess, nontraumatic epidural hematoma, vascular malformations, and spinal cord infarction.

Neck infections are fairly common in the emergency setting, affecting a broad spectrum of the patient population. Care should be taken not only to distinguish these conditions from other noninfectious origin such as malignancy but also to guide acute clinical management. A familiarity with neck anatomy, the imaging modalities used for investigation of such conditions, as well as common findings on imaging are critical to the care of affected patients. Cross-sectional imaging is a mainstay in this setting. This article presents the most common neck infections, and details some of their most prominent findings on cross-sectional imaging.

This article summarizes current state-of-the-art techniques used in the management of pediatric neurologic emergencies. Solutions to challenges faced by the radiologist, including the selection of an appropriate modality for an individual patient, are discussed. Imaging appearances of specific entities are described with an emphasis on conditions unique to the pediatric population.

Foreword

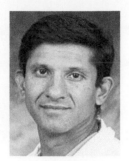

Suresh K. Mukherji, MD
Consulting Editor

I think we can all agree that one of the most challenging areas we all face in our practices is interpretation of "Middle of the Night" neuroradiology studies. How and who interprets these studies are very variable. The ultimate goal however is to ensure that the studies are interpreted both promptly and accurately. It is with this in mind that I invited Alisa Gean from the University of California, San Francisco to edit this important issue of *Neuroimaging Clinics of North America*.

Alisa has assembled a very experienced group of authors to provide a comprehensive update on the most common disease entities that may be encountered in the middle of the night. The topics include stroke, traumatic head injuries, infections, seizures, and spinal pathology In addition, there are articles dedicated to CNS emergencies in children and head and neck... (of course!).

I strongly encourage you to read Dr Gean's Preface---I certainly did!! I am not quite sure if anyone has ever read one of my Forewords, but "hope springs eternal." I still wanted to write this Foreword even if it goes unread by the *masses*, as this provides me the opportunity to formally and publicly thank Alisa for her outstanding issue. Alisa has worked tirelessly on this edition, and I am very grateful for her enthusiasm to make this such an outstanding issue. Thank you, Alisa!!

Suresh K. Mukherji, MD
Department of Radiology
University of Michigan Health System
1500 East Medical Center
Ann Arbor, MI 48109-0030, USA

E-mail address:
mukherji@med.umich.edu

Neuroimag Clin N Am 20 (2010) xiii
doi:10.1016/j.nic.2010.09.002
1052-5149/10/$ — see front matter © 2010 Elsevier Inc. All rights reserved.

neuroimaging.theclinics.com

Preface

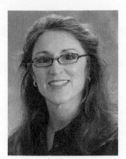

Alisa D. Gean, MD
Guest Editor

To be honest, I'm not sure if I have ever taken the time to read a book's preface, so I'll keep this short and sweet. The current issue is devoted to the imaging diagnosis of neurologic emergencies. The authors are experts in their fields. The illustrations are top-notch; the references are up-to-date, and the discussions are clinically relevant. I guarantee that it's worth more than a brief look!

Thank you and enjoy!

Alisa D. Gean, MD
Department of Radiology
University of California, San Francisco
San Francisco General Hospital
1001 Potrero Avenue
San Francisco, CA 94110, USA

E-mail address:
alisa.gean@radiology.ucsf.edu

Neuroimag Clin N Am 20 (2010) xv
doi:10.1016/j.nic.2010.09.001

Neuroimaging Clinics of N Am

Preface

Alisa D. Gean, MD

To be honest, I'm not sure if I have ever taken the time to read a book's preface, so I'll keep this short and sweet. The current issue is devoted to the imaging diagnosis of neurologic emergencies. The authors are experts in their fields. The illustrations are top-notch, the references are up-to-date, and the discussions are clinically relevant. I guarantee that it is worth more than a brief look.

Thank you and enjoy!

Alisa D. Gean, MD
Department of Radiology
University of California, San Francisco
San Francisco General Hospital
1001 Potrero Avenue
San Francisco, CA 94110-3518

Neuroimaging Clin N Am 20 (2010) xv
doi:10.1016/j.nic.2010.09.001
1052-5149/10/$ – see front matter © 2010 Elsevier Inc. All rights reserved.

Imaging of Acute Ischemic Stroke

Carlos Leiva-Salinas and Max Wintermark*

KEYWORDS

- Stroke • MRI • CT • DW imaging
- Perfusion • Thrombolysis

Stroke is the third leading cause of death in the United States, Canada, Europe, and Japan. The American Heart Association and the American Stroke Association estimate that approximately 800,000 new strokes occur each year, resulting in more than 130,000 annual deaths in the United States alone.[1] Direct and indirect costs related to stroke are estimated to be $70 billion annually, and will likely increase in the next decades.[2] Stroke is the leading cause of adult disability in North America.[1]

Ischemic stroke is caused by a reduction in the blood supply to the brain (usually a clot occluding a cerebral artery), which subsequently disrupts the supply of oxygen and nutrients to brain tissue. Ischemic strokes account for more than 80% of strokes[1] and can be further subdivided into cardiogenic, atherosclerotic, lacunar, hemodynamic, or cryptogenic sources.[3] Another 15% of strokes are related to the disruption of a cerebral artery, resulting in intracerebral hemorrhage (ICH).[1] Other rare causes of stroke-like symptoms include subarachnoid hemorrhage, cerebral venous sinus thrombosis, chronic subdural hematoma, neoplasms, inflammatory disease, migraine, reversible cerebral vasoconstriction syndrome, seizure, and hypoglycemia. Some of these subjects are discussed in other articles elsewhere in this issue.

Imaging has revolutionized acute ischemic stroke diagnosis and management. Previously, structural imaging modalities, typically noncontrast computed tomography (NCT), were used to assess the presence and extent of acute ischemic stroke and exclude stroke mimics. With the development of functional imaging modalities such as perfusion CT (PCT) and perfusion magnetic resonance (MR) imaging, stroke has been redefined from an all-or-none to a dynamic and evolving process. In particular, the advent of effective thrombolytic therapies, such as intravenous tissue plasminogen activator (tPA),[4] has motivated us to better define the so-called ischemic penumbra and improve patient selection for reperfusion therapy. Studies have indicated favorable clinical outcomes with thrombolytic therapies administered to patients selected by imaging criteria in an extended time window.[5]

In this article, the individual components of multimodal CT and multimodal MR imaging are discussed, the current status of neuroimaging for the evaluation of the acute ischemic stroke is presented, and the potential role of a combined multimodal stroke protocol is addressed.

PHYSIOPATHOLOGY: THE CONCEPT OF PENUMBRA

When a cerebral artery is occluded, a core of brain tissue dies rapidly. Surrounding this infarct core is an area of brain that is hypoperfused, but still viable because of collateral blood flow. This area of at-risk, but potentially salvageable, tissue is called the ischemic penumbra.[6–8]

Studies in primates and positron emission tomography studies in humans[9–12] have shown that brain parenchyma can compensate for hypoperfusion through an increase in oxygen extraction

The authors have nothing to disclose.

Division of Neuroradiology, Department of Radiology, University of Virginia, 1215 Lee Street-New Hospital, 1st Floor, Room 1011, PO Box 800170, Charlottesville, VA 22908, USA

* Corresponding author.

E-mail address: Max.Wintermark@virginia.edu

Neuroimag Clin N Am 20 (2010) 455–468

doi:10.1016/j.nic.2010.07.002

down to a cerebral blood flow (CBF) threshold of approximately 20 to 23 mL/100 g tissue/min. If the CBF decreases below this threshold, neuronal function is impaired. The affected neurons remain viable and recover without injury after normalization of the CBF as long as it remains more than approximately 10 to 15 mL/100 g tissue/min. If the CBF decreases below this point, a shortage of metabolites occurs, causing an Na^+/K^+ channel failure in the ischemic cells. This membrane channel failure results in an uncontrolled net shift of extracellular water in the intracellular space. The consequence is cytotoxic edema and irreversible damage to the neuronal cells.[6] The extent and severity of the CBF reduction and the neuronal integrity determine the size of the core and the penumbra.[9–12]

The rate of change in the size of the core and penumbra is a dynamic process that depends mainly on the reperfusion of the ischemic brain. If the occlusion is not removed, the infarct core may grow and progressively replace the penumbra. In early recanalization, either spontaneously or resulting from thrombolysis, the penumbra may be salvaged from infarction.[13]

WHY IMAGE A PATIENT WITH ACUTE STROKE?

The central premise of acute stroke treatment is to rescue the ischemic penumbra. The current guidelines[14] neglect the fact that the portion of potentially salvageable ischemic tissue is not only dependent on the time window, but also on the individual patient's collateral blood flow. The presence and extent of the ischemic penumbra are *time-dependent*, but are especially *patient-dependent*. From patient to patient, survival of the penumbra can vary from less than 3 hours to well beyond 48 hours. Of patients with supratentorial arterial occlusion, 90% to 100% show ischemic penumbra in the first 3 hours of a stroke, but 75% to 80% of patients still have penumbral tissue at 6 hours after stroke onset.[13,15,16]

The only drug treatment of acute stroke approved by the US Food and Drug Administration is intravenous thrombolysis with recombinant tPA. It is limited to the first 3 to 4.5 hours after symptom onset, and after intracranial hemorrhage has been ruled out by NCT or gradient echo MR imaging.[17] Only 3% to 8.5% of potentially eligible patients are treated because few are medically evaluated at an early enough stage,[18] and there is the widespread concern of hemorrhagic conversion resulting from overly aggressive reperfusion therapy. However, it has been suggested[19,20] that intravenous thrombolytic therapy can be safely administered beyond 3 to 4.5 hours in selected patients with a sufficient amount of salvageable brain tissue, thereby affording a safe treatment to a larger percentage of patients with stroke. This situation strongly emphasizes the need for an improved delineation of the salvageable ischemic penumbra by imaging in patients with acute stroke.[21]

The negative results of thrombolysis trials between 3 to 6 hours[16] may be because no method of penumbral imaging was used to select patients for therapy, despite penumbra being the target for treatment and despite the high percentage of patients with penumbra within this time window. Please see the article Acute Neuro-Interventional Therapies elsewhere in this issue for additional information regarding neurointerventional therapy for acute ischemic infarction.

A tissue clock that determines the presence and relative extent of both infarct and penumbra would be an ideal guide to patient selection for thrombolysis, rather than a rigid time window as is recommended by the current guidelines.[14] During the last decade, several models for ischemic penumbra delineation using MR imaging, and increasingly, CT, have been developed to predict the outcome of ischemic brain tissue.

ACUTE STROKE MR IMAGING
Multimodal MR Imaging Stroke Protocol

A typical stroke MR imaging protocol consists of T2/fluid attenuated inversion recovery (FLAIR), T2*, diffusion-weighted (DW) and perfusion-weighted (PW) images (Table 1) and MR angiography (MRA).[22] This protocol can be performed in less than 30 minutes. It achieves reliable information about the site of vessel occlusion, the extent of potentially salvageable brain tissue, and the exclusion of differential diagnoses of ischemic stroke.

The MR Imaging Protocol Sequence by Sequence

T2 and FLAIR imaging
On T2-weighted and FLAIR images, ischemic infarction appears as a hyperintense lesion usually seen within the first 3 to 8 hours after stroke onset (Fig. 1).[23–25] In a recent study of patients with acute ischemic stroke studied by MR imaging within 6 hours of symptom onset, patients without a visible hyperintense lesion on FLAIR images had greater than 90% probability of being imaged within the first 3 hours of symptom onset. Thus, a mismatch between positive DW imaging and negative FLAIR images appears to be useful in

Table 1
Recommended acquisition protocol for perfusion-weighted MR imaging

Sequence	Single-shot Gradient Echo Echoplanar Imaging
Image acquisition parameters	TR ≤1500 ms TE = 35 to 45 ms at 1.5 T TE = 25 to 30 ms at 3 T Flip angle = 60° to 90° at 1.5 T Flip angle = 60° at 3 T
Image acquisition duration	90 to 120 s Image acquisition started 10 s before initiation of bolus injection to achieve at least 10 baseline images
Coverage and slice thickness	Field of view ≈ 24 cm Whole brain coverage using ≥12 slices Gap 0 to 1 mm Slice thickness 5 mm Matrix size 128 × 128
Slice orientation	Parallel to hard palate
Contrast material	Standard gadolinium-based contrast material
Contrast volume	Single dose (for half molar agent ≈ 20 mL for 100 kg person) followed by 20 to 40 mL saline flush
Injection rate	4 to 6 mL/s; same rate for saline
IV access	18- to 20-gauge IV line; right antecubital vein preferred

Abbreviations: IV, intravenous; TE, echo time; TR, repetition time.

the identification of patients who are likely to benefit from thrombolysis.[24]

FLAIR images are also highly sensitive to subarachnoid hemorrhage[26] as well as acute cerebral venous sinus thrombosis.[27,28] In the setting of hyperacute stroke, T2-weighted images can be useful to detect the loss of the arterial signal flow void in occluded vessels within minutes of the stroke onset.[25] T2-weighted and FLAIR images are both used to assess older cerebral infarctions and the extent of concomitant small vessel disease.[25]

Diffusion-weighted imaging and apparent diffusion coefficient

Diffusion MR imaging provides image contrast that is dependent on the molecular motion of water.[29] Cerebral ischemia leads to energy metabolism disruption with the failure of the Na^+/K^+ and other ionic pumps. This situation induces a loss of ionic

gradients and a net transfer of water from the extracellular to the intracellular compartment causing a cytotoxic edema.[6] Excessive intracellular water accumulation leads to a reduced extracellular volume, which usually facilitates water mobility, and therefore to a reduction of water diffusion in the extracellular matrix.[29] This phenomenon is detected with DW imaging within minutes of vessel occlusion[13,29] and can be measured quantitatively with the apparent diffusion coefficient (ADC).

DW imaging is the most sensitive method for the depiction of ischemia in the hyperacute stage (see **Fig. 1; Fig. 2**).[30,31] However, DW imaging lesions can be at least partially reversible in the early phase of ischemia, and the size of the DW imaging abnormality does not necessarily reflect irreversibly damaged tissue. A recent series of 68 acute patients with ischemic stroke[32] showed that 20% of the patients had ADC normalization in greater than 5 mL of brain tissue. The partial normalization was predominantly seen in the basal ganglia and white matter in patients with distally located vessel occlusions, and it was associated with a trend toward a better clinical outcome. This study suggests that patients with a perfusion/diffusion match within 3 hours of symptom onset may still have salvageable tissue at risk and might benefit from thrombolysis.

Noncontrast MR angiography
The most commonly used noncontrast MRA technique is time-of-flight (TOF) imaging. This sequence depicts vascular flow by repeatedly applying a radiofrequency pulse to a volume of tissue, followed by dephasing and rephasing gradients. Stationary tissue in the volume becomes saturated by the repeated excitation pulses and has low signal. Conversely, inflowing blood protons are not saturated and therefore produce increased signal intensity.[25,33] The vessel contrast is proportional to the blood velocity (ie, flow-related enhancement). For selective imaging of arteries, saturation bands are applied on the venous side of imaging sections to null signal from the venous flow.[33]

Three-dimensional (3D) TOF-MRA is the preferred technique for the examination of intracranial vessels. MRA is particularly useful in the detection of vascular occlusion and/or stenosis in patients with ischemic stroke (see **Fig. 2**).[25] Technical improvements such as parallel imaging and higher magnetic fields allow high spatial isotropic resolution, fast acquisition times, and reduced artifacts.[25]

Perfusion-weighted MR imaging
PW imaging allows the measurement of capillary perfusion to the brain. The bolus passage of a paramagnetic intravascular MR imaging contrast

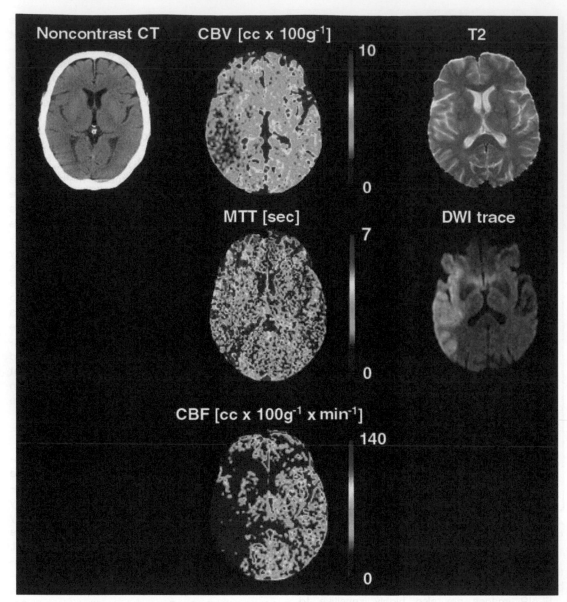

Fig. 1. 75-year-old man presenting with sudden onset of a left face-arm-leg hemisyndrome. Physical examination revealed a left hemianopsia, rightward gaze deviation, dysarthria, and left hemineglect. CT and MR examination were obtained 2 and 3 hours after admission, respectively. PCT (cerebral blood volume [CBV], mean transit time [MTT], CBF), and DW imaging trace images clearly depict an acute stroke extending to the superficial right middle cerebral artery territory. Note how the lesion is far more subtle on the corresponding T2-weighted image, and especially on the NCT, where it features a cortical ribbon loss sign.

agent through the cerebral capillaries causes a nonlinear signal loss on T2* images.[34] This dynamic contrast-enhanced technique tracks the tissue signal changes caused by the susceptibility effect to create a hemodynamic time-to-signal intensity curve.[35]

Gradient recalled echo (T2) weighted imaging*
Hyperacute stroke imaging demands the differentiation between ischemic stroke and hemorrhagic stroke (*discussed in the article* Hemorrhagic Stroke and Non-traumatic Intracranial Hemorrhage *elsewhere in this issue*), which is impossible by clinical means only. Although CT is the standard method for the diagnosis of ICH, studies have shown that hyperacute ICH can be identified on MR (mainly FLAIR and gradient-recalled echo [GRE] imaging) with excellent accuracy.[36]

Moreover, microbleeds (small hemosiderin deposits) not apparent on CT can be detected by

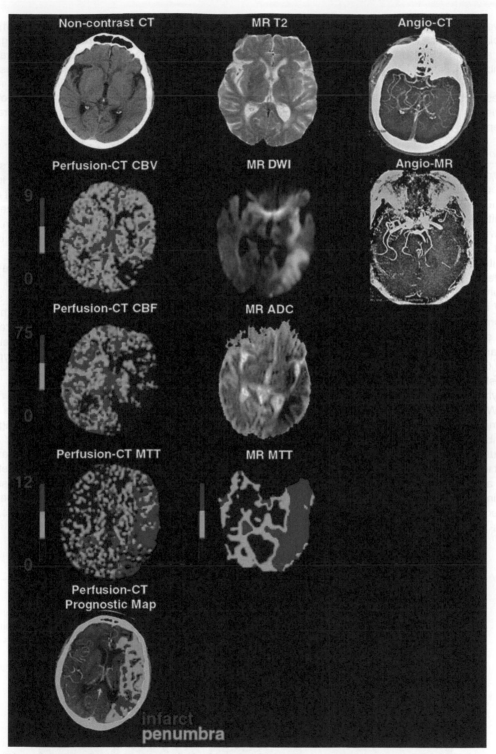

Fig. 2. 71-year-old woman presenting with sudden onset of a right face-arm-leg hemisyndrome and nonfluent aphasia. Noncontrast cerebral CT/PCT and DW/PW MR imaging were performed 2 and 2.3 hours after symptom onset, respectively. The NCT shows a left insular ribbon sign and subtle left parietal hypodensity. The cerebral infarct and cerebral blood volume CBV abnormality on PCT (mL/100 g) show a similar size to the DW imaging-MR imaging abnormality. However, the size of the CBF/MTT abnormality on PCT ([mL/100 g/min]/[s]) and on the MR MTT image involves the entire left MCA territory (ie, mismatched defect with penumbral tissue in the anterior MCA territory). The corresponding M1 occlusion is clearly identified on both the CTA and MRA. The patient underwent unsuccessful thrombolysis.

T2*-weighted images.[37] These chronic lesions are associated with an increased risk of spontaneous ICH and may also be a risk factor for thrombolysis-related hemorrhage.[38,39]

In suspected acute stroke, T2*-weighted images can detect an intraluminal thrombus as a linear low signal region of magnetic susceptibility.[25]

Alternative Sequences for Selected Conditions

Susceptibility-weighted imaging

Susceptibility-weighted (SW) imaging is a high-resolution 3D gradient echo sequence that uses magnitude and phase information to create a new source of contrast. It offers information about any tissue that has a different susceptibility than its surrounding structures, such as deoxygenated blood, hemosiderin, ferritin, and calcium.[40]

SW imaging is exquisitely sensitive in detecting hemorrhage.[40] Studies have shown that it is more sensitive in detecting hemorrhagic conversion and old microbleeds than CT and conventional GRE sequences.[40,41]

Fresh clots contain a high concentration of deoxyhemoglobin, and thus appear hypointense on SW images. As a complementary sequence, SW imaging may be useful to depict distal branch thrombi that are not well visualized by MRA.[40] Because of a decrease in arterial flow, and subsequent increase in the proportion of deoxyhemoglobin, acute thromboembolism may result in prominent hypointensity in the draining veins located in hypoperfused areas on SW imaging. In suspected acute stroke, therefore, SW imaging could also have a potential role by assessing areas of hypoperfusion without the need of contrast.[40]

Despite its many potential advantages, this technique is not available on all major MR manufacturers' systems and, despite the technical advances, approximately 5 minutes are still needed to image the entire brain.[40]

Fat-saturated T1-weighted imaging

Fat-saturated T1 (T1-FS)-weighted images should be considered if cervical artery dissection is suspected. Vascular dissection is an important cause of acute infarction, causing up to 20% of cerebral infarctions in young patients. It occurs when blood extends into the wall of a vessel through an intimal tear.[42]

Dissection occurs most frequently in the distal extracranial portion of the internal carotid artery and vertebral artery. It causes ischemic stroke primarily through embolization rather than through hemodynamic flow limitation.[25] The intramural blood appears hyperintense on T1-FS-weighted images when met-hemoglobin develops, typically within 2 to 3 days after dissection (**Fig. 3**).[42]

Contrast-enhanced MRA of the cervical arteries

Contrast-enhanced MRA (CE-MRA) is the technique of choice for extracranial artery imaging.[29] It relies on injection of a paramagnetic agent such as gadolinium to reduce the T1 relaxation time of tissue and to generate contrast between the intravascular lumen and surrounding tissues.[43] Unlike TOF-MRA, vascular contrast is therefore relatively independent of flow dynamics, and

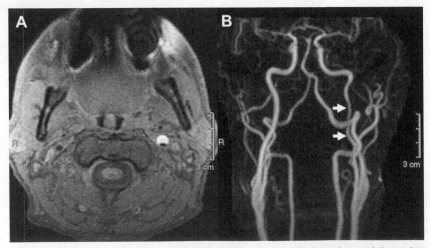

Fig. 3. 40-year-old man presenting with left-sided neck pain and right-sided weakness. (*A*) Axial T1 fat-saturated (T1-FS)-weighted MR image shows a large crescent of hyperintense signal (representing intramural met-hemoglobin) within the cervical portion of the left ICA, consistent with a carotid dissection. (*B*) Coronal contrast-enhanced MRA maximum intensity projection image shows narrowing of the left ICA at the site of dissection (*arrows*).

artifacts associated with saturation effects are substantially reduced. Vessels from the aortic arch to the circle of Willis can be obtained in less than 1 minute. This sequence enables potential assessment of stenosis or vessel occlusion.[43] CE-MRA is also used to show luminal narrowing in acute dissection (see Fig. 3).[44]

MR Imaging for the Differentiation of Infarct Core and Penumbra

It has been hypothesized that DW imaging reflects the irreversibly damaged infarct, whereas PW imaging reflects the overall area of hypoperfusion.[45] The volume difference between these techniques, termed the PW/DW imaging *mismatch*, represents the MR imaging correlate of the ischemic penumbra (see Figs. 1 and 2). Conversely, if there is no difference in PW and DW imaging volumes, or even a negative difference (PW < DW imaging), this is termed a PW/DW imaging *match*. This matched defect is seen in the patient who does not have penumbral tissue either because of normalization of previous hypoperfusion or because of completion of the infarction and the total loss of penumbra.[45–47] It may be argued that this model does not take into account that the PW imaging lesion also assesses areas of oligemia that are not in danger and that DW imaging abnormalities do not necessarily turn into infarction.[32,48] It is not yet clear which parameter gives the best approximation to critical hypoperfusion and allows differentiation of infarct from penumbra. However, most investigators agree that in current clinical practice, T_{max} and mean transit time (MTT) seem to give the best results.

Stroke MR Imaging in Clinical Trials

Stroke MR imaging has been investigated in the clinical setting to evaluate its role for thrombolysis in an extended time window. The DIAS (Desmoteplase in Acute Ischemic Stroke) and DEDAS (Dose Escalation of Desmoteplase for Acute Ischemic Stroke) trials[19,20] used a new fibrinolytic drug, desmoteplase, in patients with acute ischemic stroke within a 3- to 9-hour time window after symptom onset. Patient screening was based on clinical examination and medical history and guided by stroke MR imaging. Only patients showing a clear DW/PW imaging mismatch were randomized. The patients who received a placebo or an ineffective dosage showed a lower recanalization rate and an unfavorable outcome. Patients who achieved early vessel recanalization and reperfusion of penumbral tissue showed a significant clinical benefit, and 60% of the patients from the most

effective dose tier had an excellent clinical outcome.[19]

In the DIAS 2 study,[49] patients were enrolled based on a mismatch diagnosed either by MR imaging or by PCT. The intention-to-treat analysis found no significant difference between the groups in clinical response rates, contrasting with their previous findings with desmoteplase in the DIAS and DEDAS trials. Clinical response rate was 46.0% in the placebo group, 47.4% in the group who received 90 μg/kg, and 36.4% in the group who received 125 μg/kg.

The DEFUSE trial[5] was designed to determine whether a mismatch between perfusion and diffusion could be used to predict clinical outcome in patients with early reperfusion after treatment with recombinant tPA during the 3- to 6-hour time window after symptom onset. Patients with a baseline mismatch between PW and DW imaging of at least 20% and a reduction in perfusion abnormality volume of at least 10 mL had a better clinical outcome. The trial thus showed that baseline MR imaging findings can be used to identify groups of patients who are more likely to benefit from thrombolytic therapy and, potentially, other forms of reperfusion therapy. Data from this study suggested that a larger difference, a mismatch ratio (PW imaging volume-DW imaging volume/DW imaging volume) of 2.6, provided the highest sensitivity and specificity for identifying patients in whom reperfusion was associated with a favorable response. However, even in the presence of a large PW/DW imaging mismatch, no benefit could be expected if early recanalization of the occluded vessel failed.[50]

Other trials have studied the role of early MR imaging changes for the prediction of thrombolysis outcome. Large ischemic lesions on DW imaging are predictive of poor outcome regardless of whether thrombolysis is performed.[51] A prospective study in patients with anterior circulation ischemic stroke treated with tPA within 3 hours of stroke onset compared the baseline DW imaging findings using the Alberta Stroke Program Early CT Score (ASPECTS) with patient clinical outcome at 7 days.[51] Clinical worsening and poor outcome were noted more frequently in patients with ASPECTS 5 or less. The investigators suggested that these patients should be excluded from studies of thrombolysis beyond the 3-hour time window.

ACUTE STROKE CT
Multimodal CT Stroke Protocol

Modern CT imaging, including NCT, PCT (Table 2), and CT angiography (CTA), fulfills all

Table 2 Recommended acquisition protocol for PCT	
Image acquisition rate	Image acquisition 6–7 s after start of injection of the contrast bolus 2 phases: First phase: 1 image per s, duration 30 to 45 s Second phase: 1 image per 2 or 3 s, duration 30 to 45 s Total duration at least 70 s
Image acquisition parameters	80 kVp, 100 mAs
Coverage and slice thickness	Field of view ≈ 24 cm Maximal coverage possible based on CT scanner configuration (minimal coverage of 20 mm slab per bolus injection preferable. Two boluses injection is possible to double coverage in scanners with less than 40 mm detector length under precluded by contrast dose considerations)
Slice orientation	Parallel to hard palate
Contrast material	High concentration (350–370 mg/mL) low/iso osmolar contrast preferred
Contrast volume	35 to 50 mL, followed by 20 to 40 mL saline flush
Injection rate	4 to 6 mL/s; same rate for saline
IV access	18- to 20-gauge IV line. Right antecubital vein preferred

the requirements for hyperacute stroke imaging.[52] NCT can exclude hemorrhage; PCT can differentiate between penumbra and irreversibly damaged brain tissue[52]; and CTA identifies intracranial thrombus and vascular narrowing. Multimodal CT offers rapid data acquisition and can be performed with conventional CT equipment.

The CT Protocol Sequence by Sequence

Noncontrast CT

With its widespread availability, short scan time, noninvasiveness and safety, NCT has been the traditional first-line imaging modality for the evaluation of acute ischemic stroke. In this setting, NCT is typically used to rule out intracranial hemorrhage and other stroke mimics. Occasionally, NCT can provide information that supports the diagnosis of hyperacute infarction.[53–55] Early CT signs of brain ischemia include

1) *Insular ribbon sign.* The insular cortex is particularly vulnerable to a proximal middle cerebral artery (MCA) occlusion because it is the region most distal from the potential anterior and posterior collateral circulation, and therefore it is a watershed arterial zone. When ischemic, the insular region shows loss of definition of the gray-white interface, or loss of the insular ribbon (see **Figs. 1** and **2**).[53]

2) *Obscuration of the lentiform nucleus.* Because of their blood supply via end arteries, the basal ganglia are also particularly vulnerable to early infarction.[54] When ischemic, an obscured outline or partial disappearance of the lentiform nucleus can be seen on NCT (**Fig. 4**).

3) *Hyperdense artery sign.* The presence of an acute thrombus in the MCA creates a linear hyperattenuation on NCT, the so-called hyperdense artery sign (see **Fig. 4**; **Fig. 5**).[55] Contrary to the other early CT signs, this one represents not an infarction but a thrombotic event.[55] Although it is highly specific for ischemia, its sensitivity is poor,[56] and false-positive results such as high hematocrit level or atherosclerotic calcification should be excluded. However, in those cases the hyperattenuation is usually bilateral.[57]

Although these early signs can be helpful in stroke detection, they are subtle, difficult to detect, and exhibit limited sensitivity in the hyperacute stage of ischemic stroke (approximately 25% during the first 3 hours) when compared with DW MR imaging.[58] Moreover, the relationship between early ischemic changes on CT and adverse outcomes after tPA treatment is not straightforward.[59,60]

In contrast to these early ischemic changes, obvious hypoattenuation is highly specific for irreversible tissue damage,[61] and its extent is predictive of the risk of hemorrhagic transformation.[62] In the European Cooperative Acute Stroke Study trials (ECASS I and II), involvement of more than one-third of the MCA territory on NCT was used as a criterion for patient exclusion from reperfusion therapy because of the potential increased risk for hemorrhagic transformation.[63] Despite its many advantages, NCT provides solely anatomic (and not physiologic) information and it cannot reliably differentiate between irreversibly damaged brain tissue and penumbral tissue.

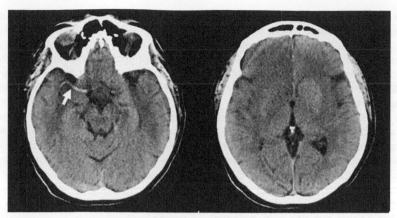

Fig. 4. Acute MCA infarction with hyperdense MCA. Noncontrast brain CT in a 62-year-old man obtained 4 hours after the onset of symptoms shows a hyperdense right MCA (*arrow*), obscuration of the right lentiform nucleus, and subtle loss of gray-white differentiation within the right orbitofrontal lobe.

Perfusion CT

PCT imaging, using standard nonionic iodinated contrast, relies on the speed of modern helical CT scanners, which can sequentially trace the entry and washout of a bolus of contrast injected into an arm vein through an intravenous line.[64] The relationship between contrast concentration and signal intensity of CT data is linear. Thereby, analysis of the signal density first increasing then decreasing during the passage of the contrast provides information about brain perfusion.[65]

More specifically, the PCT evaluation of brain perfusion consists of 3 types of parametric maps: cerebral blood volume (CBV), MTT, and CBF. CBV reflects the blood volume per unit of

brain (4–6 mL/100g in gray matter). MTT designates the average time required by a bolus of blood to cross the capillary network (4 seconds in gray matter). CBF relates to the volume of blood flowing per brain mass during a time interval of 1 minute (50–60 mL/100 g/min in gray matter).[64,65] The relationship between CBV, MTT and CBF is expressed by the equation CBF = CBV/MTT.[64,65] Recently, CBF values from PCT imaging have been shown to be highly accurate in humans when compared with the gold standard (PET).[66]

CT angiography

Advances in multidetector row CT technology have made CTA a valid alternative to conventional

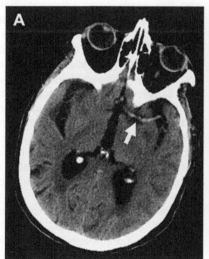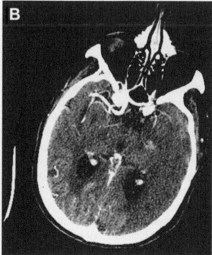

Fig. 5. 86-year-old woman admitted to the emergency department after sudden onset of right face-arm-leg hemisyndrome. (*A*) NCT of the brain shows a hyperdense left MCA (*arrow*). (*B*) Concurrent CTA shows nonfilling of the left MCA, consistent with intraluminal thrombus. Note how the margins of the infarct are more conspicuous on the CTA source image.

catheter-based cerebral angiography.[67,68] With current CT scanners, the region from the aortic arch up to the circle of Willis can be covered in a single data acquisition with excellent, isotropic spatial resolution, in less than 5 seconds. Multiplanar reformatted images, maximum-intensity projection images, and 3D reconstructions of source images provide images comparable with those obtained with conventional angiography.[69,70]

CTA allows a detailed evaluation of the intra- and extracranial vasculature.[70,71] Its usefulness in acute stroke lies not only in its ability to detect large vessel thrombi within intracranial vessels (see Fig. 2), and to evaluate the carotid and vertebral arteries in the neck[71] but also in its potential for guiding therapy. In particular, the exact location and the extent of vascular occlusion have been shown to have prognostic value in the response to thrombolytics and the determination of collateral circulation and possible risk of subsequent recanalization.[72] For example, patients with a top-of-carotid occlusion, proximal MCA branch occlusion, or significant thrombus burden might be poor candidates for intravenous thrombolytics, and may be better candidates for intra-arterial or mechanical thrombolysis.[73]

CT in Differentiation of Infarct Core and Penumbra

PCT distinction of the infarct core from the penumbra is based on the concept of cerebral vascular autoregulation.[65,74,75] In hypoperfused areas of brain parenchyma, there are typically high MTT values as a result of supply via collateral circulation. Autoregulation attempts to preserve CBF values by inducing vasodilatation, which results in an increased CBV. Brain regions characterized by such PCT values are considered areas of ischemic penumbra that could benefit from reperfusion. Conversely, when ischemic injury is more severe and prolonged, autoregulation is unable to maintain the CBV above the threshold for neuronal death, and the tissue experiences irreversible hypoxic damage with a subsequent decrease in CBV; this area represents the infarct core, where tissue no longer viable does not benefit from reperfusion and is at risk for hemorrhage (see Figs. 1 and 2).[65,74]

Large prospective studies on patients with acute ischemic infarction have proved the validity of this theory and have provided evidence about the optimal approach to defining the infarct core and penumbra.[76] The PCT parameter that most accurately describes the tissue at risk of infarction is the relative MTT, with an optimal threshold of 145%. The parameter that most accurately describes the infarct core on admission is the absolute CBV, with an optimal threshold of 2.0 mL/100g. The mismatch between these 2 parameters affords the most accurate delineation of the tissue at risk of infarction in the absence of recanalization.

Therefore, by combining MTT and CBV results, PCT has the ability to reliably identify the reversible ischemic penumbra and the irreversible infarct core in patients with acute stroke immediately after admission.[76] *In the infarct core, MTT is prolonged and CBV values are lowered, whereas in the penumbra, cerebral vascular autoregulation attempts to compensate for a reduced CBF by a local vasodilatation, resulting in increased CBV values.*[65,74]

The penumbra, as described by PCT, has been shown to be accurate when compared with acute and delayed DW/PW imaging (see Fig. 2).[75,77]

CT or MR: Which One to Choose?

CT and MR imaging provide similar information. The infarct core and the ischemic penumbra, as shown by DW/PW imaging and by PCT, are comparable.[74,77] In addition to the similarity of their results, both CT and MR imaging techniques have respective advantages and drawbacks to be considered in the special setting of acute stroke.

Stroke MR imaging is still available only in a limited number of hospitals. Depending on each individual setting, it is difficult to conduct stroke MR imaging without losing too much time before treatment onset. The main advantages of MR imaging are the direct visualization of the full extent of infarction that is seen on DW imaging and the whole brain coverage that allows the detection of small but clinically relevant hypoperfusion areas. Visualization of the circle of Willis can be performed in ~3 minutes with a TOF-MRA. No additional radiograph dosage or iodinated contrast agent is needed and hence no nephrotoxicity or relevant allergic reactions are expected. However, the control of vital signs and the access to the patient during the MR imaging study are limited by the magnet. In addition, it takes some effort to train technicians to conduct a stroke MR imaging in a short period to establish an adequate work flow during the hyperacute phase of an ischemic stroke.

CT is often criticized for its use of radiation and iodinated contrast material. Nevertheless, when using such parameters, the effective radiation dose associated with a single-slab PCT study is approximately equal to that of an unenhanced head CT, roughly 2 to 3 mSv,[78] and no renal failure has yet been reported following a PCT examination.[79] However, because of limited spatial resolution, PCT cannot detect small lacunas, and NCT is not so sensitive to microbleeds as GRE or SW MR imaging. Further, PCT has a limited spatial coverage (usually 20 to 40 mm thickness). This issue is currently been solved through the development of multidetector CT scanners with greater arrays of elements. Volumetric studies using the full width of the new 320-detector CT scanners enable full brain coverage in a single rotation. The major advantages of this technology in acute stroke are the extent of coverage and the ability to obtain combined perfusion and angiographic data from the same contrast injection. The dynamic aspect of stroke can be used to assess collateral flow based on temporal resolution.[80] Despite its many advantages, recent phantom measurements indicate that imaging with this newly introduced volumetric CT results in a higher effective radiation dose compared with a multimodal stroke protocol using a conventional 64-detector-row CT scanner dose.[81] More recently, flat-detector (FD)–equipped angiography machines have been used to obtain not only high-quality 3D rotational angiography images but also CT-like images (FD-CT) of brain parenchyma. A recent preliminary study has shown good correlation of CBV color maps and absolute values between FD-CT and standard PCT. In the future, this technology may be able to obtain both anatomic and physiologic information without the need to transfer patients from the angiography suite to a CT facility.[82]

Even now, PCT has 95% accuracy in the delineation of supratentorial strokes despite its limited spatial coverage.[83] PCT has also been shown to be equal to MR imaging for the evaluation of vertebrobasilar ischemia.[84]

The low technical requirements for performing PCT/CTA and its wide availability are key advantages. Because of the low cost and usefulness in other areas of medicine, particularly emergency medicine and trauma, CT scanners are becoming widely available, and it is foreseeable that every major emergency center will eventually be able to perform this form of imaging within minutes of the patient entering the emergency department. Another major advantage of PCT compared with MR imaging relates to its quantitative accuracy. Whereas MR perfusion imaging affords only semiquantitative comparison of one hemisphere with the other, quantitative accuracy of PCT makes it a potential surrogate marker to monitor the efficiency of acute reperfusion therapy.

The debate regarding the superiority of either CT or MR imaging for acute stroke imaging should not obscure the ultimate goal: to increase the availability and improve the efficiency of thrombolytic therapy. From this standpoint, CT and MR imaging must be considered equivalent tools, and whichever technique available at each individual institution should be used in the best interest and benefit of the patient with acute stroke.

REFERENCES

1. Lloyd-Jones D, Adams RJ, Brown TM, et al. Executive summary: heart disease and stroke statistics—2010 update: a report from the American Heart Association. Circulation 2010;121(7):948–54.
2. Kolominsky-Rabas PL, Heuschmann PU, Marschall D, et al. Lifetime cost of ischemic stroke in Germany: results and national projections from a population-based stroke registry: the Erlangen Stroke Project. Stroke 2006;37(5):1179–83.
3. Adams HP Jr, Bendixen BH, Kappelle LJ, et al. Classification of subtype of acute ischemic stroke. Definitions for use in a multicenter clinical trial. TOAST. Trial of Org 10172 in Acute Stroke Treatment. Stroke 1993;24(1):35–41.
4. Tissue plasminogen activator for acute ischemic stroke. The National Institute of Neurological Disorders and Stroke RT-PA Stroke Study Group. N Engl J Med 1995;333(24):1581–7.
5. Albers GW, Thijs VN, Wechsler L, et al. Magnetic resonance imaging profiles predict clinical response to early reperfusion: the diffusion and perfusion imaging evaluation for understanding stroke evolution (DEFUSE) study. Ann Neurol 2006;60(5):508–17.
6. Astrup J, Siesjo BK, Symon L. Thresholds in cerebral ischemia—the ischemic penumbra. Stroke 1981;12(6):723–5.
7. Hossmann KA. Viability thresholds and the penumbra of focal ischemia. Ann Neurol 1994;36(4):557–65.
8. Hossmann KA. Neuronal survival and revival during and after cerebral ischemia. Am J Emerg Med 1983;1(2):191–7.
9. Jones TH, Morawetz RB, Crowell RM, et al. Thresholds of focal cerebral ischemia in awake monkeys. J Neurosurg 1981;54(6):773–82.
10. Powers WJ, Grubb RL Jr, Darriet D, et al. Cerebral blood flow and cerebral metabolic rate of oxygen requirements for cerebral function and viability in humans. J Cereb Blood Flow Metab 1985;5(4):600–8.
11. Eastwood JD, Lev MH, Azhari T, et al. CT perfusion scanning with deconvolution analysis: pilot study in patients with acute middle cerebral artery stroke. Radiology 2002;222(1):227–36.
12. Mayer TE, Hamann GF, Baranczyk J, et al. Dynamic CT perfusion imaging of acute stroke. AJNR Am J Neuroradiol 2000;21(8):1441–9.
13. Read SJ, Hirano T, Abbott DF, et al. The fate of hypoxic tissue on 18F-fluoromisonidazole positron

emission tomography after ischemic stroke. Ann Neurol 2000;48(2):228–35.

14. Donnan GA, Davis SM. Neuroimaging, the ischaemic penumbra, and selection of patients for acute stroke therapy. Lancet Neurol 2002;1(7):417–25.

15. Darby DG, Barber PA, Gerraty RP, et al. Pathophysiological topography of acute ischemia by combined diffusion-weighted and perfusion MRI. Stroke 1999; 30(10):2043–52.

16. Hacke W, Donnan G, Fieschi C, et al. Association of outcome with early stroke treatment: pooled analysis of ATLANTIS, ECASS, and NINDS rt-PA stroke trials. Lancet 2004;363(9411):768–74.

17. Schellinger PD, Warach S. Therapeutic time window of thrombolytic therapy following stroke. Curr Atheroscler Rep 2004;6(4):288–94.

18. Bambauer KZ, Johnston SC, Bambauer DE, et al. Reasons why few patients with acute stroke receive tissue plasminogen activator. Arch Neurol 2006;63(5):661–4.

19. Hacke W, Albers G, Al-Rawi Y, et al. The Desmoteplase in Acute Ischemic Stroke Trial (DIAS): a phase II MRI-based 9-hour window acute stroke thrombolysis trial with intravenous desmoteplase. Stroke 2005;36(1):66–73.

20. Furlan AJ, Eyding D, Albers GW, et al. Dose Escalation of Desmoteplase for Acute Ischemic Stroke (DEDAS): evidence of safety and efficacy 3 to 9 hours after stroke onset. Stroke 2006;37(5): 1227–31.

21. Kaste M. Reborn workhorse, CT, pulls the wagon toward thrombolysis beyond 3 hours. Stroke 2004; 35(2):357–9.

22. Wintermark M, Albers GW, Alexandrov AV, et al. Acute stroke imaging research roadmap. AJNR Am J Neuroradiol 2008;29(5):e23–30.

23. Mohr JP, Biller J, Hilal SK, et al. Magnetic resonance versus computed tomographic imaging in acute stroke. Stroke 1995;26(5):807–12.

24. Thomalla G, Rossbach P, Rosenkranz M, et al. Negative fluid-attenuated inversion recovery imaging identifies acute ischemic stroke at 3 hours or less. Ann Neurol 2009;65(6):724–32.

25. Gonzalez RG, Schaefer P. Conventional MRI and MR angiography of stroke. In: Gonzalez RG, Hirsch JA, Koroshetz WJ, et al, editors. Acute ischemic stroke: imaging and intervention. 1st edition. Berlin: Springer; 2006. p. 115–37.

26. Fiebach JB, Schellinger PD, Geletneky K, et al. MRI in acute subarachnoid haemorrhage; findings with a standardised stroke protocol. Neuroradiology 2004;46(1):44–8.

27. Boukobza M, Crassard I, Bousser MG, et al. MR imaging features of isolated cortical vein thrombosis: diagnosis and follow-up. AJNR Am J Neuroradiol 2009;30(2):344–8.

28. Lovblad KO, Bassetti C, Schneider J, et al. Diffusion-weighted MR in cerebral venous thrombosis. Cerebrovasc Dis 2001;11(3):169–76.

29. Srinivasan A, Goyal M, Al Azri F, et al. State-of-the-art imaging of acute stroke. Radiographics 2006; 26(Suppl 1):S75–95.

30. Fiebach JB, Schellinger PD, Jansen O, et al. CT and diffusion-weighted MR imaging in randomized order: diffusion-weighted imaging results in higher accuracy and lower interrater variability in the diagnosis of hyperacute ischemic stroke. Stroke 2002;33 (9):2206–10.

31. Saur D, Kucinski T, Grzyska U, et al. Sensitivity and interrater agreement of CT and diffusion-weighted MR imaging in hyperacute stroke. AJNR Am J Neuroradiol 2003;24(5):878–85.

32. Fiehler J, Knudsen K, Kucinski T, et al. Predictors of apparent diffusion coefficient normalization in stroke patients. Stroke 2004;35(2):514–9.

33. Miyazaki M, Lee VS. Nonenhanced MR angiography. Radiology 2008;248(1):20–43.

34. Grandin CB. Assessment of brain perfusion with MRI: methodology and application to acute stroke. Neuroradiology 2003;45(11):755–66.

35. Rosen BR, Belliveau JW, Vevea JM, et al. Perfusion imaging with NMR contrast agents. Magn Reson Med 1990;14(2):249–65.

36. Fiebach JB, Schellinger PD, Gass A, et al. Stroke magnetic resonance imaging is accurate in hyperacute intracerebral hemorrhage: a multicenter study on the validity of stroke imaging. Stroke 2004;35(2): 502–6.

37. Kidwell CS, Chalela JA, Saver JL, et al. Comparison of MRI and CT for detection of acute intracerebral hemorrhage. JAMA 2004;292(15): 1823–30.

38. Fiehler J, Albers GW, Boulanger JM, et al. Bleeding risk analysis in stroke imaging before thromboLysis (BRASIL): pooled analysis of T2*-weighted magnetic resonance imaging data from 570 patients. Stroke 2007;38(10):2738–44.

39. Vernooij MW, van der Lugt A, Breteler MM. Risk of thrombolysis-related hemorrhage associated with microbleed presence. Stroke 2008;39(7):e115 [author reply: e116].

40. Mittal S, Wu Z, Neelavalli J, et al. Susceptibility-weighted imaging: technical aspects and clinical applications, part 2. AJNR Am J Neuroradiol 2009; 30(2):232–52.

41. Hermier M, Nighoghossian N. Contribution of susceptibility-weighted imaging to acute stroke assessment. Stroke 2004;35(8):1989–94.

42. Ozdoba C, Sturzenegger M, Schroth G. Internal carotid artery dissection: MR imaging features and clinical-radiologic correlation. Radiology 1996; 199(1):191–8.

43. Leclerc X, Gauvrit JY, Nicol L, et al. Contrast-enhanced MR angiography of the craniocervical vessels: a review. Neuroradiology 1999;41(12):867–74.

44. Bowen BC. MR angiography versus CT angiography in the evaluation of neurovascular disease. Radiology 2007;245(2):357–60 [discussion: 60–1].

45. Jansen O, Schellinger P, Fiebach J, et al. Early recanalisation in acute ischaemic stroke saves tissue at risk defined by MRI. Lancet 1999;353(9169):2036–7.

46. Schellinger PD, Fiebach JB, Hacke W. Imaging-based decision making in thrombolytic therapy for ischemic stroke: present status. Stroke 2003;34(2):575–83.

47. Parsons MW, Barber PA, Chalk J, et al. Diffusion- and perfusion-weighted MRI response to thrombolysis in stroke. Ann Neurol 2002;51(1):28–37.

48. Kidwell CS, Alger JR, Saver JL. Beyond mismatch: evolving paradigms in imaging the ischemic penumbra with multimodal magnetic resonance imaging. Stroke 2003;34(11):2729–35.

49. Hacke W, Furlan AJ, Al-Rawi Y, et al. Intravenous desmoteplase in patients with acute ischaemic stroke selected by MRI perfusion-diffusion weighted imaging or perfusion CT (DIAS-2): a prospective, randomised, double-blind, placebo-controlled study. Lancet Neurol 2009;8(2):141–50.

50. Marks MP, Olivot JM, Kemp S, et al. Patients with acute stroke treated with intravenous tPA 3-6 hours after stroke onset: correlations between MR angiography findings and perfusion- and diffusion-weighted imaging in the DEFUSE study. Radiology 2008;249(2):614–23.

51. Kimura K, Iguchi Y, Shibazaki K, et al. Large ischemic lesions on diffusion-weighted imaging done before intravenous tissue plasminogen activator thrombolysis predicts a poor outcome in patients with acute stroke. Stroke 2008;39(8):2388–91.

52. Latchaw RE, Yonas H, Hunter GJ, et al. Guidelines and recommendations for perfusion imaging in cerebral ischemia: a scientific statement for healthcare professionals by the writing group on perfusion imaging, from the Council on Cardiovascular Radiology of the American Heart Association. Stroke 2003;34(4):1084–104.

53. Truwit CL, Barkovich AJ, Gean-Marton A, et al. Loss of the insular ribbon: another early CT sign of acute middle cerebral artery infarction. Radiology 1990;176(3):801–6.

54. Tomura N, Uemura K, Inugami A, et al. Early CT finding in cerebral infarction: obscuration of the lentiform nucleus. Radiology 1988;168(2):463–7.

55. Tomsick TA, Brott TG, Chambers AA, et al. Hyperdense middle cerebral artery sign on CT: efficacy in detecting middle cerebral artery thrombosis. AJNR Am J Neuroradiol 1990;11(3):473–7.

56. Leys D, Pruvo JP, Godefroy O, et al. Prevalence and significance of hyperdense middle cerebral artery in acute stroke. Stroke 1992;23(3):317–24.

57. Rauch RA, Bazan C 3rd, Larsson EM, et al. Hyperdense middle cerebral arteries identified on CT as a false sign of vascular occlusion. AJNR Am J Neuroradiol 1993;14(3):669–73.

58. Barber PA, Darby DG, Desmond PM, et al. Identification of major ischemic change. Diffusion-weighted imaging versus computed tomography. Stroke 1999;30(10):2059–65.

59. Patel SC, Levine SR, Tilley BC, et al. Lack of clinical significance of early ischemic changes on computed tomography in acute stroke. JAMA 2001;286(22):2830–8.

60. Roberts HC, Dillon WP, Furlan AJ, et al. Computed tomographic findings in patients undergoing intra-arterial thrombolysis for acute ischemic stroke due to middle cerebral artery occlusion: results from the PROACT II trial. Stroke 2002;33(6):1557–65.

61. von Kummer R, Bourquain H, Bastianello S, et al. Early prediction of irreversible brain damage after ischemic stroke at CT. Radiology 2001;219(1):95–100.

62. Larrue V, von Kummer RR, Muller A, et al. Risk factors for severe hemorrhagic transformation in ischemic stroke patients treated with recombinant tissue plasminogen activator: a secondary analysis of the European-Australasian Acute Stroke Study (ECASS II). Stroke 2001;32(2):438–41.

63. Hacke W, Kaste M, Fieschi C, et al. Intravenous thrombolysis with recombinant tissue plasminogen activator for acute hemispheric stroke. The European Cooperative Acute Stroke Study (ECASS). JAMA 1995;274(13):1017–25.

64. Eastwood JD, Lev MH, Provenzale JM. Perfusion CT with iodinated contrast material. AJR Am J Roentgenol 2003;180(1):3–12.

65. Wintermark M, Maeder P, Thiran JP, et al. Quantitative assessment of regional cerebral blood flows by perfusion CT studies at low injection rates: a critical review of the underlying theoretical models. Eur Radiol 2001;11(7):1220–30.

66. Kudo K, Terae S, Katoh C, et al. Quantitative cerebral blood flow measurement with dynamic perfusion CT using the vascular-pixel elimination method: comparison with H2(15)O positron emission tomography. AJNR Am J Neuroradiol 2003;24(3):419–26.

67. Prestigiacomo CJ. Surgical endovascular neuroradiology in the 21st century: what lies ahead? Neurosurgery 2006;59(5 Suppl 3):S48–55 [discussion: S3–13].

68. Wang H, Fraser K, Wang D, et al. The evolution of endovascular therapy for neurosurgical disease. Neurosurg Clin N Am 2005;16(2):223–9, vii.

69. Lell MM, Anders K, Uder M, et al. New techniques in CT angiography. Radiographics 2006;26(Suppl 1):S45–62.

70. Prokop M. Multislice CT angiography. Eur J Radiol 2000;36(2):86–96.

71. Lev MH, Farkas J, Rodriguez VR, et al. CT angiography in the rapid triage of patients with hyperacute stroke to intraarterial thrombolysis: accuracy in the detection of large vessel thrombus. J Comput Assist Tomogr 2001;25(4):520–8.

72. Tan JC, Dillon WP, Liu S, et al. Systematic comparison of perfusion-CT and CT-angiography in acute stroke patients. Ann Neurol 2007;61(6):533–43.

73. Zaidat OO, Suarez JI, Santillan C, et al. Response to intra-arterial and combined intravenous and intra-arterial thrombolytic therapy in patients with distal internal carotid artery occlusion. Stroke 2002;33(7): 1821–6.

74. Wintermark M, Reichhart M, Thiran JP, et al. Prognostic accuracy of cerebral blood flow measurement by perfusion computed tomography, at the time of emergency room admission, in acute stroke patients. Ann Neurol 2002;51(4):417–32.

75. Heiss WD, Sobesky J, Hesselmann V. Identifying thresholds for penumbra and irreversible tissue damage. Stroke 2004;35(11 Suppl 1):2671–4.

76. Wintermark M, Flanders AE, Velthuis B, et al. Perfusion-CT assessment of infarct core and penumbra: receiver operating characteristic curve analysis in 130 patients suspected of acute hemispheric stroke. Stroke 2006;37(4):979–85.

77. Wintermark M, Reichhart M, Cuisenaire O, et al. Comparison of admission perfusion computed tomography and qualitative diffusion- and perfusion-weighted magnetic resonance imaging in acute stroke patients. Stroke 2002;33(8):2025–31.

78. Konstas AA, Goldmakher GV, Lee TY, et al. Theoretic basis and technical implementations of CT perfusion in acute ischemic stroke, part 2: technical implementations. AJNR Am J Neuroradiol 2009;30(5):885–92.

79. Smith WS, Roberts HC, Chuang NA, et al. Safety and feasibility of a CT protocol for acute stroke: combined CT, CT angiography, and CT perfusion imaging in 53 consecutive patients. AJNR Am J Neuroradiol 2003;24(4):688–90.

80. Salomon EJ, Barfett J, Willems PW, et al. Dynamic CT angiography and CT perfusion employing a 320-detector row CT: protocol and current clinical applications. Klin Neuroradiol 2009;19(3):187–96.

81. Diekmann S, Siebert E, Juran R, et al. Dose exposure of patients undergoing comprehensive stroke imaging by multidetector-row CT: comparison of 320-detector Row and 64-detector row CT scanners. AJNR Am J Neuroradiol 2010;31(6):1003–9.

82. Struffert T, Deuerling-Zheng Y, Kloska S, et al. Flat detector CT in the evaluation of brain parenchyma, intracranial vasculature, and cerebral blood volume: a pilot study in patients with acute symptoms of cerebral ischemia. AJNR Am J Neuroradiol April 8, 2010 [online].

83. Wintermark M, Fischbein NJ, Smith WS, et al. Accuracy of dynamic perfusion CT with deconvolution in detecting acute hemispheric stroke. AJNR Am J Neuroradiol 2005;26(1):104–12.

84. Nagahori T, Hirashima Y, Umemura K, et al. Supratentorial dynamic computed tomography for the diagnosis of vertebrobasilar ischemic stroke. Neurol Med Chir (Tokyo) 2004;44(3):105–10 [discussion: 110–1].

Nontraumatic Intracranial Hemorrhage

Nancy J. Fischbein[a],* and Christine A.C. Wijman[b]

KEYWORDS
- Intracranial hemorrhage • Cerebral amyloid angiopathy
- Vascular malformation • Venous infarction

Spontaneous or nontraumatic intracranial hemorrhage (ICH) accounts for approximately 10% to 15% of strokes in the United States. The hemorrhages are typically parenchymal, but may also primarily involve the subarachnoid space, subdural space, intraventricular space, or, rarely, epidural space. The clinical presentation of a parenchymal hemorrhage is usually with the sudden onset of a focal neurologic deficit, often accompanied by headache, alteration in the level of consciousness, seizure, and/or nausea and vomiting; intracranial extracerebral hemorrhage more typically presents with headache and alteration in the level of consciousness, although focal neurologic deficits may also be present, notably as a consequence of tissue shift and brain herniation.

The clinical presentations of ischemic stroke and ICH may be similar, and neuroimaging is indicated for further evaluation of the type of stroke and likely cause. Noncontrast computed tomography (CT) of the head is generally the first study performed on presentation to medical attention, because CT is rapid, widely available, and safe. CT is also highly sensitive to acute ICH, which appears dense compared with normal brain tissue and cerebrospinal fluid (CSF) (Fig. 1). Many institutions also perform CT angiography (CTA) and, less commonly, CT perfusion (CTP) as part of the assessment of acute ICH. MR with gradient-recalled echo (GRE) imaging is sensitive to acute hemorrhage, but MR (often with MR angiography [MRA], MR venography [MRV], and/or MR perfusion) is usually performed following CT to assess the cause of a known hemorrhage and to evaluate its effect on the rest of the brain parenchyma. In the setting of acute ischemic stroke with hemorrhagic transformation, MR with diffusion-weighted (DW) imaging is often key to making a diagnosis that could be missed on a non-contrast CT alone, and even on a CT that includes CTA and CTP, depending on the site and size of the infarct that underlies the hemorrhage. In the setting of spontaneous ICH, MR is generally most useful in assessing the cause of hemorrhage rather than the presence of hemorrhage itself; in addition, MR is sensitive to both acute and chronic hemorrhage, whereas CT is most sensitive to acute blood products.

The appearance of blood products is more complex on MR than on CT. On CT, acute blood is dense compared with brain tissue and CSF, and gradually decreases in density over days to weeks depending on the size of the hematoma. On MR, the appearance of the hematoma changes on T1- and T2-weighted images as the blood products evolve from oxyhemoglobin to eventually ferritin and hemosiderin.[1] The evolution of blood products on MR sequences is shown in Fig. 2 and summarized in Table 1.[2,3]

The causes of nontraumatic ICH are numerous. This review focuses on the entities most commonly associated with nontraumatic ICH, such as hypertension and cerebral amyloid angiopathy (CAA),

[a] Department of Radiology (NF), Stanford University School of Medicine, Room S-047, 300 Pasteur Drive, Stanford, CA 94305-5105, USA
[b] Department of Neurology (CW), Stanford University School of Medicine, Stanford Stroke Center, 780 Welch Road, Suite 205, Stanford, CA 94305, USA
* Corresponding author.
E-mail address: fischbein@stanford.edu

Neuroimag Clin N Am 20 (2010) 469–492
doi:10.1016/j.nic.2010.07.003

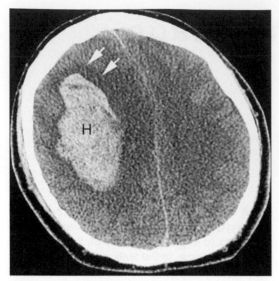

Fig. 1. Axial nonenhanced CT scan shows a large dense hematoma (H) in the right frontal lobe. Only a small amount of vasogenic edema (*arrows*) is seen around this acute intraparenchymal hemorrhage.

but some increasingly recognized less common entities such as isolated cortical vein thrombosis, moyamoya disease, and the reversible cerebral vasoconstrictive syndrome are also discussed.

HYPERTENSIVE HEMORRHAGE

Long-standing hypertension is the leading cause of spontaneous intraparenchymal hemorrhage in adults. Pathophysiologically, long-standing hypertension leads to reactive hyperplasia of smooth muscle cells in cerebral arterioles. Eventually, smooth muscle death occurs, and vascular walls are replaced by collagen. Vascular occlusion or ectasia may then result, with either ischemic or hemorrhagic consequences. Hypertensive hemorrhages may also arise at sites of previous ischemic damage to the walls of small arteries and arterioles.[4]

Hypertensive hemorrhages tend to occur in the basal ganglia, thalami, cerebellum, and pons; the lobar white matter may also be affected (Fig. 3). A homogeneous, round or ovoid hematoma in one of these locations in an older adult patient has a high likelihood of being a result of the microangiopathy associated with long-standing uncontrolled hypertension. The age of the patient (whether older than 45 years or not), the presence of a history of hypertension, and the presence of certain associated imaging findings may help determine the yield of further imaging to assess for causes other than

hypertension. On a CT scan, one may see evidence of microvascular ischemic change in the white matter as well as evidence of lacunar infarcts; these changes are common in the setting of chronic hypertension and increase the likelihood that hypertension is the underlying cause of the acute hemorrhage. On MR, one may also see evidence of white matter microvascular changes on fluid attenuated inversion recovery (FLAIR) and T2-weighted images, as well as evidence of prior lacunar infarcts or remote parenchymal hemorrhages. It is important to include a T2*-weighted sequence in the MR imaging protocol, because the presence of microbleeds in the brainstem and deep gray nuclei supports the likelihood of chronic hypertension and a hypertension-related hemorrhage (Fig. 4).[5] Brain hemorrhages related to drug abuse (typically cocaine and methamphetamine) may mimic the appearance of brain hemorrhages associated with long-standing hypertension on imaging studies, and likely share a common pathophysiology, but they tend to occur in a younger age group.

Intraparenchymal hematomas may expand by more than one-third of their original volume in up to 38% of patients who are imaged early.[6] Hematoma expansion most commonly occurs in the first few hours after symptom onset and has been associated with poor outcome. Risk factors for hematoma growth include time to initial CT scan (in that the earlier a patient is scanned after ICH onset, the more likely it is that the next CT will show ICH expansion), larger ICH volume on the initial CT, and oral anticoagulant use.[7] Other potentially important factors include hyperglycemia, renal failure, low serum cholesterol, platelet dysfunction, and persistently increased blood pressure.[8] On CTA and on the contrast-enhanced CT obtained after the CTA, the presence of focal contrast extravasation is associated with hematoma expansion,[9–11] providing potential justification for consideration of performing these studies on presentation to the hospital. Performing CTA can also help avoid the pitfall of misinterpreting hemorrhages caused by underlying pathologic conditions such as aneurysms or vascular malformations as hypertensive in patients who are older and who do have a diagnosis of hypertension (Fig. 5).

Supportive care (including blood pressure control and correction of coagulopathy) is the mainstay of management of acute intraparenchymal hemorrhage, with surgical evacuation having a more limited role in its management.[12] Most experts agree that cerebellar hematomas that are greater than 3 cm in diameter should be emergently evacuated if the patient is deteriorating neurologically or if the hematoma exerts mass effect on the brainstem or causes hydrocephalus. Furthermore,

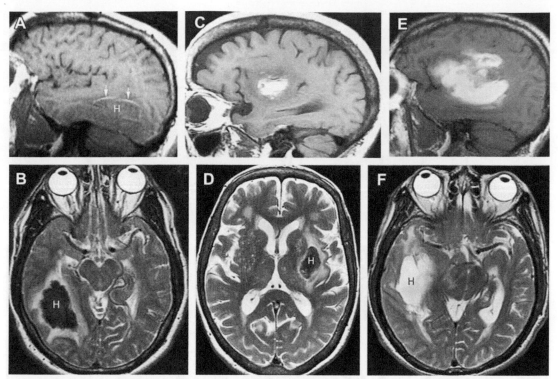

Fig. 2. Vertically paired images of acute, early subacute, and late subacute hematomas. (*A*) Sagittal T1-weighted (T1W) image shows an acute right temporal lobe hematoma (H) consisting largely of isointense deoxyhemoglobin. The beginning of transformation to methemoglobin along the periphery is seen as a thin bright line (*white arrows*). (*B*) Axial T2-weighted (T2W) image in the same patient shows low signal intensity because of deoxyhemoglobin in the hematoma (H). A surrounding rim of bright signal represents vasogenic edema. (*C*) Sagittal T1W image in a patient with an early subacute left subinsular/lateral putaminal hematoma shows high signal. (*D*) Corresponding T2W image shows central low signal intensity. This finding is consistent with intracellular methemoglobin in the hematoma (H). (*E*) Sagittal T1W image in a patient with a large right frontotemporal late subacute hematoma shows bright signal in the lesion. (*F*) Axial T2W image in the same patient also shows high signal in the hematoma (H), consistent with extracellular methemoglobin. There is surrounding vasogenic edema, as well as mass effect with uncal herniation and midbrain compression.

Table 1
MR imaging appearance of intraparenchymal hemorrhage

Timing	Blood Product	T1W Image	T2W Image
Hyperacute (<12 h)	Intracellular oxyhemoglobin	Isointense to hypointense	Hyperintense (variable hypointense rim)
Acute (hours to days)	Intracellular deoxyhemoglobin	Isointense	Hypointense
Subacute-early (few days)	Intracellular methemoglobin	Hyperintense	Hypointense
Subacute-late (week to months)	Extracellular methemoglobin	Hyperintense	Hyperintense
Chronic-early	Extracellular methemoglobin; ferritin/hemosiderin wall	Hyperintense	Hyperintense with low signal rim
Chronic-late	Hemosiderin	Isointense	Hypointense

Data from Refs.[1–3]

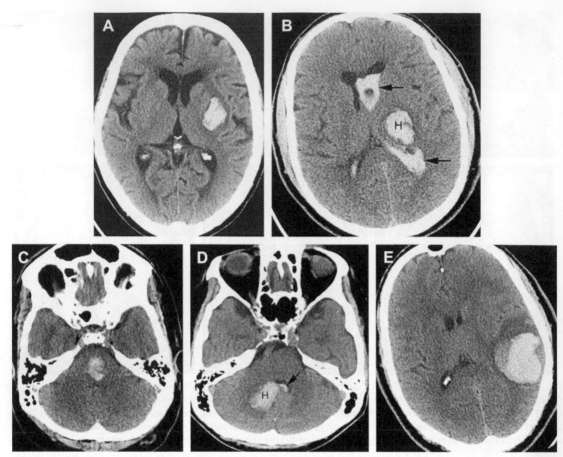

Fig. 3. Five different patients show the CT appearance of intraparenchymal hemorrhage associated with long-standing hypertension in the locations typically associated with hypertensive hemorrhage. (*A*) Acute hematoma in the left lateral putamen/external capsule. (*B*) Acute hematoma (H) in the left thalamus, complicated by intra-ventricular extension (*arrows*). (*C*) Acute hematoma in the central pons. (*D*) Acute hematoma (H) involving the deep white matter of the right cerebellum with extension into the fourth ventricle (*arrow*). (*E*) A large lobar hematoma with associated vasogenic edema. This location is less specific for ICH associated with long-standing hypertension and should raise concern for other potential causes, notably amyloid angiopathy in an elderly patient or tumor or vascular malformation in a younger patient.

based on the results of the International Surgical Trial in Intracerebral Hemorrhage (STICH), surgical evacuation may be considered for patients with superficial (<1 cm from the cortical surface) lobar hematomas.[13] Whether minimally invasive surgical techniques (using mechanical devices and/or endoscopy) to remove the hematoma offer benefit over conventional craniotomy/craniectomy is unknown and currently under investigation.

CEREBRAL AMYLOID ANGIOPATHY

CAA, a disorder that primarily affects individuals older than 60 years, is defined by the accumulation of amyloid in the walls of small and medium-sized cerebral arteries within the brain and leptome-ninges. Both inherited and sporadic forms of

CAA exist; the inherited form is less common, has an earlier onset of symptoms, and is more strongly associated with dementia.[14] Amyloid deposition in cerebral blood vessels can have several clinical consequences. First, it may be asymptomatic, as it is known that more than 50% of individuals older than 80 years have pathologic evidence of CAA. Second, it may weaken the vessel wall, leading to a rupture and ICH. Third, it can obliterate the vascular lumen, leading to ischemia and contributing to leukoencephalopathy.[15]

CAA-related hemorrhages are said to account for 5% to 20% of nontraumatic cerebral hemorrhages in elderly patients, so it is second only to hyper-tension as a cause of spontaneous ICH. The hallmark of the CAA-related hemorrhage is a lobar, cortical,

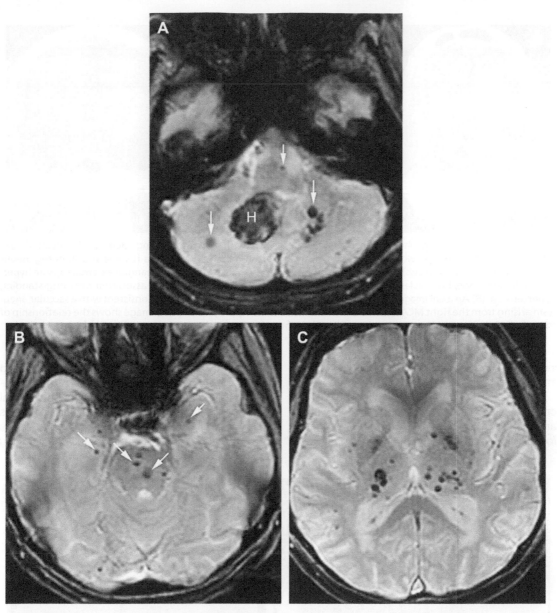

Fig. 4. (A) Axial GRE image through the posterior fossa in a patient with a cerebellar hemorrhage (H) shows multifocal microhemorrhages (*arrows*) related to chronic hypertension. (B) A more superior GRE image in the same patient shows microhemorrhages in the pons as well as a few scattered microhemorrhages in the temporal lobes. (C) An axial GRE image at the level of the deep gray nuclei shows numerous microhemorrhages with a thalamic predilection. This deep and central distribution of microhemorrhages is typical of chronic severe and uncontrolled hypertension.

or cortical-subcortical hemorrhage affecting normotensive individuals older than 55 years; the hemorrhages are frequently multiple and recurrent, and often extend to the subarachnoid space.[16] An important clue to the diagnosis of CAA is the presence of multiple petechial hemorrhages (microbleeds) in characteristic locations identified on T2*-weighted MR images (Fig. 6). Unlike the microbleeds associated with chronic hypertension, which

are typically located in the brainstem and deep gray nuclei, the microbleeds of CAA tend to be located peripherally in the cerebellum and in the cortical-subcortical region of the cerebral hemispheres. Newer MR imaging methods such as susceptibility-weighted imaging are exquisitely sensitive to chronic blood products and will likely increase the frequency of diagnosis of CAA and other hemorrhagic disorders in coming years, as will the

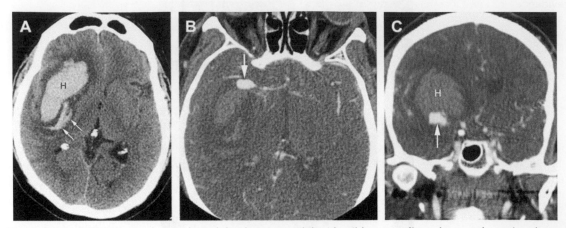

Fig. 5. (A) Axial NECT image shows a large lobar hematoma (H) with mild surrounding edema and associated mass effect in a 53-year-old man with a history of chronic hypertension. The hematoma is somewhat heterogeneous along its medial aspect (arrows), and it extends more anteriorly than a typical basal ganglia/external capsule hypertensive hemorrhage, but this lesion could potentially be diagnosed as a hemorrhage associated with long-standing hypertension. (B) An axial image from a CTA shows a lobulated, contrast-filled mass consistent with a saccular aneurysm arising from the right MCA. (C) A coronal maximum-intensity projection (MIP) image shows the relationship of the inferiorly located MCA aneurysm (arrow) to the more superior hematoma (H).

increasing prevalence of high-field (3 T and greater) imaging systems.[17]

The use of warfarin in patients with CAA is controversial. Warfarin use is associated with an annual ICH risk of 0.3% to 0.6%, and risk factors for warfarin-associated ICH include older age, leukoaraiosis, and CAA. Given the associated stroke risk of 5% to 12% per year with atrial fibrillation and 4% per year in patients with mechanical valves, most clinicians choose to place patients with atrial fibrillation or mechanical heart valves on chronic warfarin therapy despite imaging

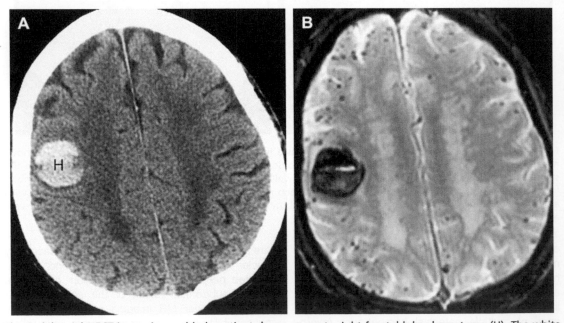

Fig. 6. (A) Axial NECT image in an elderly patient shows an acute right frontal lobar hematoma (H). The white matter shows diffuse hypodensity consistent with chronic microvascular ischemic change. (B) Axial GRE image shows the right frontal hematoma but also shows innumerable peripherally located microhemorrhages. This GRE appearance is classic for CAA.

evidence of an increased risk of warfarin-associated ICH in patients with CAA. In patients who have suffered a warfarin-associated ICH, the risk of subsequent cardioembolic complications needs to be weighed against the risk of ICH recurrence.[18]

HEMORRHAGIC TRANSFORMATION OF ISCHEMIC STROKE

Hemorrhagic transformation of an ischemic stroke (HTIS) can be misdiagnosed as a primary intraparenchymal hemorrhage if the underlying ischemic infarct is not appreciated from clinical or imaging evaluation, but in most cases it is readily recognized as a complication of prior arterial infarction (Fig. 7). HTIS has been associated with baseline stroke severity, hyperglycemia, uncontrolled hypertension,[19] advanced age, use of thrombolytics, nonrecanalization, and use of anticoagulants, among other risk factors.[20–22] HTIS may be evident on imaging studies alone (usually petechial hemorrhage), or may cause deterioration of a patient's clinical condition (parenchymal hematoma). HTIS is reported as complicating from 2% to 40% of ischemic strokes, depending how carefully one looks for it with various imaging modalities. Symptomatic intracerebral hemorrhage in the setting of ischemic infarction treated with intravenous or intraarterial thrombolytic therapy occurs in only approximately 6% to 12% of patients.

Predicting which ischemic strokes may undergo hemorrhagic transformation is of interest as use of thrombolytic agents becomes more widespread and as these agents are more frequently administered in later time windows (eg, more than 4.5 hours after symptom onset). Radiographic risk factors for hemorrhagic transformation after thrombolytic therapy include large areas of hypoattenuated brain parenchyma and a hyperdense middle cerebral artery (MCA) sign on the pretreatment head CT.[23,24] In addition, patients who do not recanalize are at higher risk for subsequent hemorrhage. On CTP, the permeability-surface area product has been suggested to be useful in identifying patients with acute ischemic stroke who are likely to develop hemorrhagic transformation.[20] On MR, a malignant pattern of large regions of DW and perfusion-weighted imaging abnormality combined with early reperfusion seemed to predict symptomatic hemorrhagic transformation and poor clinical outcome.[21,25] In addition, the cause of ischemic stroke influences whether hemorrhagic transformation occurs. Septic emboli, especially those of fungal cause, are often accompanied by parenchymal hemorrhage, and this diagnosis should be strongly considered in the appropriate clinical setting when a patient presents with multifocal ischemic infarcts associated with hemorrhage (Fig. 8).[26] Ischemic stroke is discussed in greater detail in the article Imaging of Ischemic Stroke by Leiva-Salinas and Wintermark elsewhere in this issue.

ANEURYSMAL SUBARACHNOID HEMORRHAGE

The most common cause of subarachnoid hemorrhage (SAH) is trauma, but aneurysmal SAH accounts for at least 85% of nontraumatic SAH

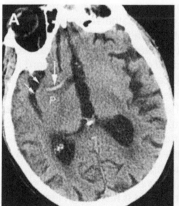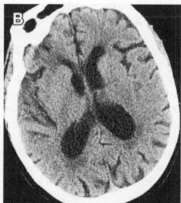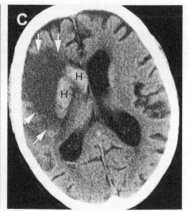

Fig. 7. (A) Axial NECT image from an elderly woman with acute onset of left hemiparesis shows a dense MCA (*large white arrow*), consistent with clot in the vessel. Signs of early arterial infarction are present, with subtle hypodensity in the right insular ribbon (*arrows*) and inferior putamen (P). (B) A more superior axial CT image from the same study shows subtle hypodensity in the right corpus striatum, as well as the insula and right frontal lobe; there is mass effect on the right lateral ventricle. (C) A follow-up NECT 3 days later shows hemorrhagic transformation (H) involving right caudate and putamen, as well as increasing hypodensity in the evolving right frontal infarct. There is increased mass effect on the right frontal horn, and a small amount of intraventricular hemorrhage.

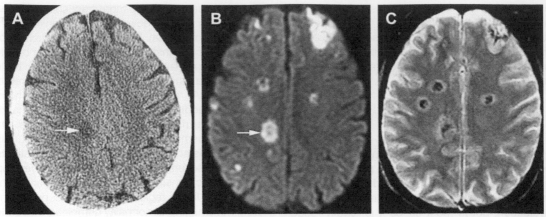

Fig. 8. (*A*) Axial NECT in a 56-year-old man after bone marrow transplant for leukemia and with new left-sided weakness shows a nonspecific hypodense lesion in the right centrum semiovale. (*B*) A brain MR image with DW imaging performed the following day shows multifocal rounded and also wedge-shaped areas of reduced diffusion, with a right posterior frontal lesion (*arrow*) corresponding to the lesion seen on the CT scan. (*C*) An axial GRE image at the same level shows that many of the lesions have central hypointensity consistent with hemorrhage. Biopsy confirmed hemorrhagic septic emboli caused by aspergillosis.

cases. Aneurysmal SAH accounts for only 5% of stroke cases, but with an associated mortality of 12% to 66% in various studies, this stroke subtype accounts for the most life-years lost to stroke.[27] Common risk factors for aneurysmal SAH are hypertension and smoking, and it affects women more frequently than men. Patients with aneurysmal SAH typically present with acute onset of severe headache, often described as the worst headache of the patient's life. Other symptoms and signs may include vomiting, seizures, nuchal rigidity, cranial nerve palsies, and alteration in the level of consciousness ranging from confusion and drowsiness to coma. The diagnosis of acute SAH is made on noncontrast CT, or by lumbar puncture when the CT scan is negative and clinical suspicion is high. The likelihood of missing acute SAH on the initial CT scan increases as the time interval between symptom onset and time of the CT scan increases. Once nontraumatic SAH has been diagnosed, the patient usually undergoes an urgent evaluation focused on identifying the cause of the SAH: saccular aneurysms are the most common cause, but dissecting intracranial aneurysms and vascular malformations (discussed in detail later) may also present with spontaneous SAH.

On nonenhanced CT (NECT) imaging, aneurysmal SAH typically presents as increased density in the basal cisterns and/or Sylvian fissures. The pattern of hemorrhage may provide insight into the likely location of the aneurysm (ie, blood in the anterior interhemispheric fissure is associated with rupture of an anterior communicating artery aneurysm).

Some patients may have an intraparenchymal hematoma in addition to blood in the subarachnoid space, and the hematoma is typically adjacent to the dome of the aneurysm. In some cases the offending aneurysm may be large enough to be identified as a mass on an NECT, or it may be seen as a relative filling defect within the dense cisternal blood; calcified aneurysms can also be identified on NECT. The most common locations for saccular aneurysms include the anterior communicating artery, posterior communicating artery, and MCA trifurcation, but many other locations (basilar tip, posterior inferior cerebellar artery, anterior choroidal artery) may also be seen.

In the past, urgent catheter angiography was generally indicated for assessment of nontraumatic SAH. In the past decade, however, CTA has evolved as the initial study of choice in many centers (**Fig. 9**). On CTA, the typical saccular aneurysm is seen as a rounded contrast-filled outpouching of the vessel wall. It is important to scrutinize both the source images and the three-dimensional (3D) reformations of the CTA carefully, because in some cases one or the other of these image sets may show the aneurysm to better advantage.

CTA can be acquired quickly and easily even in acutely ill patients, and it has a high level of diagnostic accuracy: modern multislice CT scanners have been reported to provide a sensitivity, specificity, and accuracy as high as 100% even for small aneurysms (5 mm or less) in multiple series.[27–29] Contraindications to CTA include allergy to iodinated contrast material and renal insufficiency; in addition, CTA can be degraded by patient motion

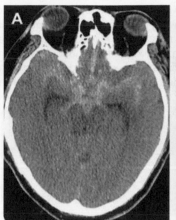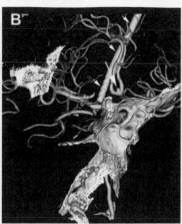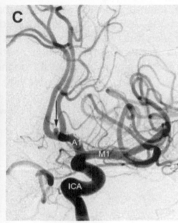

Fig. 9. (*A*) Axial NECT shows diffuse acute SAH in the suprasellar cistern, anterior interhemispheric fissure, and Sylvian fissures. Mild hydrocephalus is present, with dilatation of the temporal horns. (*B*) Oblique view of a 3D volume-rendered image from a CTA shows a saccular aneurysm of the anterior communicating artery (*large white arrow*). An intraventricular drain is also in place (*short white arrows*). (*C*) An anterioposterior view from a catheter angiogram with left ICA injection confirms the presence of the small saccular aneurysm arising from the anterior communicating artery. Also indicated are the A1 and M1 segments of the left anterior and middle cerebral arteries.

and a poor quality bolus (because of technical factors or patient factors such as poor cardiac output). CTA can also be a significant source of radiation exposure, especially if multiple studies are performed. If clinical suspicion of aneurysmal SAH is high and CTA is negative, then assessment with digital subtraction angiography (DSA), preferably accompanied by 3D rotational angiography, should be strongly considered.[30] Furthermore, although many surgeons proceed to the operating room from CTA alone, DSA may be indicated for preoperative assessment of complex aneurysms and for assessment of the presence of additional asymptomatic aneurysms. MRI/MRA may be used in selected situations for the assessment of aneurysmal SAH, but high signal intensity of the CSF on FLAIR is not specific for hemorrhage, and areas of poor CSF suppression limit overall sensitivity to hemorrhage in the subarachnoid space; MRI/MRA also takes longer than CTA, making the MR scanner a less optimal environment for a critically ill patient than the CT scanner.[31] Safety concerns regarding the MR environment also make it less appropriate for critically ill patients in whom appropriate MR safety screening cannot be performed.

Once an aneurysm has been identified, then the course of treatment is dictated to a large extent by the precise anatomy of the aneurysm, the clinical condition of the patient, the preferences of patient and family, and the availability of neurosurgical and neurointerventional services, as both surgical

clipping and endovascular coiling of aneurysms are in routine clinical use. If a patient survives the initial aneurysm rupture, then he/she must be carefully watched for the development of vasospasm; angiographic vasospasm occurs in approximately 70% of patients who survive the initial rupture, and about half of these patients develop neurologic deficits. Clinical and transcranial Doppler monitoring for development of vasospasm can often be effectively supplemented with CTA,[32] thereby avoiding unnecessary DSA in many cases, although DSA is necessary for intraarterial therapy for vasospasm. The treatment of aneurysms and aneurysmal SAH is discussed in more detail in the article Acute Neuro-Interventional Therapies by Hetts and English elsewhere in this issue.

VASCULAR MALFORMATIONS

Vascular malformations account for approximately 20% of spontaneous ICHs and are the leading cause of spontaneous ICH in young adults.[33] Vascular malformations include arteriovenous malformations (AVMs), dural arteriovenous fistulas (dAVFs), cavernous malformations (CMs), developmental venous anomalies (DVAs), and capillary telangiectasias, with AVMs and CMs accounting for most of the clinically evident hemorrhages.

An AVM is a developmental lesion characterized by abnormal connections between pial arteries and veins with no intervening capillary bed; the feeding arteries are usually branches of the internal carotid or vertebrobasilar system, and the AVM is typically located in the brain parenchyma. A central nidus that varies in size from microscopic to several centimeters represents the site of anomalous connection, and in larger lesions, enlarged feeding arteries and draining veins can be seen extending to and away from the central nidus. In the absence of hemorrhage most patients are asymptomatic, although some may have headaches or seizures that bring them to medical attention, and some AVMs are incidentally detected on imaging studies performed for other indications; however,

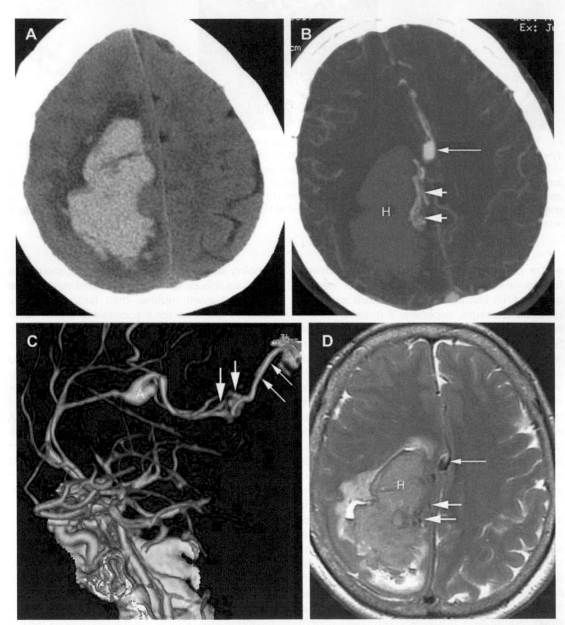

Fig. 10. (A) Axial NECT shows a large lobar hematoma with surrounding edema in a 69-year-old woman. (B) An axial MIP image from a CTA shows a nidus of abnormally enlarged vessels (*short white arrows*), consistent with an arteriovenous malformation located along the medial aspect of the hematoma (H). The thin long arrow indicates a feeding artery aneurysm arising from the right anterior cerebral artery. (C) A 3D volume-rendered image from the CTA in a roughly sagittal projection shows the feeding artery aneurysm (A), the nidus of the AVM (*thick white arrows*), and the dominant draining vein (*thin white arrows*). (D) An axial T2W image from an MR scan performed shortly after the CTA shows the large hematoma (H), as well as the anterior cerebral artery (ACA) aneurysm (*long arrow*) and the subtle flow voids associated with the nidus of the AVM (*thick white arrows*).

hemorrhage is often the initial clinical presentation of AVM.

On a noncontrast CT scan, an AVM associated with ICH may be recognized because of enlarged, serpiginous, dense feeding arteries and/or draining veins; there may also be encephalomalacia and/or mineralization of the adjacent brain parenchyma. On CTA, the abnormal vessels usually can be directly visualized (Fig. 10). Similarly, if MRI/MRA is performed, then abnormal vessels also may be directly visualized. Catheter angiography is used to diagnose small AVMs that may be occult on both CT and MR, to fully characterize an AVM, and often for therapeutic intervention. In rare instances, AVMs may be occult even on contrast angiography, generally because the abnormal vessels are compressed in the acute phase by hematoma. Repeat angiography in the chronic phase after resorption of the hematoma is appropriate in selected patients with a high index of suspicion and a negative initial cerebral angiogram. Once an AVM has been identified, treatment is often multimodality depending on the complexity of the lesion; transcatheter embolization, surgical resection, and stereotactic radiosurgery may all play a role in AVM management. The well-known Spetzler and Martin grading system for AVMs is summarized in Table 2 and attempts to predict the risk of surgical morbidity and mortality by assigning points to an AVM from several lesion characteristics.[34]

CMs affect 0.2% to 0.4% of the population, but the frequency of associated clinically evident ICH is far lower.[35] CMs are considered vascular hamartomas; these low-flow lesions consist of closely apposed endothelial-lined blood vessels without intervening brain tissue. CMs may be found in any region of the brain, and they may occur in isolation, in association with a DVA, or as part of a genetic syndrome in which numerous CMs are present. CMs may be associated with acute ICH, but many come to attention because of headache or seizure, or they are detected incidentally on imaging studies performed for unrelated indications.

On CT, CMs are often difficult to appreciate, although they may be seen as small (usually 1 cm or smaller, although some are as large as 5 cm or more), round or ovoid areas of subtle hyperdensity caused by mineralization and blood products. If a CM has recently bled, then the acute hemorrhage may be evident on the CT scan. On MR, CMs are characterized by a mixed signal intensity core with areas that are typically bright on both T1- and T2-weighted images, and a low signal intensity rim (Fig. 11). The hemosiderin rim is especially well appreciated on GRE sequences,

Graded Feature[a]	Points Assigned
Size of AVM (cm)	
Small (<3)	1
Medium (3 to 6)	2
Large (>6)	3
Eloquence of adjacent brain	
Noneloquent	0
Eloquent	1
Pattern of venous drainage	
Superficial only	0
Deep	1

Table 2
Spetzler-Martin grading system for arteriovenous malformation

[a] Grade, sum of points assigned in each of the 3 categories, and so ranges from I to V.

Data from Spetzler RF, Martin NA. A proposed grading system for arteriovenous malformation. J Neurosurg 1986;65:476–83.

and often a small CM is detectable only on this sequence. Gadolinium is usually given to look for an associated developmental venous anomaly (DVA). This is also very useful in the setting of acute hemorrhage: the underlying CM may be obliterated or compressed by an acute hematoma, but if a DVA can be identified in proximity to the hematoma, then CM is likely the underlying cause of the hemorrhage. CMs are typically angiographically occult, and catheter angiography does not play a role in their diagnostic evaluation or management.

dAVFs are a heterogeneous group of lesions that share the common feature of arteriovenous shunting within the dura: an abnormal direct connection (fistula) is present between a meningeal artery and a meningeal vein or dural venous sinus.[36] These lesions represent 6% of supratentorial and 35% of infratentorial vascular malformations. They are typically acquired and idiopathic, although some may be associated with antecedent events such as prior dural sinus thrombosis, craniotomy, or trauma[37]; rarely these lesions are congenital. They may occur at any level of the brain, skull base, and spine, but intracranially they are most common at the level of the cavernous sinus and in the posterior fossa. Several classification systems exist for dAVF, and the commonly used systems are summarized in Table 3.[38,39] These classification systems help to stratify patients according to their risk of hemorrhagic complications related to the underlying dAVF.

dAVFs may present with ICH or progressive neurologic deficits. Venous hypertension may lead to localized symptoms such as pulsatile tinnitus or cavernous-orbital syndrome depending on the precise location and drainage characteristics of the fistula, or may lead to more generalized and diffuse symptoms such as intracranial hypertension and dementia. Spontaneous ICH may also be a presenting symptom, usually in patients in whom antegrade drainage is obstructed and cortical venous drainage is present. NECT may be normal if the patient does not have ICH or hydrocephalus, but in some patients abnormal dural sinuses or transosseous vascular channels may be noted. Contrast-enhanced CT and CTA may show abnormally enlarged and tortuous feeding arteries, enlarged or occluded dural sinuses, and enlarged cortical draining veins depending on the precise angioarchitecture of the fistula (Fig. 12). MRI/MRA/MRV may show similar imaging features, and dynamic MRA may be particularly useful in fistula identification and characterization.[40] Catheter angiography plays several essential roles in the evaluation and management of dAVFs:

1. Diagnosis: the lesions may be subtle or occult on noninvasive imaging studies
2. Characterization: angiography allows complete assessment of arterial input and venous drainage
3. Treatment: many dAVFs can be treated partially or completely with endovascular methods.

DVAs and capillary telangiectasias do not typically present with ICH (except as discussed earlier, when CMs occur in association with DVAs) and are not further discussed in this article.

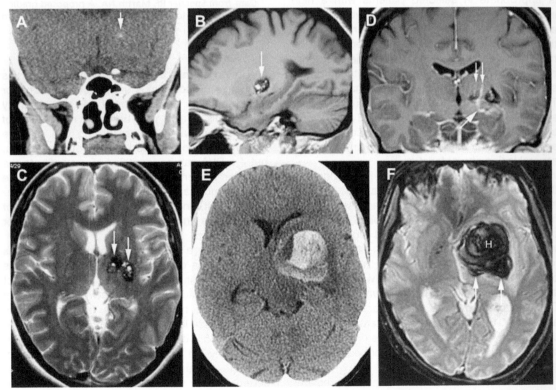

Fig. 11. (*A*) Coronal reconstructed image from an NECT obtained for assessment of sinusitis shows a subtle focus of parenchymal calcification in the region of the deep gray nuclei on the left (*arrow*). (*B*) A sagittal T1W image in the same patient shows a well-circumscribed rounded lesion with heterogeneous high signal in the center and a peripheral rim of hemosiderin staining. This appearance is typical of a CM. (*C*) An axial T2W image in the same patient shows that there are 2 CMs adjacent to each other along the margin of the left thalamus and the left internal capsule. These lesions have the popcorn or mulberrylike appearance of lobulated central T2 hyperintensity and peripheral hypointensity that is typical of CMs. (*D*) Following administration of gadolinium, a coronal T1W image shows a venous malformation adjacent to the CMs, with smaller venous radicles (*thin arrows*) draining into a larger vein (*large thick arrow*). (*E*) Axial NECT 2 years later when the patient developed acute headache and right-sided weakness shows a large acute somewhat heterogeneous hematoma centered in the left putamen and thalamus. (*F*) Axial GRE image shows the acute hematoma (H) with the lobulated CMs (*arrows*) at its posterior aspect. The patient subsequently underwent evacuation of the hematoma and resection of the CMs.

Table 3
Classification schemes for dAVF

Borden Classification	
Type I	Dural arterial supply drains antegrade into venous sinus
Type II	Dural arterial supply drains into venous sinus. High pressure in sinus results in both antegrade drainage and retrograde drainage via cortical veins
Type III	Dural arterial supply drains retrograde into cortical veins
Cognard Classification	
Type I	Drainage into a venous sinus, with normal antegrade flow in sinus
Type II	Drainage into a sinus but with insufficient antegrade venous drainage and reflux. (IIa) retrograde venous drainage into sinus(es) only; (IIb) retrograde venous drainage into cortical vein(s) only; (IIa+b) retrograde venous drainage into sinus (es) and cortical vein(s)
Type III	Direct cortical venous drainage without venous ectasia
Type IV	Direct cortical venous drainage with venous ectasia >5 mm in diameter and 3 times larger than the diameter of the draining vein
Type V	Intracranial fistula drains into spinal perimedullary veins

Data from Borden JA, Wu JK, Shucart WA. A proposed classification for spinal and cranial dural arteriovenous fistulous malformations and implications for treatment. J Neurosurg 1995;82:166–79; and Cognard C, Gobin YP, Pierot L, et al. Cerebral dural arteriovenous fistulas: clinical and angiographic correlation with a revised classification of venous drainage. Radiology 1995;194:671–80.

VENOUS THROMBOSIS

Thrombotic occlusion of the cerebral veins and dural sinuses accounts for approximately 1% to 2% of strokes in adults, but represents a higher proportion of strokes that occur in young patients. Major risk factors for cerebral venous thrombosis include oral contraceptive use and pregnancy, genetic and acquired thrombophilia, malignancy,

and infection.[41] The clinical presentation is highly variable and ranges from headache to seizures and focal neurologic deficits to impairment of the level of consciousness. The pathophysiology of injury relates to venous hypertension, which may manifest acutely as localized venous ischemia and infarction, often with complicating parenchymal hemorrhage. Brain parenchymal edema and hemorrhage in particular locations (posterior temporal lobe, parasagittal frontal or parietal lobe, bilateral thalami) should always suggest the diagnosis of venous thrombosis, and imaging studies should be carefully scrutinized for the presence of suggestive or diagnostic findings.

NECT scans are typically performed as the first line of investigation for patients who present emergently. On noncontrast CT, parenchymal edema and hemorrhage may be present if the patient has a venous infarct. Abnormal increased density may be present in thrombosed venous sinuses, as well as in thrombosed cortical veins (the so-called "cord sign").[42] This density decreases after the first week, making the thrombosis more difficult to detect on NECT. Contrast-enhanced CT and CTA are helpful in assessment of possible venous thrombosis, as thrombus appears as a filling defect or segmental lack of opacification in what should be a completely opacified vein or dural sinus.[43] This situation gives rise to the "empty delta" sign, a cardinal sign of dural sinus thrombosis (Fig. 13). MR imaging of the brain is more sensitive than CT to the parenchymal edema of venous ischemia and nonhemorrhagic venous infarction, and also shows parenchymal hemorrhage well on T2* sequences (Fig. 14). DW images show variable reduced diffusion in venous ischemia/infarction compared with acute arterial infarction, and the lack of reduced diffusion does not exclude venous ischemia/infarction.[44] Routine spin-echo images may show a lack of dural sinus flow void or may show abnormal signal intensity in a thrombosed cortical vein. Some patients may have only a thrombosed cortical vein without associated thrombosis of the dural sinus. This entity has gained more recognition in recent years, and thrombosed cortical veins may be appreciated on NECT or spin-echo or gradient-echo MR images (Fig. 15). With venous thrombosis, MRV typically shows a lack of flow-related enhancement in the affected cerebral vein or dural sinus, but one must be careful not to interpret a hypoplastic sinus as a thrombosed sinus. Following gadolinium administration, the MR equivalent of the empty delta sign may be observed in the dural venous sinuses.

The mainstay of treatment of cerebral venous thrombosis is anticoagulation, even in the setting of brain parenchymal hemorrhage. Catheter

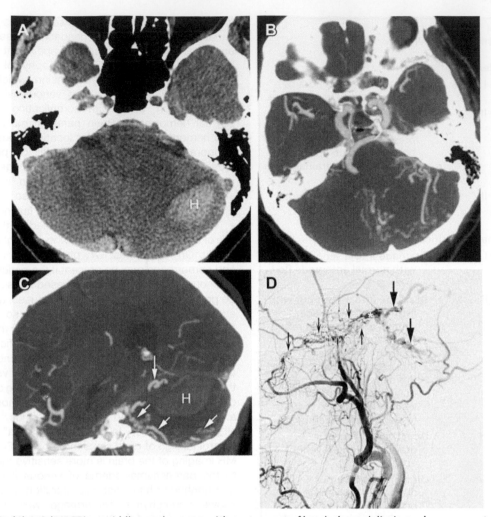

Fig. 12. (*A*) Axial NECT in a middle-aged woman with acute onset of headache and dizziness shows an acute hematoma (H) in the left lateral cerebellum. This is an atypical location for a hypertensive hemorrhage in the cerebellum, because these are usually centered in the deep white matter of the cerebellum. (*B*) Axial MIP from a CTA shows numerous tortuous, corkscrewlike vessels in the posterior fossa, without a discrete nidus. (*C*) Sagittal MIP from the CTA again shows numerous corkscrew vessels in the posterior fossa (*white arrows*), extending along the dural surfaces, as well as the cerebellar hematoma (H). (*D*) A lateral view from a catheter angiogram during injection of the left external carotid artery shows numerous small, irregular arterial feeders (*black arrows*) arising from the middle meningeal artery. The location of the fistulous communication within the dura is indicated by the asterisk (*), and associated enlarged tortuous early draining cortical veins are also seen (*large black arrows*).

angiography generally does not play a role in the diagnosis of cerebral venous thrombosis, but may be indicated for administration of intravenous thrombolytics and for mechanical clot lysis as a rescue therapy in patients with a fulminant course or in those who continue to worsen in spite of systemic anticoagulation.

NEOPLASIA

Primary and metastatic brain tumors may have associated ICH, occurring in up to 15% of patients, but rarely is hemorrhage the presenting

symptom of a previously undiagnosed brain mass.[45] In this circumstance, the diagnosis of an underlying tumor may pose diagnostic difficulties, especially if the tumor is small compared with the volume of the brain hematoma. Although many malignant gliomas show microscopic evidence of hemorrhage, acute hemorrhage as the presenting sign of a malignant glioma is most common with glioblastoma multiforme. The intracerebral metastases that are most likely to hemorrhage are those caused by choriocarcinoma, melanoma, thyroid carcinoma, and renal cell carcinoma, although most hemorrhagic

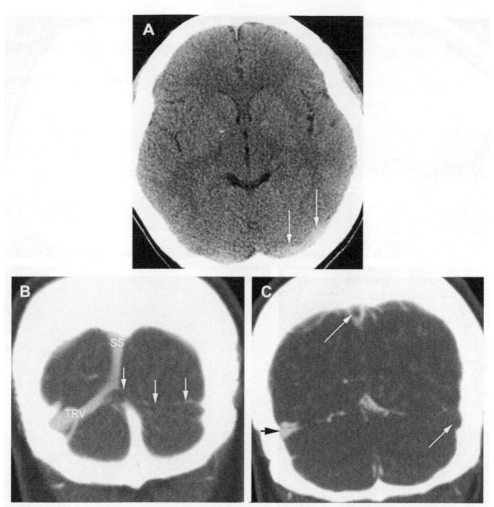

Fig. 13. (A) Axial NECT in a young woman with headache shows increased density along the course of the left trans-verse sinus. (B) A coronal reconstructed image from a CTA shows normal opacification of the superior sagittal sinus and right transverse sinus on this slice; the thrombosed left transverse sinus (*white arrows*) does not opacify with contrast, and thrombus extends medially to the torcular herophili. (C) A more anterior coronal image shows not only the thrombosis at the level of the left transverse-sigmoid junction (*lower white arrow*), but also a filling defect in the superior sagittal sinus, consistent with partial thrombosis at this level (*upper white arrow*) and demonstrating the "empty delta" sign. The normal right transverse-sigmoid junction is indicated (*black arrow*).

metastases are caused by breast and lung carci-nomas because these are more common causes of brain metastases in the general population. Another entity to consider is atrial myxoma, which may give rise to oncotic intracranial aneurysms with secondary subarachnoid and/or paren-chymal hemorrhage.

Certain imaging findings have been described as more consistent with malignant or intratumoral cerebral hemorrhage.[46] Most of these findings are applicable to MR, as CT scans most commonly show areas of nonspecific hemorrhage (**Fig. 16**). However, more perihematoma edema on the CT scan than one would expect from the ICH

alone should raise suspicion for an underlying malignancy, as should marked heterogeneity of the hematoma. On MR imaging, intratumoral hemorrhages tend to be extremely heterogeneous because of blood products in varying phases of signal evolution, debris-fluid levels, and/or the presence of edema, tumor, and necrotic tissue mixing with blood products. These lesions often show associated regions of nonenhancing or enhancing nonhemorrhagic tumor tissue (**Fig. 17**), and any surrounding hypointense rim of ferritin or hemosiderin may be incomplete or irregular. If the hematoma is followed over time because of uncer-tainty about its benign or malignant nature, then it

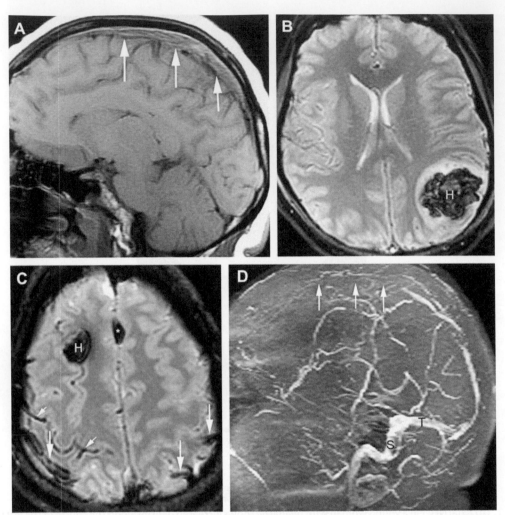

Fig. 14. (A) Sagittal T1W image shows abnormal increased signal intensity in the superior sagittal sinus (*white arrows*), consistent with thrombosis. Normally, a flow void would be expected in the sagittal sinus on a spin-echo image. (B) Axial GRE image shows a left parietal intraparenchymal hemorrhage (H) with associated edema, consistent with hemorrhagic venous infarction. (C) A more superior GRE image shows an additional hematoma (H) in the right frontal lobe, as well as areas of SAH (*small white arrows*). Several thrombosed cortical veins heading toward the sagittal sinus are also appreciated (*large white arrows*). (D) A lateral projection from an MR venogram shows a lack of flow-related enhancement in the superior sagittal sinus (*white arrows*). Flow-related enhancement is seen in the transverse (T) and sigmoid (S) sinuses.

may show delayed evolution of blood breakdown products and persistent edema and mass effect, even in late stages of evolution. The identification of additional enhancing lesions in the brain may be helpful in making the diagnosis of metastatic disease, and in some cases a systemic staging workup with body CT and/or fluorodeoxyglucose positron emission tomography CT may be indicated to assess for a primary lesion as well as other metastatic sites of disease.

VASCULITIS/VASCULOPATHY/VASOSPASM

Primary vascular abnormalities such as vasculitis, nonatherosclerotic vasculopathy, and vasoconstrictive syndromes may on occasion present with spontaneous hemorrhages that may be parenchymal or subarachnoid in location.[47] Central nervous system (CNS) vasculitis may be primary or secondary to systemic vasculitides and often presents with headache, confusion,

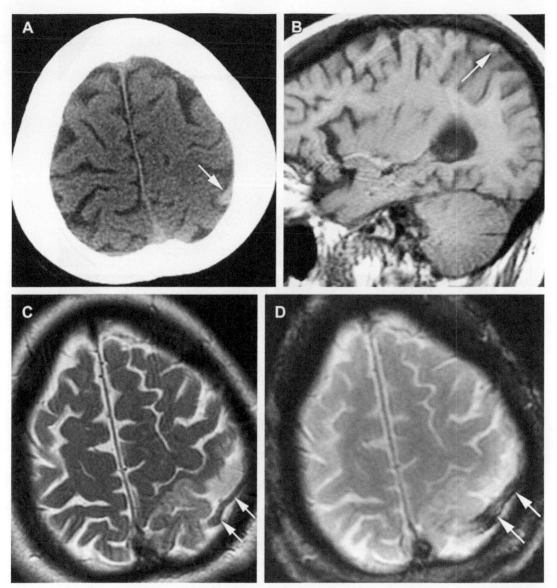

Fig. 15. (*A*) Axial NECT in a young woman with headache and right arm sensory deficits shows a tubular structure of increased density, consistent with a thrombosed cortical vein. The underlying brain parenchyma shows hypodensity and crowding of sulci, consistent with parenchymal edema caused by localized venous hypertension. (*B*) A sagittal T1W image shows high signal intensity in a thrombosed cortical vein overlying the left parietal lobe. (*C*) An axial fast spin-echo T2W image shows to better advantage the left parietal vasogenic edema, as well as the thrombosed cortical vein (*white arrows*). (*D*) An axial GRE image shows blooming of the clot within the left parietal cortical vein caused by magnetic susceptibility effects of the acute clot.

seizure, and focal neurologic deficits. MR imaging typically shows multifocal areas of T2 signal abnormality involving the deep gray nuclei and subcortical white matter, accompanied by reduced diffusion in the acute stage of injury and variable enhancement after gadolinium. CTA and MRA may show vascular irregularity, particularly if larger vessels are involved, but these modalities are relatively insensitive to small vessel involvement, and catheter angiography is often indicated for further evaluation. The hallmark of vasculitis on cerebral angiography is multifocal areas of vascular stenosis and dilatation involving small and medium-sized vessels; sometimes this can be difficult to differentiate from intracranial atherosclerosis, and the overall presentation of the

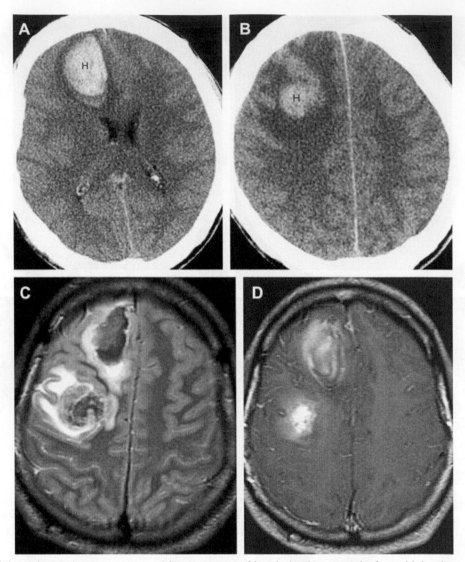

Fig. 16. (*A*) Axial NECT in a young man with acute onset of headache shows a right frontal lobar hematoma (H) with mild surrounding vasogenic edema. (*B*) A more superior NECT shows a second hematoma (H) associated with a larger amount of vasogenic edema. This amount of edema would not be expected for a hyperacute benign hematoma. (*C*) Axial T2W image from an MR scan acquired shortly after the CT shows 2 right frontal hematomas with heterogeneous signal intensity and associated vasogenic edema. (*D*) Axial T1W postgadolinium image shows heterogeneous high signal intensity associated with the hematomas, most of which was present before gadolinium administration. In this patient the suspicion for underlying neoplasia was high, and metastatic choriocarcinoma was confirmed when the lesions were surgically decompressed.

patient must be considered in assigning a diagnosis of CNS vasculitis in the absence of biopsy confirmation of this diagnosis.

Most nonatherosclerotic vasculopathies present with ischemic lesions, but intracerebral hemorrhage may be a presenting or complicating feature of these disorders. Moyamoya disease and moyamoya syndrome are characterized by progressive stenosis of the intracranial internal carotid arteries

(ICAs) and their proximal branches. Most patients in the United States present with ischemic symptoms, although hemorrhage may be the presenting sign in as many as 20% of adults.[48] These hemorrhages may be intraparenchymal (often basal ganglia), intraventricular, or subarachnoid in location (Fig. 18). Bleeding is usually attributed to rupture of fragile collateral vessels, although shifting circulation patterns may lead to formation of cerebral

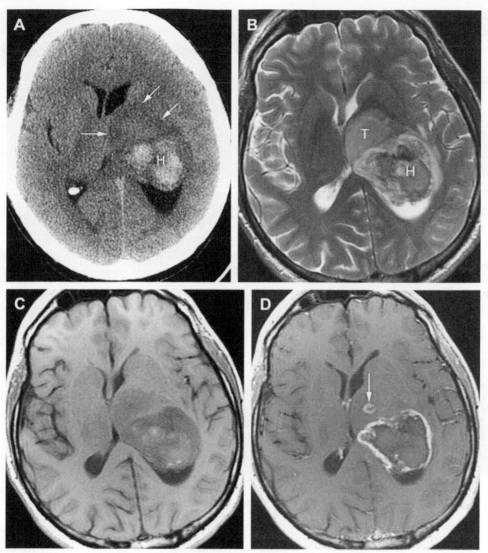

Fig. 17. (*A*) Axial NECT in a young man with headache and right-sided motor and sensory deficits shows a hematoma (H) in the posterior left thalamus. The hematoma is somewhat heterogeneous and is associated with a large area of hypodensity anteriorly (*white arrows*). Edema and mass effect are present, as well as trapping of the left ventricular atrium. (*B*) An axial T2W image shows that the hematoma (H) has heterogeneous signal intensity. More anteriorly, abnormal T2 hyperintensity is present in the thalamus, suggestive of nonenhancing infiltrative tumor (T). (*C*) An axial T1W image again shows the atypical hematoma as well as the more anterior infiltrative tissue. (*D*) Following administration of gadolinium, an axial T1W image shows irregular peripheral enhancement around the hemorrhagic component of the tumor, as well as focal nodular enhancement (*arrow*) more anteriorly within the thalamus. Subsequent hematoma evacuation and biopsy confirmed glioblastoma multiforme.

aneurysms (often of the posterior circulation) and this may be another cause of hemorrhage in patients with moyamoya. MRI/MRA studies in moyamoya typically show ischemic lesions, often in a watershed distribution, as well as unilateral or bilateral supraclinoid ICA stenosis or occlusion and dilated lenticulostriate collateral vessels; MR perfusion studies are typically abnormal, with decreased flow in the affected vascular territories.

Management of moyamoya often requires direct or indirect revascularization procedures.[49]

Reversible cerebral vasoconstriction syndrome (RCVS) is increasingly recognized as a cause of ischemic and hemorrhagic lesions of the brain.[50] It is characterized by prolonged but reversible vasoconstriction of the cerebral arteries and typically presents with thunderclap headache, with or without focal neurologic symptoms or signs.

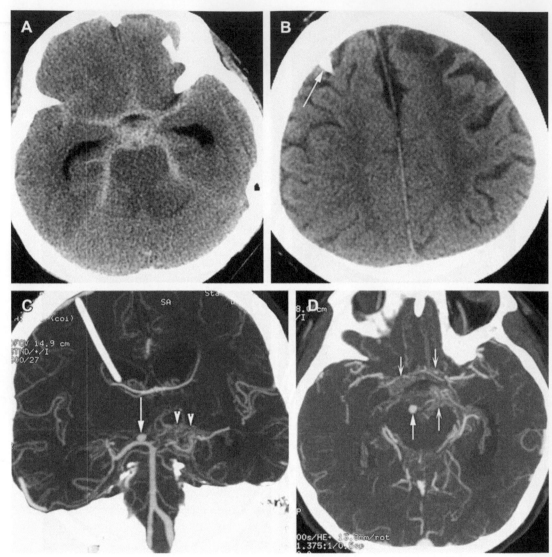

Fig. 18. (*A*) Axial NECT shows extensive SAH in the basal cisterns of a 48-year-old woman, as well as ventricular enlargement consistent with hydrocephalus. (*B*) A more superior NECT shows part of a right external ventricular drain (*arrow*), as well as left frontal encephalomalacia suggesting a remote ischemic insult, although the patient and her family reported no history of stroke. (*C*) Coronal MIP image from a CTA shows a saccular aneurysm (*large white arrow*) arising from the right P1 segment of the posterior cerebral artery, which is an unusual location for a saccular aneurysm. The image also shows poor visualization of the left P1 segment and instead shows a tangle of small collateral vascular channels (*arrowheads*). An external ventricular drain is present with its tip in the right frontal horn. (*D*) An axial MIP image from the CTA again shows the saccular right P1 aneurysm (*straight white arrow*). Numerous small collateral vessels are seen throughout the suprasellar cistern (*concave white arrows*); in addition, the proximal M1 segments of the MCAs are poorly seen bilaterally, and the A1 segments of the ACAs are diminutive. These findings are consistent with advanced moyamoya disease.

This entity has previously been known by a variety of names, including Call-Fleming syndrome and benign or reversible angiitis of the CNS. Associated conditions include eclampsia, use of amphetamines and other sympathomimetics, use of serotonergic drugs, and a history of migraine or other headache syndromes.[51] CT and MR images of these patients may show areas of ischemic infarction and/or hemorrhage (Fig. 19); CTA and MRA examinations may show diffuse vascular irregularity, although this may be difficult to differentiate from motion or a poor bolus (ie, artifactual causes of apparent vascular irregularity) on these noninvasive studies. Catheter angiography shows

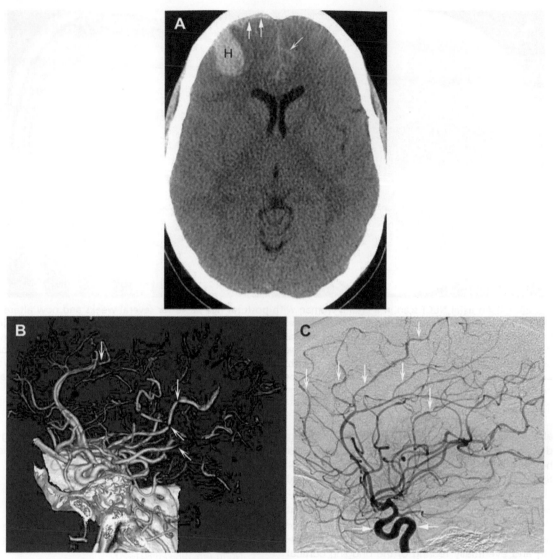

Fig. 19. (A) Axial NECT image from a middle-aged woman with acute onset of severe headache shows a right frontal lobar hematoma (H), as well as a small subdural hematoma (*straight white arrows*) and subarachnoid blood (*concave arrow*) interdigitating into frontal sulci. (B) A 3D reconstruction of the intracranial vasculature from a CTA shows numerous sites of vascular irregularity and narrowing (*arrows*), but it is difficult to be sure if the vessels are truly abnormal or if a poor bolus could be influencing the appearance of the peripheral arterial branches. (C) A lateral view from a catheter angiogram with injection of the left ICA shows normal proximal vessels, with a normal carotid siphon (*large white arrows*). Peripherally, however, MCA and ACA branches show extensive multifocal sites of vascular irregularity and narrowing (*concave white arrows*). In the past this would likely have been interpreted as CNS vasculitis, but this patient improved markedly with only supportive care and calcium channel blockers. These clinical and radiographic findings were interpreted as consistent with RCVS.

diffuse irregularity of the cerebral vasculature that mimics CNS vasculitis. However, these patients have a more benign course and often improve spontaneously in several weeks; some have improved more rapidly with calcium channel blockers. It is essential to consider RCVS in the differential diagnosis before a patient is put on aggressive therapy such as steroids and cyclophosphamide for presumed CNS vasculitis.

Vascular changes have also been described in posterior reversible encephalopathy syndrome (PRES), and the relationship between PRES and RCVS, if any, remains to be elucidated.[52]

SUBDURAL HEMORRHAGE

Spontaneous hemorrhage into the subdural space may be seen with intracranial hypotension[53,54] and

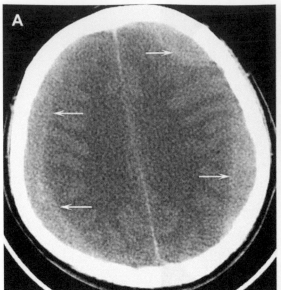 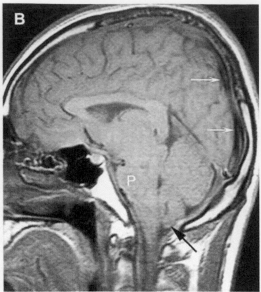

Fig. 20. (A) An axial NECT scan in a young woman with postural headache for several weeks and now altered mental status shows bilateral subacute holohemispheric subdural hematomas. (B) A midline sagittal T1W image from an MR scan in the same patient shows downward displacement of the diencephalon and mesencephalon, flattening of the pons (P) against the clivus, and crowding of the foramen magnum (black arrow). The superior sagittal sinus is patent and prominent, consistent with intracranial hypotension; if intracranial hypertension were present, then one would expect the venous sinus to be small. This patient underwent evacuation of her subdural hematomas and her intracranial hypotension resolved after 2 epidural blood patches.

also with hemorrhagic dural metastases; clotting disorders may also lead to spontaneous subdural hematoma (SDH). Spontaneous intracranial hypotension is further discussed in the article Intracranial Hypo- and Hypertension by Yuh and Dillon elsewhere in this issue, but in brief, the downward displacement of the brain that occurs in spontaneous intracranial hypotension may lead to stretching and eventually tearing of the bridging cortical veins, resulting in frank subdural hemorrhage (Fig. 20) rather than just vascular engorgement of the dura. SDH is a rare presentation of intracranial metastatic disease, but has been described in the setting of several cancers, notably breast carcinoma and choriocarcinoma.[55]

OTHER CONDITIONS ASSOCIATED WITH ICH

Many other conditions may be associated with spontaneous ICH, including the use of anticoagulants (even in the absence of trauma or hypertension), clotting factor deficiencies, hepatic dysfunction, metabolic disorders, and viral encephalitides. Excellent communication between the radiologist and the referring physician can help to determine the cause of a spontaneous ICH, although in some patients the cause remains

uncertain despite an extensive clinical and diagnostic imaging workup in the acute and chronic phase.

REFERENCES

1. Barkovich AJ, Atlas SW. Magnetic resonance imaging of intracranial hemorrhage. Radiol Clin North Am 1988;26:801–20.
2. Atlas SW, Thulborn KR. MR detection of hyperacute parenchymal hemorrhage of the brain. AJNR Am J Neuroradiol 1998;19:1471–507.
3. Parizel PM, Makkat S, Van Miert E, et al. Intracranial hemorrhage: principles of CT and MRI interpretation. Eur Radiol 2001;11:1770–83.
4. Sessa M. Intracerebral hemorrhage and hypertension. Neurol Sci 2008;29:S258–9.
5. Kinoshita T, Okudera T, Tamura H, et al. Assessment of lacunar hemorrhage associated with hypertensive stroke by echo-planar gradient-echo T2*-weighted MRI. Stroke 2000;31:1646–50.
6. Brott T, Broderick J, Kothari R, et al. Early hemorrhage growth in patients with intracerebral hemorrhage. Stroke 1997;28:1–5.
7. Cucchiara B, Messe S, Sansing L, et al. CHANT Investigators. Hematoma growth in oral anticoagulant related intracerebral hemorrhage. Stroke 2008; 39:2993–6.

8. Fujii Y, Takeuchi S, Sasaki O, et al. Multivariate analysis of predictors of hematoma enlargement in spontaneous intracerebral hemorrhage. Stroke 1998;29:1160–6.

9. Wada R, Aviv RI, Fox AJ, et al. CT angiography "spot sign" predicts hematoma expansion in acute intracerebral hemorrhage. Stroke 2007;38:1257–62.

10. Goldstein JN, Fazen LE, Snider R, et al. Contrast extravasation on CT angiography predicts hematoma expansion in intracerebral hemorrhage. Neurology 2007;68:889–94.

11. Kim J, Smith A, Hemphill JC III, et al. Contrast extravasation on CT predicts mortality in primary intracerebral hemorrhage. AJNR Am J Neuroradiol 2008;29:520–5.

12. Broderick J, Connolly S, Feldmann E, et al. Guidelines for the management of spontaneous intracerebral hemorrhage in adults: 2007 update: a guideline from the American Heart Association/American Stroke Association Stroke Council, High Blood Pressure Research Council, and the Quality of Care and Outcomes in Research Interdisciplinary Working Group. Circulation 2007;116(16):e391–413.

13. Mendelow AD, Gregson BA, Fernandes HM, et al. Early surgery versus initial conservative treatment in patients with spontaneous supratentorial intracerebral haematomas in the International Surgical Trial in Intracerebral Haemorrhage (STICH): a randomised trial. Lancet 2005;365:387–97.

14. Zhang-Nunes SX, Maat-Schieman ML, van Duinen SG, et al. The cerebral beta-amyloid angiopathies: hereditary and sporadic. Brain Pathol 2006;16:30–9.

15. Pezzini A, Padovani A. Cerebral amyloid angiopathy-related hemorrhages. Neurol Sci 2008;29:S260–3.

16. Knudsen KA, Rosand J, Karluk D, et al. Clinical diagnosis of cerebral amyloid angiopathy: validation of the Boston criteria. Neurology 2001;56:537–9.

17. Tsui YK, Tsai FY, Hasso AN, et al. Susceptibility-weighted imaging for the differential diagnosis of cerebral vascular pathology: a pictorial review. J Neurol Sci 2009;287(1–2):7–16.

18. Rosand J, Hylek EM, O'Donnell HC, et al. Warfarin-associated hemorrhage and cerebral amyloid angiopathy: a genetic and pathologic study. Neurology 2000;55:947–51.

19. Tsivgoulis G, Frey JL, Flaster M, et al. Pre-tissue plasminogen activator blood pressure levels and risk of symptomatic intracerebral hemorrhage. Stroke 2009;40:3631–4.

20. Aviv RI, D'Esterre CD, Murphy BD, et al. Hemorrhagic transformation of ischemic stroke: prediction with CT perfusion. Radiology 2009;250:867–77.

21. Lansberg MG, Thijs VN, Bammer R, et al. Risk factors of symptomatic intracerebral hemorrhage after tPA therapy for acute stroke. Stroke 2007;38:2275–8.

22. Albers GW, Thijs VN, Wechsler L, et al. Magnetic resonance imaging profiles predict clinical response to early reperfusion: the diffusion and perfusion imaging evaluation for understanding stroke evolution (DEFUSE) study. Ann Neurol 2006;60:508–17.

23. Khatri P, Wechsler LR, Broderick JP. Intracranial hemorrhage associated with revascularization therapies. Stroke 2007;38(2):431–40.

24. Lansberg MG, Albers GW, Wijman CA. Symptomatic intracerebral hemorrhage following thrombolytic therapy for acute ischemic stroke: a review of the risk factors. Cerebrovasc Dis 2007;24:1–10.

25. Singer OC, Humpich MC, Fiehler J, et al. Risk for symptomatic intracerebral hemorrhage after thrombolysis assessed by diffusion-weighted magnetic resonance imaging. Ann Neurol 2008;63:52–60.

26. Ruttmann E, Willeit J, Ulmer H, et al. Neurological outcome of septic cardioembolic stroke after infective endocarditis. Stroke 2006;37:2094–9.

27. Chen W, Wang J, Xin W, et al. Accuracy of 16-row multislice computed tomographic angiography for assessment of small cerebral aneurysms. Neurosurgery 2008;62:113–22.

28. McKinney AM, Palmer CS, Truwit CL, et al. Detection of aneurysms by 64-section multidetector CT angiography in patients acutely suspected of having an intracranial aneurysm and comparison with digital subtraction and 3D rotational angiography. AJNR Am J Neuroradiol 2008;29:594–602.

29. Yoon DY, Lim KJ, Choi CS, et al. Detection and characterization of intracranial aneurysms with 16-channel multidetector row CT angiography: a prospective comparison of volume-rendered images and digital subtraction angiography. AJNR Am J Neuroradiol 2007;28:60–7.

30. Hochmuth A, Spetzger U, Schumacher M. Comparison of three-dimensional rotational angiography with digital subtraction angiography in the assessment of ruptured cerebral aneurysms. AJNR Am J Neuroradiol 2002;23:1199–205.

31. White PM, Teasdale EM, Wardlaw JM, et al. Intracranial aneurysms: CT angiography and MR angiography for detection. Prospective blinded comparison in a large patient cohort. Radiology 2001;219:739–49.

32. Chaudhary SR, Ko N, Dillon WP, et al. Prospective evaluation of multidetector row CT angiography for the diagnosis of vasospasm following subarachnoid hemorrhage: a comparison with digital subtraction angiography. Cerebrovasc Dis 2008;25:144–50.

33. Al-Shahi R, Warlow C. A systematic review of the frequency and prognosis of arteriovenous malformations of the brain in adults. Brain 2001;124:1900–26.

34. Spetzler RF, Martin NA. A proposed grading system for arteriovenous malformation. J Neurosurg 1986;65:476–83.

35. Al-Shahi Salman R, Berg MJ, Morrison L, et al. Hemorrhage from cavernous malformations of the brain. Stroke 2008;39:3222–30.

36. Wilson M, Enevoldson P, Menezes B. Intracranial dural arterio-venous fistula. Pract Neurol 2008;8:362–9.

37. Zipfel GJ, Shah MN, Refai D, et al. Cranial dural arteriovenous fistulas: modification of angiographic classification scales based on new natural history data. Neurosurg Focus 2009;26:E14.

38. Borden JA, Wu JK, Shucart WA. A proposed classification for spinal and cranial dural arteriovenous fistulous malformations and implications for treatment. J Neurosurg 1995;82:166–79.

39. Cognard C, Gobin YP, Pierot L, et al. Cerebral dural arteriovenous fistulas: clinical and angiographic correlation with a revised classification of venous drainage. Radiology 1995;194:671–80.

40. Farb RI, Agid R, Willinsky RA, et al. Cranial dural arteriovenous fistula: diagnosis and classification with time-resolved MR angiography at 3T. AJNR Am J Neuroradiol 2009;30:1546–51.

41. English JD, Fields JD, Le S, et al. Clinical presentation and long-term outcome of cerebral venous thrombosis. Neurocrit Care 2009;11(3):330–7.

42. Linn J, Pfefferkorn T, Ivanicova K, et al. Noncontrast CT in deep cerebral venous thrombosis and sinus thrombosis: comparison of its diagnostic value for both entities. AJNR Am J Neuroradiol 2009;30:728–35.

43. Linn J, Ertl-Wagner B, Seelos KC, et al. Diagnostic value of multidetector-row CT angiography in the evaluation of thrombosis of the cerebral venous sinuses. AJNR Am J Neuroradiol 2007;28:946–52.

44. Makkat S, Stadnik T, Peeters E, et al. Pathogenesis of venous stroke: evaluation with diffusion- and perfusion-weighted MRI. J Stroke Cerebrovasc Dis 2003;12:132–6.

45. Salmaggi A, Erbetta A, Silvani A, et al. Intracerebral haemorrhage in primary and metastatic brain tumours. Neurol Sci 2008;29:S264–5.

46. Atlas SW, Grossman RI, Gomori JM, et al. Hemorrhagic intracranial malignant neoplasms: spin-echo MR imaging. Radiology 1987;164:71–7.

47. Refai D, Botros JA, Strom RG, et al. Spontaneous isolated convexity subarachnoid hemorrhage: presentation, radiological findings, differential diagnosis, and clinical course. J Neurosurg 2008;109:1034–41.

48. Scott RM, Smith ER. Moyamoya disease and moyamoya syndrome. N Engl J Med 2009;360:1226–37.

49. Guzman R, Lee M, Achrol A, et al. Clinical outcome after 450 revascularization procedures for moyamoya disease. J Neurosurg 2009;111(5):927–35.

50. Santos E, Zhang Y, Wilkins A, et al. Reversible cerebral vasoconstriction syndrome presenting with haemorrhage. J Neurol Sci 2009;276:189–92.

51. Ducros A, Boukobza M, Porcher R, et al. The clinical and radiological spectrum of reversible cerebral vasoconstriction syndrome. A prospective series of 67 patients. Brain 2007;130:3091–101.

52. Bartynski WS, Boardman JF. Catheter angiography, MR angiography, and MR perfusion in posterior reversible encephalopathy syndrome. AJNR Am J Neuroradiol 2008;29:447–55.

53. Gordon N. Spontaneous intracranial hypotension. Dev Med Child Neurol 2009;51:932–5.

54. Schievink WI. Spontaneous spinal cerebrospinal fluid leaks. Cephalalgia 2008;28:1345–56.

55. Rocque BG, Baskaya MK. Spontaneous acute subdural hematoma as an initial presentation of choriocarcinoma: a case report. J Med Case Reports 2008;2:211.

Acute Neurointerventional Therapies

Steven W. Hetts[a],[*] and Joey D. English[b]

KEYWORDS

- Interventional neuroradiology • Endovascular treatment
- Acute ischemic stroke • Brain aneurysm

CEREBRAL ISCHEMIC DISEASE
Acute Ischemic Stroke

As mentioned in Imaging of Acute Ischemic Stroke by Carlos Leiva-Salinas and Max Wintermark, acute ischemic stroke (AIS) affects 780,000 people each year in the United States, is the third leading cause of death, and is the leading cause of long-term disability. Costs to the US health care system are in excess of $56 billion annually.[1] Although few therapies for AIS existed before the 1990s, the past 2 decades have seen a proliferation in both noninvasive and invasive image-guided treatments for ischemic stroke. Thrombolytic therapies for AIS trace their roots to the 1980s, when the widespread availability of computed tomography (CT) scanning first permitted rapid differentiation between hemorrhagic and ischemic strokes. Intravenous tissue plasminogen activator (IV tPA) (Genentech, South San Francisco, CA, USA) was approved in 1996 for use in patients during the first 3 hours of AIS.[2] The time window for IV tPA use was recently expanded to 4.5 hours for many AIS patients.[3,4] Both small-vessel and large-vessel ischemic strokes can be treated successfully with IV tPA.

Endovascular therapies for AIS began in the 1980s with off-label use of urokinase, streptokinase, and tPA all delivered intraarterially via a microcatheter into thromboemboli occluding the large (>1 mm luminal diameter) arteries at the base of the brain. Streptokinase research was later abandoned, and intraarterial (IA) tPA became the principal endovascular AIS treatment of patients who either could not receive IV tPA (Box 1 IV tPA exclusion criteria[5]), arrived too late in the time course of AIS to receive IV tPA, or whose symptoms failed to improve sufficiently following IV tPA administration. The PROACT-I (Prolyse in Acute Cerebral Thromboembolism), PROACT-II, and IMS (Interventional Management of Stroke) trials of the late 1990s and early 2000s confirmed the usefulness of IA lytic therapies in AIS up to at least 6 hours following symptom onset.[6–9]

Despite the success of IA tPA in improving AIS outcome for many patients with small-vessel (lacunar) or large-vessel occlusion (LVO) strokes, many patients with LVO show persistent occlusion following microcatheter-directed thrombolysis. This finding served as the impetus for developing mechanical thrombectomy devices in the 2000s, a process that continues today. Initial experience using balloon angioplasty of intracranial large-vessel thrombosis was of mixed success, with some centers reporting favorable outcomes (vessel recanalization and improved clinical status) and others reporting a high rate of vascular perforation. In 2004, a wire-based thrombectomy device (Merci X retriever, Concentric Medical, Mountain View, CA, USA) was approved by the US Food and Drug Administration (FDA) for use in AIS.[10] Further iterations of this device (L series and V series) added suture material to the corkscrew-shaped wire device, with improved results at intravascular clot extraction and vessel recanalization.[11,12]

[a] UCSF Medical Center, 505 Parnassus Avenue, L-352, San Francisco, CA 94143, USA
[b] UCSF Neurocritical Care and Stroke, 400 Parnassus Avenue, San Francisco, CA 94143, USA
* Corresponding author.
E-mail address: steven.hetts@radiology.ucsf.edu

Neuroimag Clin N Am 20 (2010) 493–510
doi:10.1016/j.nic.2010.07.009

In 2008, the Penumbra device (Penumbra, Alameda, CA, USA) was approved by the FDA for treatment of LVO AIS.[13] The Penumbra is a mechanical thrombectomy device consisting of an aspiration catheter attached to a suction pump coupled with a bulbous tipped separator wire. It is designed to macerate clot within the catheter and just beyond the catheter tip. Initial results of the Penumbra device were similar to those of the Merci device with regards to recanalization of the internal carotid artery (ICA), middle cerebral artery (MCA), and basilar artery, as well as with regards to clinical outcomes. Two case examples of mechanical thrombectomy in AIS are illustrated in **Fig. 1**.

In addition to FDA-approved wire- and aspiration-based thrombectomy devices, several devices based on intracranial stent technology are currently under investigation. The fundamental observation that deployment of a stent can sometimes open a completely occluded artery has led to off-label use of intracranial stents in patients in whom IA lytics and/or approved mechanical thrombectomy devices have not achieved vessel recanalization. Balloon-expandible and open-cell self-expanding stents can be deployed permanently and closed-cell self-expanding stents can be deployed either permanently or temporarily. Transient deployment of a stent to open a vessel during stroke treatment with recapture and removal of the stent at the end of the procedure has an inherent advantage over permanent stent placement: if no stent is left in situ, then the patient does not have to be placed on long-term dual antiplatelet therapy (typically aspirin and clopidogrel).[14,15] This finding is of particular importance in patients with atrial fibrillation, as the addition of multiple antiplatelet agents to a warfarin regimen can lead to an increased rate of delayed intracranial hemorrhage (ICH).

Although there is great enthusiasm for mechanical thrombectomy devices, such devices have limitations with regards to stiffness and size that prevent their safe use in vessels beyond the base of the brain. In addition, a comparison of data from the Multi-MERCI (Mechanical Embolus Removal in Cerebral Ischemia) trial and PROACT-II trial suggests that, once baseline patient enrollment characteristics are factored out, mechanical thrombectomy and microcatheter-directed IA thrombolysis seem to result in similar rates of good clinical outcome in LVO AIS.[16]

The stroke treatment algorithm and therapeutic windows currently in place at the authors' institution are illustrated in **Fig. 2** and **Table 1**,

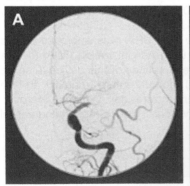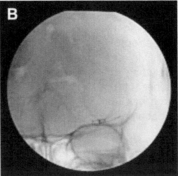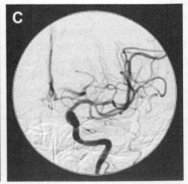

Fig. 1. Intracranial arterial thrombectomy in AIS. 62-year-old woman developed acute right hemiparesis and aphasia, which did not improve following administration of IV tPA. Initial catheter angiogram of the left ICA (*A*, anteroposterior [AP] projection) shows embolic occlusion of the left M1 MCA segment. A Merci thrombectomy device is deployed in the M1 MCA (*B*) to remove the embolus. Postthrombectomy angiography (*C*) shows successful recanalization and normal antegrade runoff to the distal MCA branches.

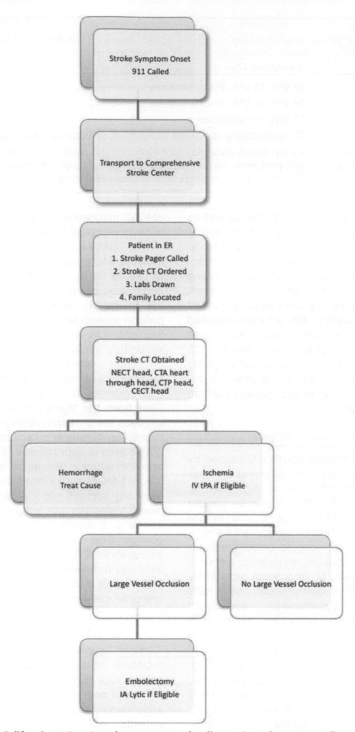

Fig. 2. University of California at San Francisco acute stroke diagnosis and treatment flow diagram.

respectively. Despite the time windows for AIS therapy listed in Table 1, exceptions to these guidelines exist. Some patients have poor outcomes despite prompt institution of AIS therapy, and others have good clinical outcomes even when treated beyond 8 hours after onset of stroke symptoms. The latter is particularly important when patients awaken with stroke symptoms. In this setting, the clinical standard is to assign the time the patient was last seen well (ie, when the patient went to sleep), even if the true onset of ischemia might have been moments before the

Table 1
Time windows for interventional treatment of AIS at University of California at San Francisco

Time	Treatment Options
0–3 h	IV tPA, IA tPA, thrombectomy
0–4.5 h	IV tPA, IA tPA, thrombectomy
0–6 h	IA tPA, thrombectomy
0–8 h	Thrombectomy (posterior circulation or dominant hemisphere)
Unknown symptom onset or beyond 8 h	CT perfusion data may be helpful in clinical decision making MR perfusion and diffusion data may be helpful in clinical decision making Thrombectomy at discretion of interventionalist

patient awoke. These wake-up strokes, as well as the more routine presentation of patients to the emergency room beyond 3 to 8 hours, has led to an intense interest in the use of magnetic resonance (MR) and CT-based physiologic imaging to better assess which patients would benefit from aggressive stroke treatment and which would not.[17] Techniques such as MR diffusion-weighted imaging and CT perfusion imaging hold great promise in improving patient selection for AIS therapy, leading some to declare that ischemic stroke treatment is moving from a clinical paradigm of time is brain to an image-guided paradigm of physiology is brain.[18–21]

Intracranial Atherosclerotic Disease

Although LVO AIS is most commonly caused by a carotid or cardiac embolus lodging at an intracranial arterial bifurcation or at a preexisting vascular stenosis, LVO AIS can also be caused by atherosclerotic plaque rupture and in situ thrombosis. High-grade but nonocclusive intracranial stenoses can also lead to blood pressure-dependent acute, subacute, and chronic ischemic symptoms. Treatment of intracranial atherosclerotic disease (ICAD) is controversial. The WASID (Warfarin-Aspirin Symptomatic Intracranial Disease) trial recently compared aspirin with warfarin for the secondary prevention of stroke in patients with a previous brain infarct or transient ischemic attack (TIA).[22,23] WASID confirmed that ICAD is a bad actor: the rate of a second stroke was similar between the aspirin and warfarin groups (approximately 20% in each at 1 and 2 years after enrollment). In addition, there was an increased risk of ICH associated with warfarin therapy. WASID has led not only to conversion of ICAD patients from warfarin to aspirin therapy but also has increased interest in endovascular treatments for ICAD. WASID also suggested that the highest risk for a second ischemic stroke is within the first 30 days after the initial ischemic stroke. Consideration of urgent revascularization

of ICAD lesions following stroke or TIA thus seems to be appropriate for at least some patients.

The SAMMPRIS (Stenting vs Aggressive Medical Management for Preventing Recurrent Stroke in Intracranial Stenosis) trial is currently under way, comparing intracranial stenting (using the Wingspan stent and Gateway angioplasty balloon system [Boston Scientific Neurovascular, Fremont, CA, USA]) with medical therapy for secondary stroke prevention.[24] This work builds on earlier uncontrolled case series and device registries describing the use of intracranial stents and coronary stents in the treatment of ICAD. Data from the Wingspan registry suggest that, whereas the 6-month restenosis rate for posterior circulation (basilar and intracranial vertebral artery [VA]) stents is approximately 20%, the restenosis rate for anterior circulation stents (supraclinoid ICA, M1 MCA) is approximately 50%.[25,26] Patients receiving supraclinoid ICA stents had a 66% 6-month restenosis rate; subgroup analysis revealed an 89% 6-month restenosis rate in patients younger than 55 years. It is not certain why the supraclinoid ICA has such a high restenosis rate, although turbulence resulting from the tortuosity of the carotid siphon has been hypothesized as one potential explanation.

Cerebral Vasospasm

Cerebral vasospasm (CV) is a special form of subacute ischemia in patients with subarachnoid hemorrhage (SAH). CV is the leading cause of mortality and morbidity for patients surviving aneurysmal SAH. Approximately 15% to 20% of patients with aneurysmal SAH develop an ischemic stroke or die because of CV. Typical CV usually starts about 5 days after aneurysm rupture, peaks between 5 and 7 days after aneurysm rupture, and resolves by 10 days to 2 weeks after ictus.[27,28] However, in some patients vasospasm can be severe and long lasting (Table 2). Rebleeding resets the CV clock, and thus patients with multiple episodes of SAH can have prolonged

Table 2
Risk factors for cerebral vasospasm in aneurysmal SAH

Risk Factor	Effect on Risk of Vasospasm
Amount of SAH on nonenhanced CT (Fisher grade)	More blood, higher risk
Clinical symptom severity (Hunt and Hess grade)	Worse grade, higher risk
Age	Younger age, higher risk
Gender	Female gender, higher risk
Sympathomimetic drug abuse	Drug abuse, higher risk

courses of vasospasm. After the ruptured aneurysm is secured with surgical clip ligation or endovascular embolization, intensive care unit (ICU) management is switched from relative hypotension (to reduce risk of aneurysm rerupture) to deliberate hypertension (to overcome the ischemic effect of reduced arterial caliber caused by CV). Patients with SAH at our hospital receive HHH therapy (hypertension, hemodilution, hypervolemia) in addition to oral nimodipine to optimize cerebral blood flow and thus counteract CV. Efforts to secure the ruptured aneurysm are made as soon as possible within the first 5 days so that management can be redirected at mitigation of CV.

In patients in whom standard ICU measures to prevent vasospasm fail to prevent new or worsening focal neurologic deficits or increasing obtundation (and other causes of declining clinical status such as hydrocephalus, rehemorrhage, salt wasting, or swelling of completed infarction have been ruled out), endovascular techniques can be used successfully to treat CV. Intraarterial vasodilators such as the calcium channel blocker verapamil and the phosphodiesterase inhibitor milrinone cause preferential dilatation of cerebral arteries (vs systemic arteries) when administered by transcatheter infusion into the cervical ICAs, cervical vertebral arteries, or cerebral arteries themselves.[29–31] The durability of pharmaceutical vasodilator treatments is limited. Angioplasty of the large intracranial arteries, including the supraclinoid ICA, M1 MCA, and basilar artery, is a safe and effective means for increasing cerebral blood flow.[32–34] Angioplasty of other arterial segments, such as the intracranial vertebral arteries, A1 anterior carotoid artery (ACA), or P1 posterior carotid artery (PCA), is possible when these specific segments are not hypoplastic, as judged by comparison with an angiogram performed before the onset of vasospasm. At our institution, we use angioplasty for the treatment of moderate and severe vasospasm involving the large arteries at the base of the brain and intraarterial verapamil infusion for treating vasospasm involving smaller arteries or mild vasospasm of the large arteries.[28]

CEREBRAL HEMORRHAGIC DISEASE
Aneurysmal SAH

Aneurysmal SAH afflicts about 30,000 people annually in the United States, thus constituting about 5% of all strokes and about 30% of all hemorrhagic strokes.[35,36] Aneurysmal SAH constitutes 80% of cases of nontraumatic SAH, with the remaining 20% divided between perimesencephalic hemorrhage, arteriovenous fistulas (dural and pial), arteriovenous malformations (AVMs), and cavernous malformations that come to the surface of the brain.[37] Perimesencephalic SAH is believed to be caused by a ruptured vein, and thus angiographically occult, and should therefore be a diagnosis of exclusion.[38] Approximately half of patients with aneurysmal SAH die because of the rupture, with most of these deaths occurring within the first 2 weeks after initial hemorrhage. Mortality is front-loaded: 10% die before arrival at the hospital and 25% die within the first 24 hours after aneurysm rupture.[37]

Ruptured brain aneurysms are highly unstable and prone to rerupture. There is at least a 4% rerupture rate within the first 24 hours, and a 30% rerupture rate within the first month.[35] Dissecting aneurysms of the intracranial VA are even more friable and prone to reruptune than other intracranial aneurysms, with rebleeding rates within the first 24 hours exceeding 40% in some case series.[39] Rebleeding of a brain aneurysm carries up to 70% risk of death. In ruptured aneurysms left untreated for long periods of time, risk of rerupture has been reported to decline to about 3% per year, although such natural history studies are few in an era of safe and effective surgical and endovascular aneurysm therapy.[35]

Beyond being life-threatening, aneurysmal SAH also causes long-term disability in many survivors. Between one-third and one-half of SAH survivors have chronic cognitive deficits and concomitantly reduced quality of life.[36,37] Focal neurologic deficits are less common, as is chronic hydrocephalus requiring ventriculoperitoneal shunting.

The International Subarachnoid Aneurysm Trial (ISAT) of 2143 patients with aneurysmal SAH reported that endovascular coiling of ruptured brain aneurysms geometrically amenable to either coiling or surgical clipping resulted in a lower rate of death or dependency at 1 year after treatment (23.7% for coiling and 30.4% for clipping) such that the trial was halted early because of the superiority of coiling over clipping.[40] More recent long-term follow-up of patients from ISAT (6–14 years, mean 9 years follow-up) confirmed that 5-year survival was superior for patients receiving endovascular coiling versus surgical clipping (14% vs 11%, respectively), but that dependency rates were similar (83% independent vs 82% independent, respectively).[41] There was an overall low (but higher) rate of recurrent SAH after 1 year for the treated aneurysm in coiled patients as opposed to clipped patients (10 vs 3, respectively). 40% of new SAH (11 of 24) were from previously untreated second aneurysms seen at the time of the initial (index) aneurysm treatment, or from entirely new aneurysms not previously detected. Based on ISAT and other data, endovascular therapy has become the treatment of choice for an increasing number of brain aneurysms in the past decade. A recent study of US hospitalizations for treatment of ruptured and unruptured intracranial aneurysms has also concluded that clipping, compared with coiling, was associated with significantly longer lengths of hospitalization and significantly higher total hospital charges for patients with both ruptured and unruptured aneurysm.[42]

Several factors are ideally taken into account in the selection of endovascular versus surgical treatment of any given ruptured aneurysm:

1. Location of the aneurysm
2. Geometry of the aneurysm
3. Age of the patient
4. SAH clinical grade
5. Patient comorbidities
6. Experience of the interventionalist and surgeon
7. Preferences of the patient or patient's family.

In general, the deeper the location of the aneurysm and more brain retraction that is required to reach it surgically, the more likely that endovascular therapy offers treatment with lower risk of side effects.

Aneurysm geometry is generally defined as narrow-necked saccular, broad-necked saccular, or fusiform. Aneurysms with narrow necks that tend to self-retain coils within the aneurysm sac often are also favorable for straightforward surgical clipping. An additional aspect of aneurysm geometry that should be taken into account is overall size of the aneurysm. Aneurysms less than 2 mm in diameter can be challenging to coil because of their small size, given that the smallest detachable aneurysm coils are 1.5 mm to 2 mm in diameter. However, in a large series of aneurysms 3 mm or less in diameter receiving endovascular coiling, procedural success and complication rates were similar to coiling of larger aneurysms, with a slightly higher procedural rupture rate (mostly asymptomatic) and lower rate (5%) of need for subsequent retreatment.[43] Giant aneurysms (25 mm or greater in diameter), which can be difficult to treat surgically because of their large size, can also be challenging to treat with primary coiling, as they often require many coils to achieve adequate aneurysm occlusion.[44] Endovascular therapy with stents, flow diverters, or liquid embolics (see later discussion) may offer advantages over coiling alone, including a potential reduction in the overall cost of therapy.

Saccular aneurysms with broad necks often require adjuncts for successful endovascular therapy. Balloon-assisted coiling involves temporary inflation of a balloon in the parent artery to encourage coils to assume a self-sustainable stable configuration within the aneurysm.[45] Patients with broad-necked coiled aneurysms are often placed on aspirin following the procedure to reduce parent artery embolic phenomena derived from clots forming on the large coil mass facing the parent artery. Stent-supported coiling consists of positioning a stent in the parent artery across the aneurysm neck to hold coils separately placed in the aneurysm (either through the stent or around the stent).[46] The disadvantage of stent placement for treatment of acutely ruptured aneurysms is the requirement for dual antiplatelet therapy, including both aspirin and clopidogrel, to reduce the risk of stent thrombosis and distal thromboembolization. Although aspirin is generally well tolerated, clopidogrel may increase the risk for secondary hemorrhage during external ventricular drain (EVD) placement.[47] However, at least one center has reported a large series of ruptured aneurysms treated with primary stent coiling without noting any increased frequency of secondary hemorrhage.[48] Early EVD placement to relieve hydrocephalus before surgical or endovascular aneurysm occlusion is prudent for the relief of increased intracranial pressure (ICP) and has a secondary benefit of allowing potentially safer use of clopidogrel or gpIIb/IIIa inhibitors (such as abciximab or eptafibitide) in patients in whom a stent is necessary to achieve stable coil position.

In patients in whom the parent artery can be sacrificed without risking major infarction, endovascular and surgical occlusion of a fusiform aneurysm (and thus the parent artery), is straightforward. For example, fusiform dissecting aneurysms of the intracranial VA below the ipsilateral posterior inferior cerebellar artery (PICA) origin can be successfully treated with detachable coil occlusion of the VA (and, therefore the aneurysm) below the PICA origin (Fig. 3). This technique can be used when the ipsilateral VA anastomoses with the basilar artery, and thus can retrogradely supply

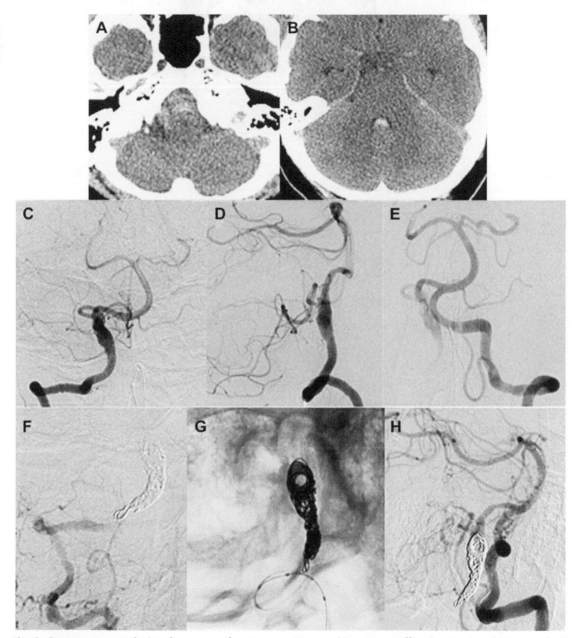

Fig. 3. **Parent artery occlusion for ruptured aneurysm.** 40-year-old woman suffered a Hunt and Hess grade III SAH. Noncontrast CT shows SAH anterior and lateral to the medulla (A) and intraventricular hemorrhage within the fourth ventricle (B). Catheter angiography of the right VA in the AP (C) and lateral (D) projections shows a fusiform dissecting pseudoaneurysm of the intracranial segment of the right VA just proximal to, and involving, the origin of the right posterior inferior cerebellar artery. Injection of the left VA shows that the vertebral arteries are codominant (E, AP projection), thus permitting coil occlusion of the right VA in the aneurysmal segment (F, G). Preservation of flow to the right PICA retrogradely across the vertebrobasilar junction is confirmed by postembolization injection of the left VA in an off-lateral projection (H).

the PICA on the side of VA sacrifice. For a fusiform dissecting VA aneurysm involving the dominant VA in which the other VA is diminutive or does not anastomose with the basilar artery, stent coiling

the aneurysm to preserve patency of the parent artery is the preferred approach (Fig. 4).

Large dolichoectatic fusiform aneurysms are often difficult to treat by endovascular and surgical

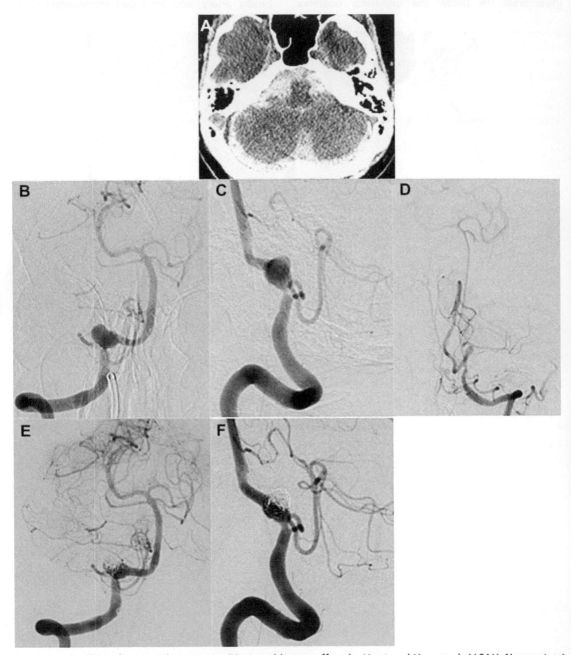

Fig. 4. **Stent coiling of ruptured aneurysm.** 50-year-old man suffered a Hunt and Hess grade V SAH. Noncontrast CT shows extensive SAH surrounding the medulla and cerebellum (A). Catheter angiography of the right VA in the AP (B) and lateral (C) projections shows a fusiform dissecting pseudoaneurysm of the intracranial right VA segment just superior to the right PICA origin. The right VA is the dominant supply to the basilar artery, as confirmed by injection of the left VA (D, AP projection), thus contraindicating right VA occlusion as a treatment of the pseudoaneurysm. Following stent-assisted coiling of the right VA pseudoaneurysm, catheter angiography of the right VA (E, AP projection, F, lateral projection) shows preservation of flow to the basilar artery and right PICA and occlusion of the aneurysm.

techniques if preservation of patency of the parent vessel is essential. It is difficult to place coils circumferentially around a stent placed in a fusiform aneurysm, as visualization of coil placement becomes increasingly challenging after several coils have already been placed. Recently, the concept of placing multiple overlapping stents or stents with a large number of struts (eg, Pipeline stent, Chestnut Medical, Menlo Park, CA, USA) to form a flow diverter and cause thrombosis in fusiform aneurysms but maintain a patent central lumen has become an area of great interest. In these patients, flow diversion may cause enough stasis in an aneurysm to cause thrombosis of the aneurysm even without placement of coils. Risks of occluding small perforating arteries arising from the aneurysm, as well as risk of aneurysm rupture, remain important open questions. An additional downside of such stent-based therapies is the need for dual antiplatelet medication. Bypass trapping is the primary surgical technique for the treatment of fusiform aneurysms in which distal flow must be preserved. In this technically demanding method, clips are placed proximal and distal to the aneurysmal segment (trapping) and a bypass graft (superficial temporal artery, radial artery transposition, or venous transposition) is placed distal to the trapped aneurysm.

Liquid embolic therapy for brain aneurysms has long been an area of interest, and the FDA has recently approved of one agent, and there has been research in others. Onyx HD500 (EV3, Irvine, CA, USA), a more viscous version of the liquid embolic already widely used in preoperative embolization of brain AVMs, has been approved in the United States for humanitarian use in the treatment of intracranial, saccular, sidewall aneurysms that present with a wide neck (4 mm or >) or with a dome/neck ratio less than 2 that are not amenable to treatment with surgical clipping.[49–53] Aneurysm treatment with a liquid embolic entails placing an embolization catheter in the aneurysm and temporarily inflating a balloon in the parent artery to prevent escape of embolic materials during intraaneurysmal injection. Because many embolic agents face the parent artery in an aneurysm with a broad neck, antiplatelet agents are used in a similar fashion for stent coiling and flow diversion techniques. Liquid embolics can be used either alone or in combination with coils and stents. The most widespread use of Onyx HD500 is not in acutely ruptured aneurysms, but instead in the treatment of aneurysms that have partially recanalized after prior coiling, in essence using the liquid embolic as a caulking agent between the in situ coils. Neucrylate (Valor Medical, San Diego, CA, USA) is another liquid embolic agent currently undergoing preclinical evaluation in the United States and clinical testing overseas. It may ultimately have advantages over other agents because of its faster delivery into aneurysms, which is of particular importance in critically ill patients with SAH. Long-term data on the durability of liquid embolics in the treatment of aneurysms are lacking; until those data exist, coils and coils in combination with adjunctive devices are likely to remain the standard of endovascular care.

Patient demographics and clinical status also play a role in determining optimal aneurysm therapy. The International Study of Unruptured Intracranial Aneurysms (ISUIA) trial comparing clipping with coiling of unruptured aneurysms suggested that patients older than 50 years had poorer surgical outcomes.[54] Patients with higher-grade SAH (Hunt and Hess grades IV and V) and comorbidities such as cardiac stun syndrome are often preferentially coiled because of their tenuous clinical status. Endovascular aneurysm treatment has only existed since the 1970s, and coiling since the early 1990s has been limited by a lack of long-term follow-up. This is not the case for surgical clipping, which has been performed since the 1930s.[55–61] Thus, for very young patients, a discussion of the relative advantages of endovascular versus surgical aneurysm treatment should include a discussion of the known and expected durability of each treatment. Endovascular approaches to pediatric aneurysms have been highly successful, but extension of the ISAT data to this age group should be tempered by the lack of long-term follow-up data. As a parallel to the ISAT data in which second aneurysms were more likely to be the source of recurrent SAH after clipping or coiling of an index aneurysm, we found that 6 of 77 (8%) children who were treated surgically or endovascularly for an index brain aneurysm developed new or enlarging aneurysms warranting treatment ~5 years after index aneurysm therapy.[62] Considering the long-expected lifetimes of these patients, long-term follow-up imaging surveillance is essential; MR angiography is our preference given its lack of ionizing radiation. In contrast, adult patients with a previous aneurysmal SAH develop new aneurysms at a rate of 2% per year and have a 6-fold increased risk of recurrent SAH over baseline (6:10,000 persons per year in patients with prior SAH vs 1:10,000 persons per year in the general population).[36] Ruptured brain aneurysms should be regarded as a potentially chronic disease, not just a one-time event. Please refer to the article by Nancy Fischbein and Christine Wijman, Hemorrhagic Stroke and Non-traumatic Intracranial Hemorrhage, in this publication, for additional information about the imaging diagnosis of SAH.

CEREBRAL VENOUS THROMBOSIS

Cerebral venous thrombosis (CVT) is an uncommon, but life-threatening, condition in which occlusion of the dural sinuses and/or cortical veins can lead to venous congestion, edema, and venous hemorrhage, with associated impairment of cerebrospinal fluid resorption. These derangements can collectively result in both cerebral infarction and increased ICP. If unrecognized and untreated, CVT carries a high risk of neurologic morbidity and mortality. Despite advances in understanding and treating this disease, CVT nonetheless remains challenging to diagnose, largely because of its protean clinical manifestations and its diverse radiographic findings (see also article on Hemorrhage, by Nancy Fischbein and Christine Wijman, in this publication).

The demographics of patients with CVT have been well characterized in multiple case series.[63,64] Overall, most patients are young healthy women (average age is about 40 years, with a 2:1 female/male ratio). Identifiable hypercoagulable risk factors are noted in approximately 80% of patients, with hormonal risk factors (eg, pregnancy, oral contraceptives) noted in up to 70% of women. Other common risk factors include inherited thrombophilia (eg, factor V Leiden or prothrombin 20210 mutation), underlying malignancy, and infection.

CVT can present in many diverse clinical patterns, including headache, nausea, and vomiting (from increased ICP), delirium, seizures and/or focal neurologic deficits (both abrupt onset to slowly progressive). These presentations can mimic those of demyelinating disease, infection, arterial stroke, and tumor. However, the classic presentation is of persistent headache, nausea, and vomiting followed by the onset of focal neurologic deficits and/or seizures, all evolving in days to weeks.

Cross-sectional imaging with CT or MR, with vascular imaging, typically allows for rapid identification of CVT, with multidetector CT angiography approaching 100% sensitivity and specificity. CVT most often involves superior sagittal and transverse sinuses, and multifocal sinus involvement is common. Parenchymal areas of edema or hemorrhage are frequently noted, with up to 50% of patients having evidence of hemorrhage at presentation.[65] These abnormalities are usually not confined to an arterial territory, and such atypical vascular distributions offer an important clue to the underlying cause. As a general rule, CVT should always be considered in young patients with unexplained, atypical parenchymal edema and/or hemorrhage.

A variety of neurointerventional techniques are now available for endovascular treatment of CVT. However, multiple studies and large cases series strongly support the use of acute anticoagulation with IV heparin as the first-line treatment of patients with symptomatic CVT. Although some have argued that concurrent ICH is a contraindication for heparin therapy and thus an indication for neurointerventional revascularization, the safety and efficacy of heparin in these patients is well established and remains the treatment of choice. True contraindications to IV heparin therapy in patients with CVT are uncommon (eg, blood dyscrasias with bleeding disorders, trauma with skull fracture, need for decompressive craniectomy).

Patients with CVT treated with anticoagulation have an excellent long-term prognosis, with approximately 90% of patients (including patients presenting with severe neurologic deficits and ICH) having a favorable long-term neurologic outcome (defined by a modified Rankin scale of 0–2).[64] Heparin failure is uncommon, and most likely occurs in patients in whom the diagnosis is delayed and significant irreversible injury has occurred before the initiation of therapy.

Given the safety and efficacy of IV heparin therapy for patients with CVT, including those with ICH, endovascular procedures should thus be reserved for those rare patients who have either failed heparin therapy or have true contraindications for this treatment. In general, endovascular options for patients with CVT are based on transvenous access to the intracranial dural segments, either from transfemoral or transjugular approaches. Reported techniques include the use of declotting catheters (eg, Angiojet rheolytic thrombectomy[66] or Penumbra aspiration catheters), balloon catheter sweeps (eg, Fogarty balloon), or prolonged intrasinus microcatheter infusions of thrombolytic agents[67] or antithrombotic medications (eg, heparin).[68] The overall safety and efficacy of such approaches remain difficult to assess given the small numbers reported, but most seem relatively safe and are likely useful treatments in selected cases of patients with CVT with true contraindications to heparin therapy.

HEAD AND NECK EMERGENCIES
Epistaxis

Epistaxis is a common and often self-limited condition. Only about 6% of all epistaxis requires medical attention, and 95% of those cases are controllable by direct nasal pressure, chemical or electrical cautery, anterior and/or posterior nasal cavity packing, and correction of coagulopathy if present.[69] In the remaining 5% of medically refractory nosebleeds, surgical ligation or endovascular occlusion of the blood supply to the nose and/or paranasal sinuses may be necessary to prevent multiple blood transfusions or frank exsanguination.

Blood supply to the nose and paranasal sinuses is primarily from the external carotid artery (ECA) via the internal maxillary artery (IMAX) and facial artery. Complete diagnostic catheter angiography of the bilateral ECA and ICA is necessary not only to diagnose the source of epistaxis and provide roadmapping for microcatheter-based therapy but also to identify any ECA-ICA anastomoses that might lead to nontarget embolization, the primary risk of epistaxis embolization procedures. These potentially dangerous ECA-ICA anastomoses have been reviewed extensively elsewhere.[70] It is incumbent on the interventionalist to be aware of possible ECA-ICA and ECA-vertebrobasilar anastomoses to achieve a good therapeutic result and avoid complications. The use of large particulate embolic agents such as polyvinyl alcohol in particle sizes of 350 to 500 μm is prudent. Smaller particulate embolics and liquid embolics penetrate more deeply into small arteries and arterioles, potentially compromising blood supply to cranial nerves and other tissues, risking necrosis and loss of function. Conversely, proximal coil embolization of the IMAX, for example, should be avoided; if rebleeding occurs, then it can be difficult to repeat the embolization procedure if the proximal arteries providing access are occluded and bleeding is occurring through small collateral branches that cannot be catheterized directly. Only in patients in whom a discrete ECA pseudoaneurysm or resectable sinonasal tumor is identified should coils be used. In patients with ICA sources for epistaxis (eg, carotid cavernous fistula or petrocavernous ICA pseudoaneurysm eroding into the sphenoid sinus), use of detachable coils is dictated by carotid cavernous sinus fistula (CCF) or pseudoaneurysm architecture and the potential need to preserve ICA patency.

CERVICAL CEREBROVASCULAR TRAUMA

Traumatic injury to the blood vessels of the neck is uncommon, occurring in approximately 1% to 2% of all trauma patients. Motor vehicle accidents remain the leading cause of cerebrovascular trauma, with most patients being young men in their 20s and 30s. Although uncommon, these injuries nonetheless carry significant risk of morbidity and mortality, mostly related to either cerebral ischemia or life-threatening hemorrhage (eg, uncontrolled epistaxis). Prompt detection and treatment of both symptomatic and asymptomatic cerebrovascular injury are thus critical components of the initial triage of all trauma patients.

Cerebrovascular trauma is typically triaged according to the mechanism of injury: blunt force versus penetrating injury. Algorithms for evaluating and treating these patients have evolved dramatically in the past decade because of advances in both cross-sectional imaging and endovascular treatment options. In particular, CT angiography allows for less invasive and more timely vascular imaging compared with conventional cerebral angiography, and has become the preferred screening imaging modality in this patient population. Endovascular techniques can afford less invasive repair of vascular lesions compared with open surgery, as well as the ability to more easily access difficult locations (eg, thoracic outlet, skull base, cervical VA). The next sections discuss evolving approaches to both blunt force and penetrating cerebrovascular trauma, with a focus on the role of neurointerventional management.

Blunt Force Cervical Cerebrovascular Trauma

Early reports of blunt force injury to either the carotid or vertebral arteries (blunt cerebrovascular injury [BCVI]) suggested that they were rare, occurring in only 0.1% of hospitalized trauma patients. However, these injuries were detected in most patients after symptomatic cerebral ischemia was noted.[71,72] When screening protocols are used, the incidence of BCVI increases to approximately 1% in all patients with asymptomatic trauma, and up to 3% in patients with more severe trauma.[73] Furthermore, although it has been argued that screening for asymptomatic BCVI is futile,[74] several recent studies have reported that such screening is cost-effective, with early identification and treatment of BCVI lowering subsequent complications (particularly cerebral ischemia).[75–77] Many algorithms have recently been proposed for identifying which trauma patients merit vascular imaging.[78] However, the best treatment of such injuries (medical therapy, surgical repair, endovascular treatment) remains controversial.

Blunt force carotid artery injury can occur following direct cervical spine trauma, cervical hyperextension or hyperflexion with rotation, intraoral trauma, or fractures of the skull base involving the sphenoid and petrous bones of the carotid canal. Blunt force VA injury is usually caused by cervical spine subluxation/dislocation, fractures of the foramen transversarium, or rotational motion around the atlantoaxial joint. All such mechanisms can lead to arterial intimal injury with secondary subintimal dissection and intramural hematoma formation.[79] The severity of BCVI can be categorized by a useful 5-point grading scale introduced by Biffl and colleagues.[80] Grade I injuries have luminal irregularity or dissection with less than 25% luminal narrowing, whereas grade II injuries have more than 25% luminal narrowing, intraluminal thrombus, or a raised luminal flap. Grade III injuries are characterized by the presence of a pseudoaneurysm. Grade IV is used to describe total vessel occlusion, and a grade V lesion is a transected vessel with free extravasation.

The primary complication of grade I to IV injuries is thromboembolism from the site of intimal injury to the intracranial circulation resulting in cerebral infarction. Grade V lesions can produce life-threatening soft tissue hemorrhage (eg, airway compromise) or, if via an open wound, exsanguination. The known sequelae of grade I to V lesions form the basis of the initial clinical survey for hard signs of BCVI in patients presenting with blunt force trauma to the head and neck region:

- Expanding cervical pulsatile hematoma or arterial hemorrhage for the neck, mouth or nose (both findings suggestive of a grade V lesion)
- Focal neurologic deficit (including isolated Horner syndrome)
- Infarct noted on screening CT or MR imaging
- Cervical bruit in a patient younger than 50 years
- Neurologic deficit unexplained by surveillance brain imaging (these latter signs suggestive of a grade I–IV BCVI).

Any patient found to have one or more of these findings warrants emergent vascular imaging, ideally with CT angiography.[78]

Patients with blunt force injury to the head and neck who do not exhibit any of these hard signs may still have worrisome but asymptomatic BCVI. Most trauma centers use algorithms based on risk factors for BCVI to identify high-risk but asymptomatic patients, and then selectively obtain urgent vascular imaging in this population. One such algorithm recently published by the Western Trauma Association recommends screening for asymptomatic BCVI in patients with known trauma and any of the following[78]:

- Evidence of LeFort II or III fractures
- Basilar skull fractures with carotid canal involvement

- Traumatic brain injury with a Glasgow Coma Scale score less than 6
- Any fracture involving a cervical vertebral body or transverse foramen
- Any injury with subluxation or ligamentous injury
- Any fracture at C1, C2, or C3
- Near hanging with anoxic injury
- Clothesline-type injury (eg, seat belt) with significant pain or swelling.

Patients without any evidence of hard signs of injury and no high-risk features can then likely be followed conservatively without the need for vascular imaging.

Untreated grade I to IV BCVIs have high rates of such thromboembolic stroke, from 20% to 25% for vertebral injury to as high as 50% for carotid injury.[81] Once these BCVIs have been discovered, conservative observation is typically not warranted. Treatment options include antiplatelet agents such as aspirin, anticoagulants such as unfractionated heparin, open surgical repair, and endovascular repair. Although no level I data exist to guide therapy, multiple retrospective studies support the use of antithrombotic agents (either antiplatelet agents or anticoagulants) as first-line treatment. One recent study by Cothren and colleagues[76] reported a 21% stroke rate in patients with untreated BCVI, compared with a 0.5% stroke rate in patients with BCVI treated with antithrombotic agents. In practice, antiplatelet agents are often selected over anticoagulants in the polytrauma patient with BCVI, although the relative safety and efficacy of the 2 approaches in such patients are not well established.

Open surgical or endovascular repair of grade I to IV BCVI is typically not indicated, given the apparent safety and efficacy of antithrombotic therapy. Some advocate repair of grade III lesions (pseudoaneurysm formation), although many centers also treat such lesions with long-term antithrombotic therapy. Grade I to III lesions that progress despite antithrombotic therapy (eg, enlarging pseudoaneurysm noted on serial imaging) or fail medical therapy (eg, new thromboembolic event despite adequate antithrombotic therapy) should probably be considered for repair. As most BCVI lesions tend to be located near the skull base, and thus are not easily accessed surgically, endovascular repair is usually the favored approach. Early experience with endovascular stenting without aggressive use of concurrent antiplatelet agents was notable for a high rate (45%) of stent thrombosis compared with a thrombosis rate of only 5% in similar patients treated with antithrombotic medications. The long-term patency and clinical outcomes of patients with BCVI treated with endovascular stenting and ongoing antiplatelet agents is less well characterized. However, a recent analysis of conservative and operative management of blunt carotid injuries from the National Trauma Data Bank showed no benefit for either open surgery or endovascular repair compared with more conservative medical management.[82] Overall, both surgical and endovascular repair of grade I to III BCVI lesions should likely be reserved for the special situations described earlier.

Grade V BCVI lesions are life-threatening injuries that require immediate surgical and/or endovascular treatment. Endovascular approaches for such lesions are discussed along with the endovascular management of life-threatening penetrating neck injuries, because treatment options are similar for both.

Penetrating Cervical Cerebrovascular Trauma

Although penetrating neck trauma (eg, gunshot and stab wounds) is much less common than blunt force cerebrovascular trauma, the associated vascular injuries tend to be more severe in nature, with early life-threatening consequences. As with BCVI, obvious hard signs of cerebrovascular injury include expanding cervical pulsatile hematoma; active arterial hemorrhage from the neck, mouth, or nose with hemodynamic instability; focal neurologic deficit; infarct noted on screening CT or MR imaging; and cervical bruit in patient younger than 50 years. Any patient with penetrating neck trauma and one or more of these signs needs emergent surgical or endovascular treatment. CT angiography should be obtained only if the patient is medically stable. Although low-risk asymptomatic patients with blunt force trauma can likely be followed conservatively without vascular imaging, essentially all patients with penetrating neck trauma merit surveillance vascular imaging.

The mechanism of vascular injury produced by penetrating neck injury differs from that of BCVI. Whereas blunt force injury primarily produces intimal injury and risk of thromboembolism, penetrating trauma typically leads to direct injury to the outer arterial wall, commonly producing an unstable pseudoaneurysm at high risk for rupture and hemorrhage. Given these differences, management approaches to the 2 types of traumatic injury are different.[79,83,84] As a general rule, whereas BCVI injuries tend to be managed conservatively with antithrombotic agents, vascular injuries from penetrating neck trauma are more often approached with surgical or endovascular repair.

For management considerations of penetrating vascular injuries, the neck is divided into 3 anatomic zones: zone I extends from the cricoid cartilage inferiorly below the clavicle (thus containing the aortic arch and proximal great vessels), zone II runs from the cricoid cartilage to the angle of the mandible (containing much of the common carotid artery [CCA] and proximal ICA), and zone III extends for the angle of the mandible to the skull base (containing the high cervical ICA). Zones I and III are difficult to access surgically, and penetrating vascular trauma in these regions is typically managed with endovascular techniques. Injuries within zone II are more surgically accessible and have traditionally been approached with open surgery (although the VA remains relatively inaccessible for open surgery in zone II as well).

In the clinically stable patient, vascular imaging (usually with CT angiography) can be obtained and the patient triaged accordingly. Modern multidetector CT scanners approach 100% sensitivity for detecting penetrating vascular injury, and most trauma centers no longer perform mandatory exploration of zone II penetrating neck trauma in clinically stable patients with normal vascular imaging.[85–87]

Endovascular treatment of traumatic pseudoaneurysms of the cervical vertebral or carotid arteries caused by penetrating trauma remains particularly challenging. The primary goal is to maintain normal patency of the cerebral circulation while repairing the pseudoaneurysm. The 2 main options include stent-assisted coil embolization of the pseudoaneurysm and the use of stent grafts or covered stents placed across the pseudoaneurysm. Both treatments require long-term use of antiplatelet medications (likely dual antiplatelet agents), and their long-term efficacy and patency are largely unknown. Nonetheless, such approaches are the best option for zone I and III pseudoaneurysms caused by penetrating trauma. Severe life-threatening injuries to the ICA or VA (eg, pseudoaneurysm or transection with active bleeding) outside zone II may be treatable only with endovascular vessel takedown (Fig. 5).

Endovascular treatment of traumatic pseudoaneurysms involving arteries other than the CCA, ICA, or VA (eg, branches of the ECA) is more straightforward, because maintaining vessel patency is not usually a primary concern. Such pseudoaneurysms can be addressed with pushable or detachable coils, Gelfoam, or liquid embolic agents such as N-butyl cyanoacrylate.[79,84]

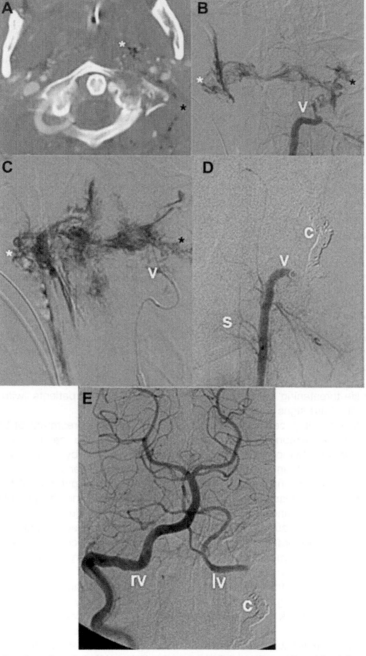

Fig. 5. **Penetrating head and neck trauma.** 24-year-old woman was shot with a pistol from the inside of the mouth. CT angiography (*A*) shows nonvisualization of the left VA and shattering the lateral mass of the C1 vertebral body. The entry site (white *) and air-filled bullet tract (between white and black *) can be seen. The left ICA is slightly irregular, likely as a result of acute vasospasm, because it was found to be normal on conventional catheter angiography (not shown). Catheter angiography (*B–E*) confirms transection of the left VA (v), with active contrast extravasation from the artery to the bullet tract and oral cavity corresponding to massive hemorrhage (*B–C*). Detachable coils (c) were rapidly placed endovascularly to occlude the left VA at C1, preserving the more proximal supply to the anterior spinal artery (s, *D*). Retrograde perfusion of the intracranial left VA (lv) across the vertebrobasilar junction from the right VA was confirmed (*E*). The patient received halo fixation for her C1 fracture. Six months later, she had no neurologic deficits.

REFERENCES

1. Gonzalez RG. Imaging-guided acute ischemic stroke therapy: from "time is brain" to "physiology is brain". AJNR Am J Neuroradiol 2006;27(4):728–35.
2. Tissue plasminogen activator for acute ischemic stroke. The National Institute of Neurological Disorders and Stroke rt-PA Stroke Study Group. N Engl J Med 1995;333(24):1581–7.
3. Hacke W, Kaste M, Bluhmki E, et al. Thrombolysis with alteplase 3 to 4.5 hours after acute ischemic stroke. N Engl J Med 2008;359(13):1317–29.
4. Wahlgren N, Ahmed N, Davalos A, et al. Thrombolysis with alteplase 3-4.5 h after acute ischaemic stroke (SITS-ISTR): an observational study. Lancet 2008;372(9646):1303–9.
5. Del Zoppo GJ, Saver JL, Jauch EC, et al. Expansion of the time window for treatment of acute ischemic stroke with intravenous tissue plasminogen activator: a science advisory from the American Heart Association/American Stroke Association. Stroke 2009;40(8):2945–8.
6. del Zoppo GJ, Higashida RT, Furlan AJ, et al. PROACT: a phase II randomized trial of recombinant prourokinase by direct arterial delivery in acute middle cerebral artery stroke. PROACT Investigators. Prolyse in Acute Cerebral Thromboembolism. Stroke 1998;29(1):4–11.
7. Furlan A, Higashida R, Wechsler L, et al. Intra-arterial prourokinase for acute ischemic stroke. The PROACT II study: a randomized controlled trial. Prolyse in Acute Cerebral Thromboembolism. JAMA 1999;282(21):2003–11.
8. Combined intravenous and intra-arterial recanalization for acute ischemic stroke: the Interventional Management of Stroke Study. Stroke 2004;35(4):904–11.
9. The Interventional Management of Stroke (IMS) II Study. Stroke 2007;38(7):2127–35.
10. Gobin YP, Starkman S, Duckwiler GR, et al. MERCI 1: a phase 1 study of Mechanical Embolus Removal in Cerebral Ischemia. Stroke 2004;35(12):2848–54.
11. Smith WS, Sung G, Saver J, et al. Mechanical thrombectomy for acute ischemic stroke: final results of the Multi MERCI trial. Stroke 2008;39(4):1205–12.
12. Smith WS, Sung G, Starkman S, et al. Safety and efficacy of mechanical embolectomy in acute ischemic stroke: results of the MERCI trial. Stroke 2005;36(7):1432–8.
13. Bose A, Henkes H, Alfke K, et al. The Penumbra System: a mechanical device for the treatment of acute stroke due to thromboembolism. AJNR Am J Neuroradiol 2008;29(7):1409–13.
14. Hauck EF, Mocco J, Snyder KV, et al. Temporary endovascular bypass: a novel treatment for acute stroke. AJNR Am J Neuroradiol 2009;30(8):1532–3.
15. Kelly ME, Furlan AJ, Fiorella D. Recanalization of an acute middle cerebral artery occlusion using a self-expanding, reconstrainable, intracranial microstent as a temporary endovascular bypass. Stroke 2008;39(6):1770–3.
16. Josephson SA, Saver JL, Smith WS. Comparison of mechanical embolectomy and intraarterial thrombolysis in acute ischemic stroke within the MCA: MERCI and Multi MERCI compared to PROACT II. Neurocrit Care 2009;10(1):43–9.
17. Nogueira RG, Liebeskind D, Gupta R, et al. DWI/PWI and CTP assessment in the triage of wake-up and late presenting strokes undergoing neurointervention: the DAWN Trial. International Stroke Conference. vol. San Francisco, February 17, 2009.
18. Hetts S. Interventional MRI: the revolution begins. Appl Radiol 2005;34(Suppl 1):S84–91.
19. Schaefer PW, Hassankhani A, Putman C, et al. Characterization and evolution of diffusion MR imaging abnormalities in stroke patients undergoing intraarterial thrombolysis. AJNR Am J Neuroradiol 2004;25(6):951–7.
20. Schaefer PW, Roccatagliata L, Ledezma C, et al. First-pass quantitative CT perfusion identifies thresholds for salvageable penumbra in acute stroke patients treated with intra-arterial therapy. AJNR Am J Neuroradiol 2006;27(1):20–5.
21. Wintermark M, Smith WS, Ko NU, et al. Dynamic perfusion CT: optimizing the temporal resolution and contrast volume for calculation of perfusion CT parameters in stroke patients. AJNR Am J Neuroradiol 2004;25(5):720–9.
22. Chimowitz MI, Lynn MJ, Howlett-Smith H, et al. Comparison of warfarin and aspirin for symptomatic intracranial arterial stenosis. N Engl J Med 2005;352(13):1305–16.
23. Kasner SE, Lynn MJ, Chimowitz MI, et al. Warfarin vs aspirin for symptomatic intracranial stenosis: subgroup analyses from WASID. Neurology 2006;67(7):1275–8.
24. Derdeyn CP, Chimowitz MI. Angioplasty and stenting for atherosclerotic intracranial stenosis: rationale for a randomized clinical trial. Neuroimaging Clin N Am 2007;17(3):355–63.
25. Fiorella DJ, Levy EI, Turk AS, et al. Target lesion revascularization after wingspan: assessment of safety and durability. Stroke 2009;40(1):106–10.
26. Turk AS, Levy EI, Albuquerque FC, et al. Influence of patient age and stenosis location on wingspan in-stent restenosis. AJNR Am J Neuroradiol 2008;29(1):23–7.
27. Komotar RJ, Zacharia BE, Otten ML, et al. Controversies in the endovascular management of cerebral vasospasm after intracranial aneurysm rupture and future directions for therapeutic approaches. Neurosurgery 2008;62(4):897–905 [discussion: 905–7].

28. Jun P, Ko NU, English JD, et al. Endovascular treatment of medically-refractory cerebral vasospasm following aneurysmal subarachnoid hemorrhage. AJNR Am J Neuroradiol 2010. [Epub ahead of print].

29. Joshi S, Meyers PM, Ornstein E. Intracarotid delivery of drugs: the potential and the pitfalls. Anesthesiology 2008;109(3):543–64.

30. Lavine SD, Wang M, Etu JJ, et al. Augmentation of cerebral blood flow and reversal of endothelin-1-induced vasospasm: a comparison of intracarotid nicardipine and verapamil. Neurosurgery 2007;60(4):742–8 [discussion: 748–9].

31. Keuskamp J, Murali R, Chao KH. High-dose intraarterial verapamil in the treatment of cerebral vasospasm after aneurysmal subarachnoid hemorrhage. J Neurosurg 2008;108(3):458–63.

32. Haque R, Kellner CP, Komotar RJ, et al. Mechanical treatment of vasospasm. Neurol Res 2009;31(6):638–43.

33. Higashida RT, Halbach VV, Cahan LD, et al. Transluminal angioplasty for treatment of intracranial arterial vasospasm. J Neurosurg 1989;71(5 Pt 1):648–53.

34. Higashida RT, Halbach VV, Dormandy B, et al. New microballoon device for transluminal angioplasty of intracranial arterial vasospasm. AJNR Am J Neuroradiol 1990;11(2):233–8.

35. Bederson JB, Connolly ES Jr, Batjer HH, et al. Guidelines for the management of aneurysmal subarachnoid hemorrhage: a statement for healthcare professionals from a special writing group of the Stroke Council, American Heart Association. Stroke 2009;40(3):994–1025.

36. Schievink WI. Intracranial aneurysms. N Engl J Med 1997;336(1):28–40.

37. Suarez JI, Tarr RW, Selman WR. Aneurysmal subarachnoid hemorrhage. N Engl J Med 2006;354(4):387–96.

38. Brinjikji W, Kallmes DF, White JB, et al. Inter- and intraobserver agreement in CT characterization of nonaneurysmal perimesencephalic subarachnoid hemorrhage. AJNR Am J Neuroradiol 2010;31(6):1103–5.

39. Santos-Franco JA, Zenteno M, Lee A. Dissecting aneurysms of the vertebrobasilar system. A comprehensive review on natural history and treatment options. Neurosurg Rev 2008;31(2):131–40 [discussion: 140].

40. Molyneux A, Kerr R, Stratton I, et al. International Subarachnoid Aneurysm Trial (ISAT) of neurosurgical clipping versus endovascular coiling in 2143 patients with ruptured intracranial aneurysms: a randomised trial. Lancet 2002;360(9342):1267–74.

41. Molyneux AJ, Kerr RS, Birks J, et al. Risk of recurrent subarachnoid haemorrhage, death, or dependence and standardised mortality ratios after clipping or coiling of an intracranial aneurysm in the International Subarachnoid Aneurysm Trial (ISAT): long-term follow-up. Lancet Neurol 2009;8(5):427–33.

42. Hoh BL, Chi YY, Lawson MF, et al. Length of stay and total hospital charges of clipping versus coiling for ruptured and unruptured adult cerebral aneurysms in the Nationwide Inpatient Sample database 2002 to 2006. Stroke 2010;41(2):337–42.

43. van Rooij WJ, Keeren GJ, Peluso JP, et al. Clinical and angiographic results of coiling of 196 very small (< or = 3 mm) intracranial aneurysms. AJNR Am J Neuroradiol 2009;30(4):835–9.

44. van Rooij WJ, Sluzewski M. Endovascular treatment of large and giant aneurysms. AJNR Am J Neuroradiol 2009;30(1):12–8.

45. Moret J, Cognard C, Weill A, et al. [Reconstruction technic in the treatment of wide-neck intracranial aneurysms. Long-term angiographic and clinical results. Apropos of 56 cases]. J Neuroradiol 1997;24(1):30–44 [in French].

46. Higashida RT, Smith W, Gress D, et al. Intravascular stent and endovascular coil placement for a ruptured fusiform aneurysm of the basilar artery. Case report and review of the literature. J Neurosurg 1997;87(6):944–9.

47. Fiorella D, Thiabolt L, Albuquerque FC, et al. Antiplatelet therapy in neuroendovascular therapeutics. Neurosurg Clin N Am 2005;16(3):517–40.

48. Tahtinen OI, Vanninen RL, Manninen HI, et al. Wide-necked intracranial aneurysms: treatment with stent-assisted coil embolization during acute (<72 hours) subarachnoid hemorrhage—experience in 61 consecutive patients. Radiology 2009;253(1):199–208.

49. Cekirge HS, Saatci I, Ozturk MH, et al. Late angiographic and clinical follow-up results of 100 consecutive aneurysms treated with Onyx reconstruction: largest single-center experience. Neuroradiology 2006;48(2):113–26.

50. Molyneux AJ, Cekirge S, Saatci I, et al. Cerebral Aneurysm Multicenter European Onyx (CAMEO) trial: results of a prospective observational study in 20 European centers. AJNR Am J Neuroradiol 2004;25(1):39–51.

51. Murayama Y, Vinuela F, Tateshima S, et al. Endovascular treatment of experimental aneurysms by use of a combination of liquid embolic agents and protective devices. AJNR Am J Neuroradiol 2000;21(9):1726–35.

52. Piske RL, Kanashiro LH, Paschoal E, et al. Evaluation of Onyx HD-500 embolic system in the treatment of 84 wide-neck intracranial aneurysms. Neurosurgery 2009;64(5):E865–75 [discussion: E875].

53. Weber W, Siekmann R, Kis B, et al. Treatment and follow-up of 22 unruptured wide-necked intracranial aneurysms of the internal carotid artery with Onyx HD 500. AJNR Am J Neuroradiol 2005;26(8):1909–15.

54. Wiebers DO, Whisnant JP, Huston J 3rd, et al. Unruptured intracranial aneurysms: natural history,

clinical outcome, and risks of surgical and endovascular treatment. Lancet 2003;362(9378):103–10.

55. Guglielmi G. The beginning and the evolution of the endovascular treatment of intracranial aneurysms: from the first catheterization of brain arteries to the new stents. J Neurointerv Surg 2009;1(1):53–5.

56. Guglielmi G, Vinuela F, Dion J, et al. Electrothrombosis of saccular aneurysms via endovascular approach. Part 2: preliminary clinical experience. J Neurosurg 1991;75(1):8–14.

57. Guglielmi G, Vinuela F, Sepetka I, et al. Electrothrombosis of saccular aneurysms via endovascular approach. Part 1: electrochemical basis, technique, and experimental results. J Neurosurg 1991;75(1):1–7.

58. Fa S. Balloon catheterization and occlusion of major cerebral blood vessels. J Neurosurg 1974;41:125–45.

59. Romodanov AP, Shcheglov VI. Intravascular occlusion of saccular aneurysms of the cerebral arteries by means of a detachable balloon catheter. In: Krayenbühl H, editor. Advances and technical standards in neurosurgery, vol. 9. Berlin: Springer; 1982. p. 25–48.

60. Hieshima GB, Grinnell VS, Mehringer CM. A detachable balloon for therapeutic transcatheter occlusions. Radiology 1981;138(1):227–8.

61. Dandy WE. Intracranial aneurysm of the internal carotid artery: cured by operation. Ann Surg 1938;107(5):654–9.

62. Hetts SW, Narvid J, Sanai N, et al. Intracranial aneurysms in childhood: 27-year single-institution experience. AJNR Am J Neuroradiol 2009;30(7):1315–24.

63. Ferro JM, Canhao P, Stam J, et al. Prognosis of cerebral vein and dural sinus thrombosis: results of the International Study on Cerebral Vein and Dural Sinus Thrombosis (ISCVT). Stroke 2004;35(3):664–70.

64. English JD, Fields JD, Le S, et al. Clinical presentation and long-term outcome of cerebral venous thrombosis. Neurocrit Care 2009;11(3):330–7.

65. Linn J, Ertl-Wagner B, Seelos KC, et al. Diagnostic value of multidetector-row CT angiography in the evaluation of thrombosis of the cerebral venous sinuses. AJNR Am J Neuroradiol 2007;28(5):946–52.

66. Dowd CF, Malek AM, Phatouros CC, et al. Application of a rheolytic thrombectomy device in the treatment of dural sinus thrombosis: a new technique. AJNR Am J Neuroradiol 1999;20(4):568–70.

67. Rahman M, Velat GJ, Hoh BL, et al. Direct thrombolysis for cerebral venous sinus thrombosis. Neurosurg Focus 2009;27(5):E7.

68. La Barge DV III, Bishop FS, Stevens EA, et al. Intrasinus catheter-directed heparin infusion in the treatment of dural venous sinus thrombosis. AJNR Am J Neuroradiol 2009;30:1672–8.

69. Willems PW, Farb RI, Agid R. Endovascular treatment of epistaxis. AJNR Am J Neuroradiol 2009;30(9):1637–45.

70. Geibprasert S, Pongpech S, Armstrong D, et al. Dangerous extracranial-intracranial anastomoses and supply to the cranial nerves: vessels the neurointerventionalist needs to know. AJNR Am J Neuroradiol 2009;30(8):1459–68.

71. Davis JW, Holbrook TL, Hoyt DB, et al. Blunt carotid artery dissection: incidence, associated injuries, screening, and treatment. J Trauma 1990;30(12):1514–7.

72. Cogbill TH, Moore EE, Meissner M, et al. The spectrum of blunt injury to the carotid artery: a multicenter perspective. J Trauma 1994;37(3):473–9.

73. Biffl WL, Moore EE, Ryu RK, et al. The unrecognized epidemic of blunt carotid arterial injuries: early diagnosis improves neurologic outcome. Ann Surg 1998;228(4):462–70.

74. Mayberry JC, Brown CV, Mullins RJ, et al. Blunt carotid artery injury: the futility of aggressive screening and diagnosis. Arch Surg 2004;139(6):609–12 [discussion: 612–3].

75. Miller PR, Fabian TC, Croce MA, et al. Prospective screening for blunt cerebrovascular injuries: analysis of diagnostic modalities and outcomes. Ann Surg 2002;236(3):386–93 [discussion: 393–5].

76. Cothren CC, Biffl WL, Moore EE, et al. Treatment for blunt cerebrovascular injuries: equivalence of anticoagulation and antiplatelet agents. Arch Surg 2009;144(7):685–90.

77. Cothren CC, Moore EE, Ray CE Jr, et al. Screening for blunt cerebrovascular injuries is cost-effective. Am J Surg 2005;190(6):845–9.

78. Biffl WL, Cothren CC, Moore EE, et al. Western Trauma Association critical decisions in trauma: screening for and treatment of blunt cerebrovascular injuries. J Trauma 2009;67(6):1150–3.

79. Krings T, Geibprasert S, Lasjaunias PL. Cerebrovascular trauma. Eur Radiol 2008;18(8):1531–45.

80. Biffl WL, Moore EE, Offner PJ, et al. Blunt carotid arterial injuries: implications of a new grading scale. J Trauma 1999;47(5):845–53.

81. Biffl WL, Ray CE Jr, Moore EE, et al. Treatment-related outcomes from blunt cerebrovascular injuries: importance of routine follow-up arteriography. Ann Surg 2002;235(5):699–706 [discussion: 706–7].

82. Li W, D'Ayala M, Hirshberg A, et al. Comparison of conservative and operative treatment for blunt carotid injuries: analysis of the National Trauma Data Bank. J Vasc Surg 2010;51(3):593–9, 599.e591–2.

83. Kesser BW, Chance E, Kleiner D, et al. Contemporary management of penetrating neck trauma. Am Surg 2009;75(1):1–10.

84. Radvany MG, Gailloud P. Endovascular management of neurovascular arterial injuries in the face and neck. Semin Intervent Radiol 2010;27:44–54.

85. Woo K, Magner DP, Wilson MT, et al. CT angiography in penetrating neck trauma reduces the need for operative neck exploration. Am Surg 2005;71(9): 754–8.

86. Stuhlfaut JW, Barest G, Sakai O, et al. Impact of MDCT angiography on the use of catheter angiography for the assessment of cervical arterial injury after blunt or penetrating trauma. AJR Am J Roentgenol 2005;185(4):1063–8.

87. Inaba K, Munera F, McKenney M, et al. Prospective evaluation of screening multislice helical computed tomographic angiography in the initial evaluation of penetrating neck injuries. J Trauma 2006;61(1): 144–9.

Orbital and Intracranial Complications of Acute Sinusitis

Joseph M. Hoxworth[a] and Christine M. Glastonbury[b,c,d,*]

KEYWORDS

- Sinusitis • Orbit • Intracranial complications
- Cellulitis • Abscess

RHINOSINUSITIS: COMPLICATIONS IN A COMMON CONDITION

Rhinosinusitis is a relatively common clinical condition affecting both children and adults. It is typically readily treated with nasal decongestants, with or without oral antibiotics. Rarely, sinus infection can result in vision loss or even life-threatening orbital and intracranial complications. Orbital extension of acute infection most commonly occurs in pediatric patients who typically present with proptosis, periorbital swelling, and erythema. When found in immunocompromised patients, such as those with diabetes, lymphoreticular malignancies, human immunodeficiency virus infection, chronic renal failure, or liver failure, intracranial infection is more likely to be secondary to acute invasive fungal sinusitis. However, orbital and/or intracranial complications may also occur in immunocompetent children, teenagers, and adults who are untreated or incompletely treated for bacterial rhinosinusitis. Although the consequences of sinogenic infections can be catastrophic, the imaging findings may be extremely subtle. Early detection of orbital and intracranial complications by the radiologist requires dedicated imaging protocols, knowledge of key imaging findings, and an understanding of disease pathogenesis.

IMAGING CONSIDERATIONS

Although radiographs may still be used to confirm the clinical impression of sinusitis, computed tomography (CT) is more accurate for making this diagnosis.[1,2] Indeed, whenever orbital or intracranial complications of sinusitis are suspected, contrast-enhanced CT should be the initial imaging modality of choice. In the current era of more actively minimizing radiation exposure, particularly for pediatric patients, it is imperative that the study be performed with the lowest radiation dose possible, although this must not be at the expense of a diagnostic study. Sinogenic complications, especially in children and immunocompromised patients, may rapidly progress. It is imperative that referring clinicians indicate their concern for complications or clinical features that might suggest orbital or intracranial infection so that the scan protocol is correct.

Most of the published reports evaluating the role of CT for diagnosing orbital complications of

[a] Department of Radiology, Mayo Clinic, 5777 East Mayo Boulevard, Scottsdale, AZ 85259, USA
[b] Department of Radiology & Biomedical Imaging, University of California San Francisco, 505 Parnassus Avenue, San Francisco, CA 94143-0628, USA
[c] Department of Otolaryngology-Head & Neck Surgery, University of California San Francisco, 505 Parnassus Avenue, San Francisco, CA 94143-0628, USA
[d] Department of Radiation Oncology, University of California San Francisco, 505 Parnassus Avenue, San Francisco, CA 94143-0628, USA
* Corresponding author. Department of Radiology & Biomedical Imaging, University of California San Francisco, 505 Parnassus Avenue, San Francisco, CA 94143-0628.
E-mail address: Christine.Glastonbury@radiology.ucsf.edu

Neuroimag Clin N Am 20 (2010) 511–526
doi:10.1016/j.nic.2010.07.004
1052-5149/10/$ — see front matter © 2010 Elsevier Inc. All rights reserved.

sinusitis were based on CT imaging with what is now outdated technology.[3–7] In addition to technologic constraints, such as slower acquisition times, decreased resolution, and nonvolumetric imaging, another limitation included the lag time between performing the CT and subsequent progression of symptoms in many of the reported cases. Despite these limitations, CT was still found to improve diagnostic accuracy relative to clinical judgment alone, a conclusion that certainly remains true today with improved CT technology.

With the continuous advancement of imaging, there are no prospective studies comparing current generation multidetector CT scanners with magnetic resonance (MR) imaging for the detection of orbital complications of sinusitis. McIntosh and Mahadevan[8,9] recently reported the benefit of MR imaging over CT, but the MR imaging in their case report was performed after a delay during which the patient's subperiosteal abscess likely progressed, as the abscess depicted with MR imaging would almost certainly have been visible with CT had it been performed simultaneously. Nevertheless, if follow-up imaging is deemed necessary to assess clinical deterioration or treatment response, MR imaging should be considered to spare the patient additional radiation exposure.

In evaluating the orbits, contrast-enhanced helical CT is best acquired in the axial plane using submillimeter collimation for isotropic voxels to allow for high-quality image reconstruction in the coronal and sagittal planes. Image data should be rendered using both soft tissue and bone algorithms to optimally assess the orbital contents as well as the thin osseous structures in the orbital and sinonasal regions. This multiplanar approach allows for more effective detection and localization of intraorbital pathology (particularly thin subperiosteal collections along the orbital roof or floor, which are more easily overlooked in the axial plane) and simultaneously provides a high-quality sinus CT that is equally necessary in this clinical context. With increased public awareness of iatrogenic radiation exposure, CT vendors are now offering radiation reduction options that include active dose modulation and improved iterative reconstruction techniques, both of which can maintain image quality while reducing dose. Although we typically use bismuth shielding to the orbits for head CT scans, this is not used at our institution for sinus CT studies because it prevents the use of the CT scan as an intraoperative stereotactic guide, and the patient would require additional scanning and thus further radiation.

Orbital MR imaging seems to be more sensitive for the detection of fungal sinusitis, with or without orbital or intracranial complications. In performing orbital MR imaging, specific imaging parameters vary based on equipment manufacturer and field strength. In general, axial and coronal T1-weighted sequences best depict the relevant orbital anatomy, and any infiltration or stranding of the normal high-intensity orbital fat should be sought as a sign of inflammation. A short tau inversion recovery (STIR) or T2-weighted fat-suppressed series should be included to evaluate for inflammatory edema and focal purulent fluid collections. Multiplanar postcontrast T1-weighted sequences with fat suppression should be acquired to search for inflammatory enhancement, as well as rim-enhancement patterns that may distinguish phlegmon from abscess. Although the local magnetic field is frequently inhomogeneous from dental hardware and air-bone interfaces in the face, it is helpful to carefully evaluate these fat-suppressed sequences in more than one plane to help distinguish high signal from failure of fat suppression versus true abnormal enhancement. In addition, the field of view for orbital MR imaging readily includes the parasellar region so the cavernous sinus should be assessed for thrombosis.

For suspected intracranial complications of sinusitis, contrast-enhanced head CT is useful as an initial screening test.[10] Despite its limitations, CT can readily identify features that would immediately triage the patient for neurosurgical management such as significant mass effect, space-occupying brain lesions, large extraaxial collections, and hydrocephalus. Once contraindications have been ruled out, lumbar puncture can be safely performed to evaluate for meningitis while the patient awaits MR imaging to evaluate the intracranial contents with greater sensitivity and specificity than can be achieved with CT.[4,11,12] The usefulness of different MR imaging pulse sequences is illustrated in greater detail through examples of specific intracranial complications.

ORBITAL COMPLICATIONS OF RHINOSINUSITIS
Epidemiology and Pathogenesis of Orbital Spread of Infection

Largely because of proximity, orbital infection is the most common complication from acute sinusitis.[13–15] Because the frontal and sphenoid sinuses develop at a later age, it is not surprising that involvement of the ethmoid sinuses is seen most often, followed in frequency by the maxillary sinuses.[3,7,16–18] Because of anatomic, immunologic, and environmental factors, pediatric patients suffer from acute rhinosinusitis more frequently than adults, and account for the greater proportion of complicated cases.[17] Recent series suggest that the average age of children with orbital complications is 6 to 8 years, although the median age tends to be slightly younger.[13,18,19] Acute and chronic sinus disease, likewise, accounts for most cases of orbital cellulitis in adults, in whom there is a trend toward declining frequency with advancing age.[14,20] Sinusitis-related orbital infection is the most common cause of unilateral proptosis in children and the third most common cause in adults after thyroid orbitopathy and pseudotumor.[21–23] For unclear reasons, a male predominance is universally reported.[13–15,17,18,20,24]

From an anatomic perspective, there are many predisposing factors that allow for spread of paranasal sinus infection to the orbit. In terms of physical proximity, the thin bony roof, floor, and medial wall of the orbit serve to separate the orbital contents from the frontal, maxillary, and ethmoid sinuses, respectively. Clearly, aggressive infections causing osteitis might directly extend from the sinus to the orbit, but this is rare and there are multiple other potential routes for the spread of infection that do not require transgression of intact bone. The orbit is formed from 7 separate bones, and this is most relevant in considering the medial wall, which is comprised of a small portion of the sphenoid body, the ethmoid lamina papyracea, the lacrimal bone, and the frontal process of the maxilla. The union of these bones results in the presence of 3 vertical sutures appropriately termed the sphenoethmoidal, lacrimoethmoidal, and lacrimomaxillary fissures. In addition, the anterior and posterior ethmoidal foramina allow transmission of vessels and nerves along the frontoethmoidal suture line. Focal osseous defects in the orbital walls can occur secondary to areas of congenital or acquired dehiscence, with the latter including sequela from both trauma and surgery.

The veins of the orbit also play a significant role in the pathogenesis of sinusitis-related complications, as it is a valveless system that allows 2-way communication between the veins of the face, paranasal sinuses, nasal cavity, orbit, pterygoid plexus, and cavernous sinus. The dominant venous drainage of the orbit is via the superior and inferior ophthalmic veins, although there are numerous smaller vessels forming a rich venous network. Most orbital and intracranial complications of sinusitis are secondary to transmission of infection via retrograde thrombophlebitis.

Despite the aforementioned features that predispose the spread of infection from the sinus to the orbit, a protective barrier exists in the form of the periorbita (ie, the periosteum of the orbit), which is analogous to the layer of dura lining the inner table of the calvarium. The periorbita is a robust fibrous membrane that can be stripped from the bone except at suture lines where it is contiguous with the periosteum on the other side. It not only serves as a barrier to the spread of infection from the sinuses to the orbit but also forms the anterior orbital septum as it reflects into the tarsal plates anteriorly. This creates a delineation between periorbital (preseptal) and intraorbital (postseptal) tissues, shielding the orbital contents from potential pathology.

Pathology and Imaging Detection

Chandler and colleagues[25] eloquently described the role of the orbital anatomic structures in complications of sinusitis 4 decades ago. This formed the basis for their revised classification system that consists of the following groups:

1. Inflammatory edema
2. Orbital cellulitis
3. Subperiosteal abscess
4. Orbital abscess
5. Cavernous sinus thrombosis.

Although still used today, there have been suggested modifications with the advent of cross-sectional imaging.[14,26,27]

Inflammatory edema/preseptal cellulitis

Initially, the description of inflammatory edema referred to local inflammation and impaired venous drainage of the eyelids caused by increased pressure in ethmoid air cells, with or without edema of the orbits. Other investigators have subsequently revised this patient group to include those who have preseptal infection, defined as periorbital cellulitis with or without a focal abscess.[14,27] The patient typically presents with eyelid erythema, tenderness, and swelling, and a detailed ophthalmologic examination is needed to ensure that underlying vision and extraocular motion is intact. Although isolated preseptal involvement frequently does not require cross-sectional imaging, it is useful when there is concern about postseptal extension.

On CT and MR imaging, infiltration of adipose tissue is seen in all types of edema, independent of whether it is a sterile hydrostatic process or frank cellulitis. Both modalities show swelling of the eyelids along with thickening and stranding of the periorbital soft tissues in cases of cellulitis, and the radiologist should evaluate for the development of a focal fluid collection to suggest an abscess (Fig. 1). It is imperative to scrutinize the orbits to ensure that no postseptal involvement is present. The presence and extent of sinusitis should also be documented.

Preseptal cellulitis in children is less often associated with acute sinusitis than in adult patients, and is seen with greater frequency in the context of trauma (especially with a retained foreign body, laceration, or insect bite) and medical comorbidities.[19]

Orbital cellulitis/postseptal cellulitis

Orbital cellulitis refers to postseptal edema involving the intra- and/or extraconal orbital contents. Although not a circumscribed process, the inflammation can be widespread or preferentially distributed in a certain portion of the orbit, in which it tends to be located adjacent to the most severely affected sinus. Depending on the amount of inflammation, varying degrees of proptosis and impairment of the function of extraocular muscles can occur. Orbital inflammation is well demonstrated with CT and appears as stranding of the orbital fat. The corresponding MR imaging appearance of this inflammatory infiltration is one of ill-defined T2 hyperintensity consistent with edema as well as concomitant enhancement following contrast administration (Fig. 2).

Subperiosteal abscess

The subperiosteal abscess typically develops when ethmoid sinus infection spreads across the medial orbital wall or, less commonly, from the frontal or maxillary sinuses across the orbital roof or floor, respectively. The tough periorbita again serves as a barrier to free dissemination of infection throughout the orbital soft tissues; however, localized infection may evolve into an abscess that strips periorbita from bone, and displaces it inward. Typically, a thin fat plane is visible between the periorbita and the adjacent extraocular muscle. When small, a subperiosteal abscess causes minimal mass effect within the orbit and is seen as a subtle elongated rim-enhancing fluid collection (Fig. 3). Larger subperiosteal abscesses assume a lenticular shape, exert significant mass effect, and can significantly impair extraocular motion and cause proptosis with compression and/or tethering of the optic nerve, resulting in vision loss (Fig. 4). Coronal reformatted images of axial-acquired contrast-enhanced CT data should always be performed to evaluate for these collections, particularly if no cause for proptosis is evident on axial imaging. Indeed, a subperiosteal abscess arising from a frontal or maxillary sinus is most often readily identified in the coronal (or sagittal) plane.

Orbital abscess

Whether intra- or extraconal, an orbital abscess is a collection of pus that is not contained by the periorbita. Orbital abscesses usually cause proptosis, ophthalmoplegia, and visual impairment, and these clinical signs are more marked with larger abscesses or orbital apex involvement. Mass effect within the more tightly confined orbital apex is more apt to involve cranial nerves II, III, IV, and VI, as well as the ophthalmic branch of cranial nerve V, because these structures exit the optic foramen and superior orbital fissure. Unlike the poorly defined edema and enhancement

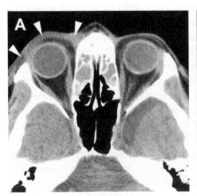
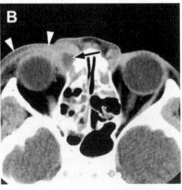

Fig. 1. Periorbital cellulitis/abscess. (*A*) 68-year-old woman with chronic frontal, maxillary, and ethmoidal sinusitis was evaluated for right eye swelling. Noncontrast CT shows right eyelid swelling with stranding of the surrounding periorbital soft tissues (*arrowheads*), consistent with periorbital cellulitis. No postseptal extension is present. Note the opacified ethmoid air cells. Incidentally noted is a small arachnoid cyst in the anterior aspect of the left middle cranial fossa. (*B*) 13-year-old boy with acute sinusitis developed right eye swelling several days before imaging. Contrast-enhanced CT shows periorbital soft tissue swelling (*arrowheads*) and a small preseptal rim-enhancing fluid collection near the medial canthus, consistent with an abscess (*arrow*). This has decompressed from the ethmoid air cells through an osseous defect.

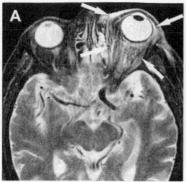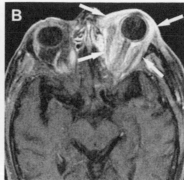

Fig. 2. Postseptal orbital cellulitis. 55-year-old man with chronic pansinusitis developed painful blurred vision in the left eye. (*A*) Axial T2-weighted fat-suppressed sequence reveals diffuse edema within the left orbital fat and extraocular muscles (*arrows*). (*B*) Axial T1 fat-suppressed contrast-enhanced sequence exhibits an infiltrative pattern of enhancement throughout the postseptal soft tissues (*arrows*). No focal abscess is present, although the patient does have left-sided proptosis.

seen with orbital cellulitis, an orbital abscess is seen as a more discrete rim-enhancing fluid collection within the orbital adipose tissue with extensive surrounding inflammation (**Fig. 5**).

Cavernous sinus thrombosis

Many cases of cavernous sinus thrombosis associated with rhinosinusitis are clinically apparent. Patients typically present with fever, headache, periorbital swelling, diplopia, chemosis, and/or

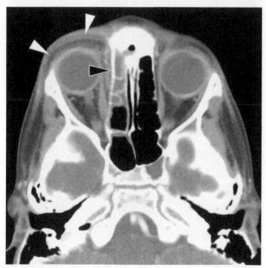

Fig. 3. Orbital cellulitis/subperiosteal abscess. 5-year-old boy with a recent upper respiratory infection was admitted to the hospital with acute right maxillary and ethmoid sinusitis complicated by periorbital cellulitis. In addition to the clinically apparent preseptal swelling (*white arrowheads*), contrast-enhanced CT also reveals the presence of a subtle subperiosteal abscess along the right lamina papyracea (*black arrowhead*) related to the adjacent infected ethmoid air cells.

proptosis.[28] Sixth nerve palsy is most commonly seen, but additional involvement of the third, fourth, fifth, or sixth cranial nerves in the context of orbital or sinus infection should heighten concern for cavernous sinus thrombosis. Contrast-enhanced CT may be unrevealing initially, but fulminate cases show a heterogeneous pattern of less than expected enhancement of the cavernous sinus, which makes the cavernous segment of the internal carotid artery more conspicuous. In addition, the cavernous sinus becomes thickened and the lateral margin assumes a convex morphology. An area of nonopacification exceeding 7 mm in maximum dimension is more common in cases of cavernous sinus thrombosis than in control patients, and this is even more suggestive when present posteriorly.[29] Indirect venous findings, which can be helpful in directing attention to the cavernous sinus, include filling defects or expansion of the superior ophthalmic vein, the inferior petrosal sinus, and sphenoparietal sinus. A similar pattern of abnormality is seen with MR imaging using a contrast-enhanced T1-weighted sequence, with the lateral convexity best demonstrated in the coronal plane (**Fig. 6**).[30] Increased dural enhancement along the lateral border of the cavernous sinus on MR imaging represents an additional indirect finding. Inflammation within the cavernous sinus can lead to narrowing or occlusion of the ipsilateral internal carotid artery, which may result in acute cerebral infarction.[31-33]

Thrombosis of the superior or inferior ophthalmic veins secondary to sinus infection may be seen as a precursor to, or as a result of, cavernous sinus thrombosis. In addition to the expected distension and incomplete enhancement of the ophthalmic veins in these patients,

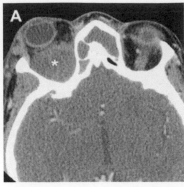
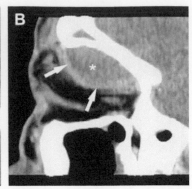

Fig. 4. **Subperiosteal orbital abscess.** 49-year-old woman with acute bacterial sinusitis presented with rapidly progressive periorbital swelling, proptosis, and vision loss. (*A*) Axial contrast-enhanced CT demonstrates sinus opacification and a large, relatively well-defined, intraorbital soft tissue mass, consistent with an abscess (*). (*B*) The sagittal reformatted image more clearly defines the subperiosteal abscess in the superior orbit (*). The distended periorbita (*arrows*) results in a lenticular morphology.

restricted diffusion may provide a clue to this diagnosis as well (Fig. 7).[34] In cases of fulminate thrombophlebitis, it is difficult to delineate whether these diffusion characteristics are secondary to the stage of intravenous blood degradation or the purulent nature of the venous contents.

Treatment, Prognosis, and Follow-up Imaging

Most cases of pre- and postseptal cellulitis are initially treated with broad-spectrum antibiotics and nasal decongestants. Empiric antibiotic coverage is directed at the typical flora of the upper respiratory tract with the caveat that the

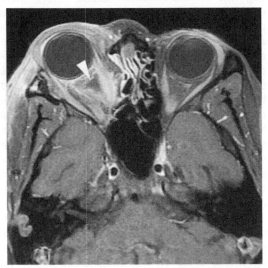

Fig. 5. **Posttraumatic orbital cellulitis/abscess (MR).** 34-year-old woman 4 days after facial trauma treated with open reduction and internal fixation. Axial T1-weighted postcontrast image with fat saturation obtained after operative placement of an orbital drain (which yielded pus), shows residual rim-enhancing intraconal fluid (*arrowhead*). Note also intense enhancement and thickening of medial rectus muscle and fractures of the lateral and medial orbital walls. The optic nerve is displaced laterally and the globe is proptotic.

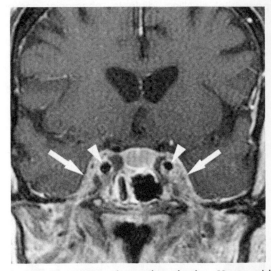

Fig. 6. **Cavernous sinus thrombosis.** 62-year-old woman with history of chronic pansinusitis was undergoing inpatient treatment of bilateral orbital cellulitis when she progressively developed ophthalmoplegia related to third, fourth, and sixth cranial nerves. Coronal contrast-enhanced T1-weighted image with fat saturation shows thickening of the cavernous sinuses with laterally convex margins (*arrows*). Note the heterogeneous enhancement of the multiple small poorly enhancing areas (ie, thrombosis). Normal caliber flow voids of the cavernous internal carotid arteries are identified (*arrowheads*).

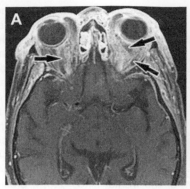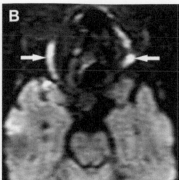

Fig. 7. Septic thrombophlebitis of the superior orbital veins. 34-year-old man with acute-on-chronic sinusitis was transferred from a community hospital following clinical deterioration while receiving empiric intravenous antibiotic therapy for bilateral orbital cellulitis. (*A*) Axial T1-weighted postcontrast image with fat saturation shows extensive infiltrative enhancement of the orbital structures, consistent with known cellulitis. Tubular, nonenhancing structures in the superior orbits represent thrombosed superior ophthalmic veins (*arrows*). (*B*) Both superior ophthalmic veins (*arrows*) exhibit restricted diffusion on an axial diffusion-weighted sequence suggesting thrombophlebitis.

microbiologic profile in complicated cases is somewhat different from routine acute bacterial sinusitis, where *Staphylococcus* and *Streptococcus* species are the most common pathogens.[35–37] With the introduction of the *Haemophilus influenzae* type b (Hib) vaccine, *H influenzae* is now much less often a cause of orbital complications of rhinosinusitis.[35,38,39] Surgical intervention may be necessary if the patient's condition fails to improve significantly within 48 hours after appropriate antibiotic administration. Additional indications for surgery include CT evidence of abscess formation, 20/60 (or worse) visual acuity on initial evaluation, and progression of orbital signs and symptoms despite therapy.[17] Increased attention has recently been given to some special considerations regarding causative agents that may contribute to inadequate response to empiric antibiotic treatment. These include the increased prevalence of methicillin-resistant *Staphylococcus aureus*, the greater recognition of the role of *Streptococcus milleri*, the contribution of polymicrobial and anaerobic infections, and the differences in flora arising from sinusitis that is chronic or related to odontogenic infection.[35,36,40]

Unlike most cases of dural sinus thrombosis (see the article Acute Neuro-Interventional Therapies by Steven Hetts and Joey English elsewhere in this issue), sinogenic cavernous sinus thrombosis is not typically treated with anticoagulants, but rather with surgical debridement of the sinuses and intravenous medical management of the infection.

Rates of blindness and mortality in patients with orbital infection secondary to sinusitis in the pre-antibiotic era were approximately 20% and 17%, respectively.[41] In recent decades, these rates have significantly declined since the advent of antibiotics, accompanied by improved imaging and less invasive endoscopic surgical techniques. For example, 2 recent series reported zero mortality and less than 3% visual morbidity, and another study reported that no patients were expected to have long-term sequela from their orbital infection.[13,15,18] In general, these outcomes still likely represent an overestimate of morbidity secondary to a selection bias, because many of these cases were derived from tertiary centers that usually treat more complicated cases.

INTRACRANIAL COMPLICATIONS OF RHINOSINUSITIS
Epidemiology and Pathogenesis of Intracranial Spread of Infection

The true incidence of intracranial complications is difficult to determine as rhinosinusitis is usually effectively treated on an outpatient basis, and reported case series are biased by selecting the most severe inpatient cases. Of patients hospitalized for sinusitis, approximately 3% to 6% may develop intracranial complications.[42–45] Although outcomes have improved, a high index of suspicion must be maintained when sinusitis fails to respond to therapy, as intracranial complications can be devastating.

Demographically, patients with intracranial complications of sinusitis, not surprisingly, share many common features with those suffering from orbital complications and these not infrequently coexist, particularly in patients older than age 7 years.[13,45,46] Both categories of complications share a striking male predominance, but patients with intracranial complications tend to have longer duration of symptoms, undergo a greater number of surgeries, and have longer hospital stays than patients with orbital complications.[13,14] In addition, intracranial complications are typically found in older patients. In studies confined to pediatric patients, this generally translates into an average patient age of 12 to 15 years.[10–13,47–51] However, the age distribution in adults is varied, particularly in older adults, in whom there seems to be a greater association with chronic sinusitis rather than the more ubiquitous acute sinusitis seen in children and adolescents.[52–54]

The frontal sinus, which does not significantly develop above the orbital ridges until around the age of 6 years and approaches adult size in late adolescence, has been singled out as having features that make it uniquely susceptible to the intracranial spread of infection.[55] The valveless diploic veins of the frontal bone drain the frontal sinus mucosa and can propagate thrombophlebitis through an intact inner table to the dural venous plexus. Further spread of infection within the intracranial venous system may result in an epidural abscess, subdural empyema, dural sinus thrombosis, meningitis, and cerebral abscess. This causal relationship is substantiated by the significantly higher prevalence of frontal sinusitis in patients with intracranial complications.[50] Less commonly, frontal sinusitis results in the development of osteomyelitis, where the calvarium allows contiguous spread of infection into the subgaleal tissues or intracranial compartment.

Pott Puffy Tumor (Forehead Subperiosteal Abscess)

Sir Percivall Pott initially described a case of subperiosteal abscess of the frontal bone presenting as a localized swelling of the forehead during the 18th century.[56] Although the infection in this index case was caused by trauma, most cases of this unusual entity represent a complication of frontal sinusitis and, in this context, are often associated with underlying osteomyelitis. Recent case series of intracranial complications of sinusitis have reported the Pott puffy tumor in 3% to 33% of these patients.[10–13,49,52,53] The association of an anterior subperiosteal abscess and intracranial complications likely reflects the bidirectional propagation of thrombophlebitis through this valveless interconnected venous network. Similarly, an epidural abscess can be seen in the context of an intact inner table, and a subdural empyema may be present without a concomitant epidural collection.

Clinically, the Pott puffy tumor typically presents with frontal scalp swelling, headache, fever, nasal

drainage, and frontal sinus tenderness.[56] More concerning features include a depressed level of consciousness and focal neurologic findings, which may represent intracranial involvement, and imaging should be tailored to evaluate for this possibility. Although contrast-enhanced CT may be performed initially, the added sensitivity and specificity of MR imaging is often needed. By definition, the Pott puffy tumor appears as a frontal subperiosteal abscess on cross-sectional imaging (Fig. 8). Frank bone destruction may be evident involving the inner or outer tables of the frontal sinus and, if present, is best seen with CT. Bone marrow edema and enhancement, indicating frontal osteomyelitis, are most readily visible with MR imaging. As described elsewhere in this article, a thorough intracranial inspection must then be performed to exclude an extraaxial fluid collection such as an epidural abscess or subdural empyema. In addition, leptomeningeal enhancement (indicating meningitis) is often subtle on CT and is more readily identifiable on MR imaging. Cerebritis, which precedes true cerebral abscess formation, is evident as focal swelling of brain parenchyma (low density on CT, high T2 signal on MR, with or without ill-defined patchy

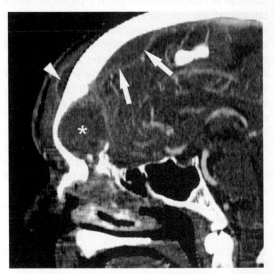

Fig. 8. Pott puffy tumor and intracranial epidural abscess. 46-year-old man with chronic sinusitis developed worsening frontal headache over the course of several weeks. Ultimately, the headache severity and new forehead fluctuant mass brought him to clinical attention. Sagittal reformatted image from a contrast-enhanced CT shows expansion of the frontal sinus (*) with erosion of the inner table, findings that were surgically confirmed to represent a pyomucocele. A lenticular-shaped collection overlying the frontal bone is consistent with a subperiosteal abscess, or Pott puffy tumor (*arrowhead*). Intracranially, an epidural abscess is also present (*arrows*).

enhancement). The cavernous and other dural sinuses should be carefully evaluated for thrombosis. The authors find this is most easily done on postcontrast imaging, with either CT or MR imaging. If MR imaging is used for initial evaluation or further characterization of contrast-enhanced CT findings, a diffusion-weighted (DWI) sequence should always be added for delineation of infected collections and detection of complicating infarcts.

Please see the article Imaging of Ischemic Stroke elsewhere in this issue, for additional information on imaging acute ischemic infarction.

In cases of relatively limited Pott puffy tumor, treatment involves empiric intravenous antibiotic coverage, drainage of the abscess and affected sinus(es), and removal of infected bone.[56,57] More radical surgery may be needed when there is extensive osteomyelitis of the frontal bone or associated intracranial complications.

Intracranial Suppuration

Extraaxial collections (epidural abscess and subdural empyema)

An epidural abscess occurs between the calvarial inner table and underlying periosteum (which is actually the outer layer of the dura). These infections may be relatively indolent because of the tight adhesion between the periosteum and inner table. Thus, they may be initially relatively asymptomatic clinically except for the presence of headache. In 1 patient cohort, nearly all patients with intracranial complications who lacked central neurologic symptoms or signs had an epidural abscess, and this correlated with improved outcome.[11] This relatively benign initial course

emphasizes the necessity of careful scrutiny of the brain as part of the evaluation of a sinusitis CT study. Similar to an epidural hematoma, an epidural abscess assumes a lenticular shape and does not cross suture lines. On CT, it is seen as a low-density collection with variable mass effect (see Fig. 8B). On MR, an epidural abscess is hyperintense on T2 with variable T1 signal intensity; the T1 signal intensity is dependent on whether there is proteinaceous or hemorrhagic content. The presence of rim enhancement is generally best appreciated on MR imaging, and restricted diffusion is characteristic (Fig. 9).

Several series report subdural empyema as the most frequent intracranial complication of rhinosinusitis.[12,51,54,58] Once the infection penetrates the dura, a subdural empyema can progress rapidly because the infection spreads easily over the convexities because of a lack of anatomic constraints. Although the collection can localize anywhere in the subdural space, the supratentorial compartment is involved in most cases.[59–61] Intracranial pressure rises rapidly, and the patient may develop seizures, focal neurologic deficits, and coma within 24 to 48 hours if untreated. CT reveals a crescent-shaped low-density collection of variable thickness that can cross sutures (Fig. 10). This may be particularly subtle on noncontrast CT scans, emphasizing the importance of a careful review of the extraaxial space and presence of subtle midline shift when a patient is particularly ill with sinusitis. On MR imaging, the signal characteristics are analogous to an epidural abscess, and thin collections that do not overlie a cranial suture can be difficult to characterize as epidural versus subdural. The presence of restricted diffusion in

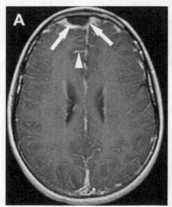 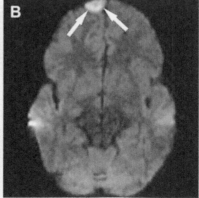

Fig. 9. Intracranial epidural abscess. 15-year-old girl receiving oral antibiotics for acute sinusitis became progressively obtunded over the course of 12 hours. (*A*) Axial T1-weighted postcontrast image reveals a small lenticular-shaped rim-enhancing fluid collection, consistent with an epidural abscess (*arrows*). The morphology and slight extension across midline support an epidural rather than subdural location. Abnormal leptomeningeal enhancement is also noted (*arrowhead*), consistent with meningitis. (*B*) Axial diffusion-weighted sequence confirms the purulent nature of the frontal epidural collection by showing restricted diffusion (*arrows*).

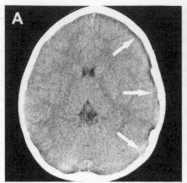
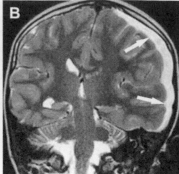
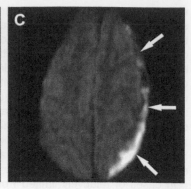

Fig. 10. **Subdural empyema.** 5-year-old boy presented with periorbital swelling and a seizure. (*A*) Axial nonenhanced CT shows diffuse cerebral swelling. Note also slight midline shift to the right; this is caused by a subtle thin left convexity intermediate- to low-density subdural collection (*arrows*). MR images was obtained the following day after further seizures. (*B*) Coronal T2-weighted image shows a left convexity subdural fluid intensity collection (*arrows*) that also showed rim enhancement (not shown). (*C*) The presence of restricted diffusion (*arrows*) distinguishes this subdural collection as an empyema rather than an effusion.

a subdural empyema can be a distinguishing characteristic from subdural effusion, which can also accompany meningitis.

Meningitis

Meningitis occurs infrequently as an isolated complication of acute rhinosinusitis and is usually seen in conjunction with subdural empyema. It classically presents with fever, headache, and meningismus, with or without signs of cerebral dysfunction, and can be rapidly progressive. The hallmark (but relatively insensitive imaging finding) is the presence of meningeal enhancement, for which MR imaging is more sensitive than CT.[11] Hydrocephalus may also be present, and there may be incomplete nulling of CSF signal intensity

within the subarachnoid space on fluid attenuation inversion recovery (FLAIR) MR images (Fig. 11).

Cerebritis and cerebral abscesses

Most brain abscesses arise secondary to rhinosinusitis.[62] The classic triad of fever, headache, and focal neurologic findings is less commonly seen in pediatric patients than in adults, and new onset seizure should heighten suspicion for intracranial infection even in the absence of symptoms suggestive of acute sinusitis.[10] Rupture into the ventricular system may precipitate a more acute clinical deterioration. Because of significant vasogenic edema and mass effect in the context of a rim-enhancing intraaxial lesion, it can be difficult to distinguish a brain abscess from a cystic

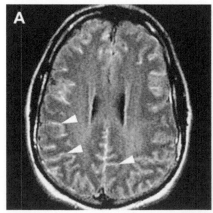
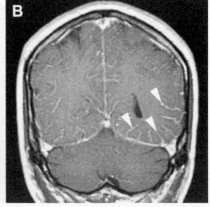

Fig. 11. **Meningitis.** 28-year-old woman who was febrile and obtunded at presentation was found to have bacterial meningitis for which the presumptive cause was acute sphenoid sinusitis. (*A*) Axial FLAIR image shows incomplete nulling of the cerebrospinal fluid (CSF) throughout the subarachnoid space (*arrowheads*; compare with normal CSF signal intensity in the lateral ventricles) reflecting increased protein and cellular content. (*B*) On the axial T1-weighted postcontrast sequence, corresponding abnormal leptomeningeal enhancement is present in most visualized sulci (*arrowheads*).

neoplasm with CT. The presence of an adjacent opacified sinus (most often frontal) should direct the radiologist to the possibility of this diagnosis. At our institution, we typically proceed to contrast-enhanced MR imaging, including dedicated imaging for stereotactic intraoperative guidance.

On MR imaging, the abscess contents and surrounding vasogenic edema are predominantly hypointense to normal brain on T1-weighted sequences and hyperintense on T2-weighted sequences (Fig. 12). Once the abscess has become organized, a capsule develops that is lower in T2 signal intensity compared with the surrounding edema. This culminates in a pattern of peripheral enhancement in which the capsule tends to be thinner on the ventricular side of the lesion. Although some tumors may exhibit restricted diffusion secondary to cellularity and necrosis, the extent of diffusion restriction is more pronounced in an abscess, usually making this a straightforward MR imaging diagnosis.[63–65] Serial diffusion-weighted MR imaging has also been shown to be useful in documenting treatment response.[66] MR perfusion can be useful in evaluating rim-enhancing cystic intraaxial lesions and typically reveals higher blood volume in tumors compared with abscesses.[63,67] If necessary, proton MR spectroscopy may demonstrate amino acid and lipid/lactate peaks and absent choline peak.[63,65,68] Please see the article Central Nervous System Infections by Ashley Aiken elsewhere in this issue, for additional imaging characteristics of intracranial infection.

Treatment, prognosis, and follow-up imaging

Suppurative intracranial complications of sinusitis (other than meningitis) are generally considered a surgical disease. Drainage of diseased sinuses is typically performed as soon as possible, and a concomitant craniotomy performed under the same anesthetic for neurosurgical drainage of intracranial abscesses in most cases, even for small lesions.[11,51,54,58] The corresponding medical management requires aggressive intravenous antibiotic therapy directed by culture and sensitivity. Infections are typically polymicrobial, often with an anaerobic contribution, and show concordance in the culture of organisms from infected sinuses and the associated intracranial pus.[37,69] Despite modern diagnosis and treatment, there is still significant morbidity and mortality, with persistent neurologic deficits in 8% to 45% of cases and death occurs in more than 10% of patients.[11,48,49,51,58]

Venous Thrombosis

Cavernous sinus thrombosis was described in more detail earlier and may accompany orbital complications of sinus infection, or arise as an intracranial complication without orbital infection. It typically presents with orbital signs and symptoms secondary to an interference in orbital venous drainage through the cavernous sinus and involvement of the cranial nerves that course through the cavernous sinus en route to the orbit.

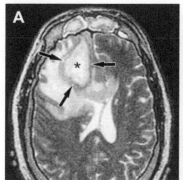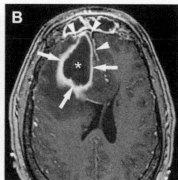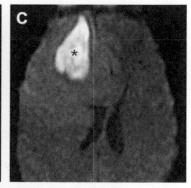

Fig. 12. **Cerebral abscess.** 55-year-old man presented to an outside institution and was initially accepted as a transfer to the neurosurgical service under the suspicion that he had a high-grade right frontal glioma. Brain MR imaging included (A) axial T2-weighted sequence, (B) axial T1-weighted postcontrast sequence, and (C) diffusion-weighted sequence. The central portion of the lesion appears cystic or necrotic based on its T2 hyperintensity and lack of enhancement (*). The rim of the lesion has T2 signal that is iso- to slightly hyperintense to normal white matter (but noticeably darker than surrounding edematous tissue) and shows associated enhancement (*arrows*). Note how the capsule is thickest and least well defined laterally. A significant amount of surrounding vasogenic edema is present, including extension across midline via the genu of the corpus callosum. The presence of frontal sinus opacification, adjacent dural enhancement (*arrowheads*), capsule enhancement characteristics, and restricted diffusion within the collection (*asterisk*) argues that this space-occupying lesion represents a sinogenic abscess, which was confirmed surgically.

Intracranial suppuration, particularly subdural empyema, causes inflammation and venous stasis that can lead to thrombosis of cortical veins and major dural venous sinuses. The resulting vasogenic edema further exacerbates increasing intracranial pressure, and venous infarction can cause focal neurologic deficits. The MR imaging findings include multifocal vasogenic edema that does not conform to an arterial distribution and the lack of the normal flow void. MR venography reveals filling defects within dural sinuses, although thrombosis of smaller cortical veins is not as readily apparent (**Fig. 13**). Postcontrast T1-weighted thin-slice volumetric imaging is often helpful for detection of more subtle filling defects in smaller vessels. Multidetector CT angiography provides a comparable assessment of the major intracranial venous structures.[70]

FUNGAL SINUSITIS

Fungal sinusitis is broadly divided into noninvasive and invasive forms, with the latter being further subdivided into granulomatous, acute fulminant, and chronic invasive forms.[71] The diagnosis of invasion requires histopathologic evidence of hyphal forms within mucosa, submucosa, blood vessels, or bone. Mucormycosis and *Aspergillus*, which represent the most common pathogens, have a propensity for angioinvasion.[72–74] Aribandi and colleagues have thoroughly reviewed the imaging features of all types of fungal sinusitis.[75] This discussion focuses on acute fulminant invasive fungal sinusitis (AFIFS), as the failure to make a prompt diagnosis can result in rapid progression and death.[73]

AFIFS is an opportunistic infection, and the patient populations at highest risk are those with impaired neutrophil function, such as those with AIDS, hematologic malignancies, insulin-dependent diabetes, and hemochromatosis. Iatrogenic immunosuppression with high-dose corticosteroids, chemotherapeutics for the treatment of malignancies, and antirejection regimens following organ or bone marrow transplantation also make patients susceptible. Although typically seen in patients with impaired immunity, immunocompetence should not exclude the diagnosis in the context of characteristic clinical and imaging features.[76–78]

Common presenting symptoms include nasal obstruction, fever, facial pain, headache, and facial swelling.[73] In susceptible patients, the presence of sinonasal symptoms and fever of unknown origin after 48 hours in spite of broad-spectrum antibiotic therapy should prompt both nasal endoscopy and imaging. Contrast-enhanced CT of the orbits and paranasal sinuses is typically the initial imaging study of choice. The most common CT findings in AFIFS include severe soft tissue edema of the nasal cavity mucosa, sinus mucoperiosteal thickening, bone erosion, orbital invasion, facial soft tissue swelling, and retroantral fat pad thickening (**Fig. 14**).[79] Bone erosion is a late finding of AFIFS and may be absent in spite of clear invasion outside of the sinonasal cavities; this is caused by extension along blood vessels. Although findings such as orbital involvement,

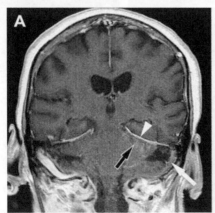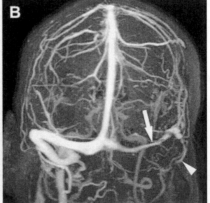

Fig. 13. **Dural venous sinus thrombophlebitis and meningitis.** 62-year-old woman with chronic pansinusitis, who initially presented with left orbital cellulitis and cavernous sinus thrombosis, continued to deteriorate clinically such that repeat imaging was pursued. (*A*) Coronal T1-weighted postcontrast image depicts abnormal signal within the left sigmoid sinus (*white arrow*) suspicious for acute dural sinus thrombosis. Note also leptomeningeal enhancement overlying the superior cerebellar hemisphere, consistent with meningitis (*black arrow*). Subtle thickening of the tentorium (*arrowhead*) is probably related to venous engorgement. (*B*) Contrast-enhanced MR venogram shows attenuation of the left transverse sinus (*arrow*) and occlusion of the left sigmoid sinus (*arrowhead*) and internal jugular vein, compatible with dural venous sinus thrombosis.

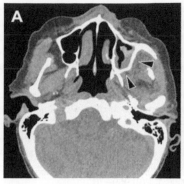 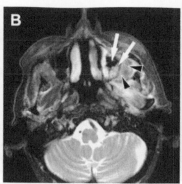 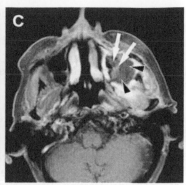

Fig. 14. **Sinogenic masticator space infection (*Aspergillus*).** 72-year-old woman undergoing chemotherapy for non-Hodgkin lymphoma developed left facial pain and trismus over the course of 48 hours. (*A*) Initial CT, which was performed without contrast because of impaired renal function, shows partial opacification of the left maxillary sinus. The posterior maxillary wall is thickened and appears intact, but there is diffuse infiltration of the retromaxillary fat (*arrowheads*). More posteriorly, the fat planes within the left masticator space are also obscured. MR imaging of the face was emergently performed, and (*B*) axial T2-weighted fat-suppressed and (*C*) axial T1-weighted postcontrast sequences are presented. Areas of opacification centrally and posterolaterally within the left maxillary sinus (*white arrows*) are lower in T2 signal and enhance less than normal mucosa. The infiltrative tissue within the left retromaxillary fat has similar signal characteristics (*black arrowheads*). More posteriorly, the left masticator space is markedly inflamed, as shown by diffuse soft tissue edema and enhancement. *Aspergillus* was recovered at the time of aggressive surgical debridement.

bone destruction, and periantral soft tissue infiltration offer greater specificity in the appropriate clinical setting, these are difficult to detect in the early stages of disease.[79,80] MR imaging may be helpful as an additional test to localize necrotic nonenhancing areas with characteristic T2 hypointensity in the thickened mucosa, and this can be useful preoperatively to help guide endoscopic biopsy.

In addition to imaging the orbits and sinonasal cavities with preoperative MR imaging, routine pre- and postcontrast imaging of the brain should also be obtained because the clinical presentation and CT do not always indicate intracranial extension.[81] The imaging spectrum of intracranial involvement can be broad, including skull base invasion, dural thickening and enhancement, cavernous sinus thrombosis, cerebritis, brain abscess, mycotic aneurysm, arterial thrombosis (**Fig. 15**), and cerebral infarction.[81,82]

Treatment and Outcome

Following histopathologic diagnosis, treatment requires reversal of the underlying predisposing condition (if possible), surgical debridement, and appropriate systemic antifungal therapy.[83] Despite prompt diagnosis and aggressive therapy, mortality in a recently reported series still exceeds 50%.[73] Poor outcome has been shown to correlate with intracranial involvement and failure to

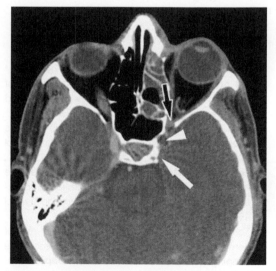

Fig. 15. **Cavernous sinus thrombophlebitis (mucormycosis).** 48-year-old woman with type 1 diabetes presented to the emergency department with an acute left middle cerebral artery territory stroke and, in retrospect, had several preceding days of blurred vision. Contrast-enhanced CT shows opacification of the left ethmoid air cells and subtle soft tissue infiltration of the left orbital apex (*black arrow*). The left cavernous sinus enhances less than the contralateral side, consistent with cavernous sinus thrombosis (*white arrow*), and the cavernous segment of the left internal carotid artery is occluded (*white arrowhead*). Mucormycosis was confirmed histopathologically.

recover from neutropenia.[74] In addition, diabetic patients have higher rates of morbidity and mortality, presumably the result of a greater prevalence of the more virulent mucor in this population, as well as delayed diagnosis because of a lower index of suspicion.[74]

AUTHORS' APPROACH TO IMAGING ACUTE SINUSITIS

The consequences of orbital or intracranial spread of sinus infection, an otherwise benign entity, are potentially devastating. When imaging a patient with acute sinusitis, particularly when orbital symptoms, altered mental status, or more sinister neurologic symptoms are present, it is important that the brain and the orbits are carefully imaged. We favor postcontrast CT with multiplanar reformats as a relatively cost-effective, fast, sensitive tool for evaluating the orbits and brain when complications are suspected clinically. In cases in which the CT abnormalities need further characterization, or when CT is unrevealing despite a high clinical suspicion for complications, or when invasive fungal infection is suspected, we do not hesitate to use the increased sensitivity and specificity of MR imaging for complete evaluation of intracranial complications and presurgical planning.

REFERENCES

1. Konen E, Faibel M, Kleinbaum Y, et al. The value of the occipitomental (Waters') view in diagnosis of sinusitis: a comparative study with computed tomography. Clin Radiol 2000;55(11):856–60.
2. Kronemer KA, McAlister WH. Sinusitis and its imaging in the pediatric population. Pediatr Radiol 1997;27(11):837–46.
3. Gutowski WM, Mulbury PE, Hengerer AS, et al. The role of C.T. scans in managing the orbital complications of ethmoiditis. Int J Pediatr Otorhinolaryngol 1988;15(2):117–28.
4. Younis RT, Anand VK, Davidson B. The role of computed tomography and magnetic resonance imaging in patients with sinusitis with complications. Laryngoscope 2002;112(2):224–9.
5. Towbin R, Han BK, Kaufman RA, et al. Postseptal cellulitis: CT in diagnosis and management. Radiology 1986;158(3):735–7.
6. Hirsch M, Lifshitz T. Computerized tomography in the diagnosis and treatment of orbital cellulitis. Pediatr Radiol 1988;18(4):302–5.
7. Weber AL, Mikulis DK. Inflammatory disorders of the paraorbital sinuses and their complications. Radiol Clin North Am 1987;25(3):615–30.
8. McIntosh D, Mahadevan M. Failure of contrast enhanced computed tomography scans to identify an orbital abscess. The benefit of magnetic resonance imaging. J Laryngol Otol 2008;122(6):639–40.
9. McIntosh D, Mahadevan M. Acute orbital complications of sinusitis: the benefits of magnetic resonance imaging. J Laryngol Otol 2008;122(3):324–6.
10. Adame N, Hedlund G, Byington CL. Sinogenic intracranial empyema in children. Pediatrics 2005; 116(3):e461–7.
11. Germiller JA, Monin DL, Sparano AM, et al. Intracranial complications of sinusitis in children and adolescents and their outcomes. Arch Otolaryngol Head Neck Surg 2006;132(9):969–76.
12. Herrmann BW, Chung JC, Eisenbeis JF, et al. Intracranial complications of pediatric frontal rhinosinusitis. Am J Rhinol 2006;20(3):320–4.
13. Oxford LE, McClay J. Complications of acute sinusitis in children. Otolaryngol Head Neck Surg 2005; 133(1):32–7.
14. Mortimore S, Wormald PJ. The Groote Schuur hospital classification of the orbital complications of sinusitis. J Laryngol Otol 1997;111(8):719–23.
15. Sultesz M, Csakanyi Z, Majoros T, et al. Acute bacterial rhinosinusitis and its complications in our pediatric otolaryngological department between 1997 and 2006. Int J Pediatr Otorhinolaryngol 2009;73(11):1507–12.
16. Schramm VL, Myers EN, Kennerdell JS. Orbital complications of acute sinusitis: evaluation, management, and outcome. Otolaryngology 1978; 86(2):ORL221–30.
17. Younis RT, Lazar RH, Bustillo A, et al. Orbital infection as a complication of sinusitis: are diagnostic and treatment trends changing? Ear Nose Throat J 2002;81(11):771–5.
18. Nageswaran S, Woods CR, Benjamin DK Jr, et al. Orbital cellulitis in children. Pediatr Infect Dis J 2006;25(8):695–9.
19. Botting AM, McIntosh D, Mahadevan M. Paediatric pre- and post-septal peri-orbital infections are different diseases. A retrospective review of 262 cases. Int J Pediatr Otorhinolaryngol 2008;72(3): 377–83.
20. Robinson A, Beech T, McDermott AL, et al. Investigation and management of adult periorbital and orbital cellulitis. J Laryngol Otol 2007;121(6):545–7.
21. Osguthorpe JD, Hochman M. Inflammatory sinus diseases affecting the orbit. Otolaryngol Clin North Am 1993;26(4):657–71.
22. Quick CA, Payne E. Complicated acute sinusitis. Laryngoscope 1972;82(7):1248–63.
23. Jackson K, Baker SR. Clinical implications of orbital cellulitis. Laryngoscope 1986;96(5):568–74.
24. Andrews TM, Myer CM 3rd. The role of computed tomography in the diagnosis of subperiosteal abscess of the orbit. Clin Pediatr (Phila) 1992;31(1): 37–43.

25. Chandler JR, Langenbrunner DJ, Stevens ER. The pathogenesis of orbital complications in acute sinusitis. Laryngoscope 1970;80(9):1414—28.

26. Schramm VL Jr, Curtin HD, Kennerdell JS. Evaluation of orbital cellulitis and results of treatment. Laryngoscope 1982;92(7 Pt 1):732—8.

27. Moloney JR, Badham NJ, McRae A. The acute orbit. Preseptal (periorbital) cellulitis, subperiosteal abscess and orbital cellulitis due to sinusitis. J Laryngol Otol Suppl 1987;12:1—18.

28. Ebright JR, Pace MT, Niazi AF. Septic thrombosis of the cavernous sinuses. Arch Intern Med 2001; 161(22):2671—6.

29. Schuknecht B, Simmen D, Yuksel C, et al. Tributary venosinus occlusion and septic cavernous sinus thrombosis: CT and MR findings. AJNR Am J Neuroradiol 1998;19(4):617—26.

30. Eustis HS, Mafee MF, Walton C, et al. MR imaging and CT of orbital infections and complications in acute rhinosinusitis. Radiol Clin North Am 1998;36(6):1165—83.

31. Perez Barreto M, Sahai S, Ameriso S, et al. Sinusitis and carotid artery stroke. Ann Otol Rhinol Laryngol 2000;109(2):227—30.

32. Wong AM, Bilaniuk LT, Zimmerman RA, et al. Magnetic resonance imaging of carotid artery abnormalities in patients with sphenoid sinusitis. Neuroradiology 2004;46(1):54—9.

33. Righini CA, Bing F, Bessou P, et al. An acute ischemic stroke secondary to sphenoid sinusitis. Ear Nose Throat J 2009;88(11):e23—8.

34. Parmar H, Gandhi D, Mukherji SK, et al. Restricted diffusion in the superior ophthalmic vein and cavernous sinus in a case of cavernous sinus thrombosis. J Neuroophthalmol 2009;29(1):16—20.

35. McKinley SH, Yen MT, Miller AM, et al. Microbiology of pediatric orbital cellulitis. Am J Ophthalmol 2007; 144(4):497—501.

36. Hwang SY, Tan KK. *Streptococcus viridans* has a leading role in rhinosinusitis complications. Ann Otol Rhinol Laryngol 2007;116(5):381—5.

37. Brook I. Microbiology and antimicrobial treatment of orbital and intracranial complications of sinusitis in children and their management. Int J Pediatr Otorhinolaryngol 2009;73(9):1183—6.

38. Barone SR, Aiuto LT. Periorbital and orbital cellulitis in the Haemophilus influenzae vaccine era. J Pediatr Ophthalmol Strabismus 1997;34(5):293—6.

39. Donahue SP, Schwartz G. Preseptal and orbital cellulitis in childhood. A changing microbiologic spectrum. Ophthalmology 1998;105(10):1902—5 [discussion: 1905—6].

40. Brook I. Microbiology of acute sinusitis of odontogenic origin presenting with periorbital cellulitis in children. Ann Otol Rhinol Laryngol 2007;116(5): 386—8.

41. Gamble RC. Acute inflammation of the orbit in children. Arch Ophthalmol 1933;10:483—97.

42. Clayman GL, Adams GL, Paugh DR, et al. Intracranial complications of paranasal sinusitis: a combined institutional review. Laryngoscope 1991;101(3): 234—9.

43. Giannoni CM, Stewart MG, Alford EL. Intracranial complications of sinusitis. Laryngoscope 1997; 107(7):863—7.

44. Lerner DN, Choi SS, Zalzal GH, et al. Intracranial complications of sinusitis in childhood. Ann Otol Rhinol Laryngol 1995;104(4 Pt 1):288—93.

45. Herrmann BW, Forsen JW Jr. Simultaneous intracranial and orbital complications of acute rhinosinusitis in children. Int J Pediatr Otorhinolaryngol 2004;68(5):619—25.

46. Reynolds DJ, Kodsi SR, Rubin SE, et al. Intracranial infection associated with preseptal and orbital cellulitis in the pediatric patient. J AAPOS 2003;7(6): 413—7.

47. Bair-Merritt MH, Shah SS, Zaoutis TE, et al. Suppurative intracranial complications of sinusitis in previously healthy children. Pediatr Infect Dis J 2005;24(4):384—6.

48. Kombogiorgas D, Seth R, Athwal R, et al. Suppurative intracranial complications of sinusitis in adolescence. Single institute experience and review of literature. Br J Neurosurg 2007;21(6):603—9.

49. Glickstein JS, Chandra RK, Thompson JW. Intracranial complications of pediatric sinusitis. Otolaryngol Head Neck Surg 2006;134(5):733—6.

50. Hakim HE, Malik AC, Aronyk K, et al. The prevalence of intracranial complications in pediatric frontal sinusitis. Int J Pediatr Otorhinolaryngol 2006;70(8): 1383—7.

51. Quraishi H, Zevallos JP. Subdural empyema as a complication of sinusitis in the pediatric population. Int J Pediatr Otorhinolaryngol 2006;70(9):1581—6.

52. Betz CS, Issing W, Matschke J, et al. Complications of acute frontal sinusitis: a retrospective study. Eur Arch Otorhinolaryngol 2008;265(1):63—72.

53. Younis RT, Lazar RH, Anand VK. Intracranial complications of sinusitis: a 15-year review of 39 cases. Ear Nose Throat J 2002;81(9):636—8, 640—2, 644.

54. DelGaudio JM, Evans SH, Sobol SE, et al. Intracranial complications of sinusitis: what is the role of endoscopic sinus surgery in the acute setting. Am J Otolaryngol 2010;31(1):25—8.

55. Goldberg AN, Oroszlan G, Anderson TD. Complications of frontal sinusitis and their management. Otolaryngol Clin North Am 2001;34(1):211—25.

56. Bambakidis NC, Cohen AR. Intracranial complications of frontal sinusitis in children: Pott's puffy tumor revisited. Pediatr Neurosurg 2001;35(2):82—9.

57. Marshall AH, Jones NS. Osteomyelitis of the frontal bone secondary to frontal sinusitis. J Laryngol Otol 2000;114(12):944—6.

58. Bayonne E, Kania R, Tran P, et al. Intracranial complications of rhinosinusitis. A review, typical

imaging data and algorithm of management. Rhinology 2009;47(1):59–65.

59. Nathoo N, Nadvi SS, van Dellen JR, et al. Intracranial subdural empyemas in the era of computed tomography: a review of 699 cases. Neurosurgery 1999;44(3):529–35 [discussion: 535–6].

60. Borovich B, Johnston E, Spagnuolo E. Infratentorial subdural empyema: clinical and computerized tomography findings. Report of three cases. J Neurosurg 1990;72(2):299–301.

61. Venkatesh MS, Pandey P, Devi BI, et al. Pediatric infratentorial subdural empyema: analysis of 14 cases. J Neurosurg 2006;105(Suppl 5):370–7.

62. Kocaeli H, Hakyemez B, Bekar A, et al. Unusual complications and presentations of intracranial abscess: experience of a single institution. Surg Neurol 2008;69(4):383–91 [discussion: 391].

63. Chiang IC, Hsieh TJ, Chiu ML, et al. Distinction between pyogenic brain abscess and necrotic brain tumour using 3-tesla MR spectroscopy, diffusion and perfusion imaging. Br J Radiol 2009;82(982):813–20.

64. Bukte Y, Paksoy Y, Genc E, et al. Role of diffusion-weighted MR in differential diagnosis of intracranial cystic lesions. Clin Radiol 2005;60(3):375–83.

65. Lai PH, Ho JT, Chen WL, et al. Brain abscess and necrotic brain tumor: discrimination with proton MR spectroscopy and diffusion-weighted imaging. AJNR Am J Neuroradiol 2002;23(8):1369–77.

66. Fanning NF, Laffan EE, Shroff MM. Serial diffusion-weighted MRI correlates with clinical course and treatment response in children with intracranial pus collections. Pediatr Radiol 2006;36(1):26–37.

67. Erdogan C, Hakyemez B, Yildirim N, et al. Brain abscess and cystic brain tumor: discrimination with dynamic susceptibility contrast perfusion-weighted MRI. J Comput Assist Tomogr 2005;29(5):663–7.

68. Pal D, Bhattacharyya A, Husain M, et al. In vivo proton MR spectroscopy evaluation of pyogenic brain abscesses: a report of 194 cases. AJNR Am J Neuroradiol 2010;31(2):360–6.

69. Brook I. Microbiology of intracranial abscesses and their associated sinusitis. Arch Otolaryngol Head Neck Surg 2005;131(11):1017–9.

70. Linn J, Ertl-Wagner B, Seelos KC, et al. Diagnostic value of multidetector-row CT angiography in the evaluation of thrombosis of the cerebral venous sinuses. AJNR Am J Neuroradiol 2007;28(5):946–52.

71. deShazo RD, O'Brien M, Chapin K, et al. A new classification and diagnostic criteria for invasive fungal sinusitis. Arch Otolaryngol Head Neck Surg 1997;123(11):1181–8.

72. Talbot GH, Huang A, Provencher M. Invasive aspergillus rhinosinusitis in patients with acute leukemia. Rev Infect Dis 1991;13(2):219–32.

73. Suslu AE, Ogretmenoglu O, Suslu N, et al. Acute invasive fungal rhinosinusitis: our experience with 19 patients. Eur Arch Otorhinolaryngol 2009;266(1):77–82.

74. Parikh SL, Venkatraman G, DelGaudio JM. Invasive fungal sinusitis: a 15-year review from a single institution. Am J Rhinol 2004;18(2):75–81.

75. Aribandi M, McCoy VA, Bazan C 3rd. Imaging features of invasive and noninvasive fungal sinusitis: a review. Radiographics 2007;27(5):1283–96.

76. Chopra H, Dua K, Malhotra V, et al. Invasive fungal sinusitis of isolated sphenoid sinus in immunocompetent subjects. Mycoses 2006;49(1):30–6.

77. Siddiqui AA, Shah AA, Bashir SH. Craniocerebral aspergillosis of sinonasal origin in immunocompetent patients: clinical spectrum and outcome in 25 cases. Neurosurgery 2004;55(3):602–11 [discussion: 611–3].

78. Sridhara SR, Paragache G, Panda NK, et al. Mucormycosis in immunocompetent individuals: an increasing trend. J Otolaryngol 2005;34(6):402–6.

79. DelGaudio JM, Swain RE Jr, Kingdom TT, et al. Computed tomographic findings in patients with invasive fungal sinusitis. Arch Otolaryngol Head Neck Surg 2003;129(2):236–40.

80. Silverman CS, Mancuso AA. Periantral soft-tissue infiltration and its relevance to the early detection of invasive fungal sinusitis: CT and MR findings. AJNR Am J Neuroradiol 1998;19(2):321–5.

81. Howells RC, Ramadan HH. Usefulness of computed tomography and magnetic resonance in fulminant invasive fungal rhinosinusitis. Am J Rhinol 2001;15(4):255–61.

82. Gabelmann A, Klein S, Kern W, et al. Relevant imaging findings of cerebral aspergillosis on MRI: a retrospective case-based study in immunocompromised patients. Eur J Neurol 2007;14(5):548–55.

83. Epstein VA, Kern RC. Invasive fungal sinusitis and complications of rhinosinusitis. Otolaryngol Clin North Am 2008;41(3):497–524, viii.

Head Trauma

Alisa D. Gean[a],* and Nancy J. Fischbein[b]

KEYWORDS

- Traumatic brain injury • Scalp • Skull • Vascular
- Hemorrhage

"No head injury is too trivial to ignore"
—Hippocrates, 460–377 BC

THE SCOPE OF THE PROBLEM

Traumatic brain injury (TBI) is termed "the silent epidemic" for good reason.[1–5] Worldwide, an estimated 10 million people are affected annually by TBI. In the United States alone, it is the leading cause of mortality and morbidity in individuals younger than 44 years, and its total direct and indirect cost to society has been estimated to exceed $60 billion annually. More than 5 million Americans currently live with long-term disability as a result of TBI and more than 1.5 million individuals sustain a new TBI each year. Furthermore, the number of victims continues to increase each year, and it has been predicted that TBI will become the third leading cause of death and disability in the world by the year 2020.

The primary etiology of head trauma varies with the age of the patient. Nonaccidental trauma (abuse) is most common in infants, whereas falls and sports-related injuries are seen in toddlers and school-aged children, respectively. Motor vehicle accidents are a frequent cause of head injury in young adults, but there is also increasing recognition of concussion in both amateur and professional athletes. The elderly population is particularly susceptible to accidental falls.

TBI CLASSIFICATION

Clinically, TBI has been traditionally divided into minor, mild, moderate, and severe injury, as judged by the widely used Glasgow Coma Scale (minor: GCS = 15; mild: GCS ≥13; moderate: GCS 9–12; severe: GCS ≤8).[6] Although the GCS has excellent interobserver reliability and correlation with outcome following severe brain injury, it fails to differentiate among different types of injury with different prognoses and fails to localize the injury.[7] Of reported TBI cases, approximately 85% are classified as mild.[7,8] It should be noted, however, that many cases of mild TBI go unreported. Unfortunately, mild TBI is the least well understood in terms of definition, imaging strategies, and correlation between imaging findings and long-term outcome. Routine structural imaging is often normal in these patients, yet studies have shown that even patients with normal imaging studies can have persistent cognitive deficits, and experience vocational and emotional distress that causes a significant socioeconomic burden to the individual and to society.[9–11]

In addition to clinical severity, TBI can also be classified chronologically into *primary* and *secondary* injuries. Primary injuries are defined as those that occur at the moment of impact (eg, immediate tissue laceration by a gunshot injury). Secondary injuries are those that occur after the initial injury (eg, cerebral swelling and herniation, ischemia, venous thrombosis, posttraumatic infection, hydrocephalus, and cerebrospinal fluid leak) as a consequence of physiologic response to injury or complications of injury.

Whereas the primary injuries are considered irreversible, secondary injuries are potentially preventable with efficient triage and stabilization, management of parameters such as brain oxygenation, intracranial pressure, and cerebral perfusion pressure, and, in some cases, decompressive

[a] Department of Radiology, University of California, San Francisco, San Francisco General Hospital, 1001 Potrero Avenue, San Francisco, CA 94110, USA
[b] Department of Radiology (NF), Stanford University School of Medicine, Room S-047, 300 Pasteur Avenue, Stanford, CA 94305-5105, USA
* Corresponding author.
E-mail address: agean@sfghrad.ucsf.edu

Neuroimag Clin N Am 20 (2010) 527–556
doi:10.1016/j.nic.2010.08.001

hemicraniectomy.[12] This classification is some-what arbitrary, however, because injury to the brain is actually more of a continuum of dynamically changing pathologies and not a single disease. For example, epidural hematoma (EDH) is classified as a primary injury, but the lesion does not necessarily present "at the moment" of injury, as it takes some time to expand. Brain injury triggers a cascade of pathophysiological events that can extend over a long period of time.[13] Indeed, TBI should be thought of not as a static event, but rather a progressive injury with varying therapeutic windows.

TBI can also be classified according to the location of the injury (intra- and/or extra-axial) and the mechanism of the injury (penetrating/open, blunt/closed, or blast). The extra-axial lesions include epidural, subdural, subarachnoid, and intraventricular hemorrhages. The intra-axial lesions include the cortical contusion, intracerebral hematoma, traumatic axonal injury (TAI), and cerebrovascular injury. Each of these lesions is reviewed later in the section "Injuries".

IMAGING TOOLS

The goals of neuroimaging are to identify treatable injuries, assist in the prevention of secondary damage, and provide useful prognostic information regarding the scope of a patient's TBI.

Skull Radiography

Conventional plain film radiography of the skull in TBI has been supplanted by computed tomography (CT), but occasional indications include (1) to better define the position of penetrating objects and radiopaque foreign bodies, and (2) to better detect skull fractures in cases of suspected child abuse.[14] In the vast majority of cases, however, the digital "scout" view of a CT scan, in combination with the CT data, is sufficient.

Computed Tomography

Noncontrast CT remains the study of choice for assessment of acute TBI because of its widespread availability, speed, safety, and compatibility with life-support and traction-stabilization devices, as well as its sensitivity to acute hemorrhage, hydrocephalus, herniation, fractures, and radiopaque foreign bodies.[15] It is an excellent tool for deciding whether the patient should be surgically or medically triaged.

A relatively recent study showed that the cost of liberal CT screening for head trauma is justified because the consequences of undiagnosed brain injury can be devastating.[16] Even with the tremendous advances in CT technology over the last 2 decades, however, most mild TBI cases show no visible abnormality on CT. Another downside of CT scanning is the radiation exposure, especially when multiple serial examinations in a young patient are necessary, as is frequently the case in the trauma setting.

Various clinical algorithms have been proposed to risk-stratify TBI patients for CT screening. In general, there is consensus that patients with moderate to severe intracranial injury (GCS ≤12) should undergo emergent noncontrast head CT. Several guidelines to determine whether patients with mild TBI (GCS >12) should undergo CT have been proposed, including the New Orleans Criteria and the Canadian CT Head Rule.[17–19] The Canadian CT Head Rule proposed scanning patients with a GCS score of 13 to 15 based on these high-risk factors:

- Failure to reach a GCS of 15 within 2 hours
- Suspected open skull fracture
- Two or more vomiting episodes
- Signs of basal skull fracture
- Age older than 65.

CT angiography

CT angiography (CTA) uses intravenous iodinated contrast to delineate the vascular structures at sub-millimeter resolution. CTA is performed best with multidetector CT (MDCT) and rapid bolus contrast injection using vessel tracking. Typical imaging parameters include a slice thickness of 1.25 mm with a 0.625-mm overlap, and a bolus injection rate between 3 and 4 mL/s. CTA plays an important role in the diagnosis of suspected vascular injuries such as pseudoaneurysm, dissection, carotid cavernous fistula, or laceration-extravasation. CTA is usually the study of choice to screen for a possible cerebrovascular injury in the setting of penetrating injury or skull base fracture traversing the carotid canal or a venous sinus.[20] If CTA is abnormal or suspicious, then conventional catheter angiography can be used to confirm and to potentially endovascularly treat the vascular injuries. Note that intravenous contrast should not be administered without a prior noncontrast examination, because intracranial contrast can both mask and mimic underlying hemorrhage.

CT perfusion

Energy consumption by the brain is high, accounting for roughly 20% of the oxygen and 25% of the glucose consumed by the body. In the uninjured brain, capillary blood flow to the brain is autonomously regulated ("autoregulation"). Insight into brain pathology can be gained through noninvasive imaging of cerebral perfusion and metabolism, and CT perfusion (CTP) is a technique that affords insight into the altered hemodynamics secondary to TBI. CTP can help clinicians distinguish between patients with preserved autoregulation and those with impaired autoregulation.

CTP is a bolus-tracking technique that involves continuous cine scanning through a limited volume of brain tissue with a scan interval of 1 second and a total scanning duration of 40 to 45 seconds. CTP measures the transient attenuation changes in the blood vessels during the first pass of an intravenously injected contrast bolus. Color maps of cerebral blood volume (CBV), mean transit time (MTT), and cerebral blood flow (CBF) are then generated from these time-attenuation curves and can be used to assess cerebral perfusion.

Although CTP is fairly routine in stroke and brain tumor imaging, it is rarely performed in TBI. Nevertheless, research studies have shown that CTP can be used to demarcate acute focal brain injury, document diffuse injury, identify areas at risk of secondary injury, and predict enlarging contusions.[21–24] Visible changes in CBV on either CTP or perfusion magnetic resonance (MR) imaging have been shown to occur in areas of contusion visible on conventional CT or MR imaging (Fig. 1). CTP can provide prognostic information regarding outcome, with normal brain perfusion or hyperemia in patients with favorable outcome and oligemia in patients with unfavorable outcome. Controversy exists, however, regarding correct selection of an arterial input vessel, the accuracy of quantitative results, and the reproducibility of results. Other limitations include CTP's limited anatomic coverage, and the additional radiation and contrast exposure that accompany this method.

Dual-energy CT

Newer CT technologies that allow for more rapid data acquisition have sparked renewed interest in dual-energy application. Knowing how a substance (eg, blood) behaves at 2 different energies can provide information about tissue composition beyond that obtainable with single-energy techniques. The current applications of dual-energy CT in head injury are unknown, but in the future are likely to include providing information about tissue structure, predicting the evolution of soft tissue injuries, the ability to generate "virtual" unenhanced images, and the improved detection of iodine-containing substances on low-energy images, thereby improving CTA and CTP in head injury at a reduced radiation dose.

Magnetic Resonance Imaging

On occasion, MR imaging may be indicated in patients with acute TBI if the patient's neurologic findings are unexplained by CT findings. MR imaging is also helpful in cases of suspected nonaccidental trauma within the first few days of injury, as it is far superior to CT in the detection of TAI and small subdural "smear" collections that might be the only clue to child abuse (Fig. 2). In general, however, MR imaging is limited in the emergency setting due to safety considerations and its relatively long imaging times; imaging time can be a significant limitation in some patients, especially if they are uncooperative, claustrophobic, or medically unstable. Furthermore, MR's incompatibility with many trauma-related or other medical devices, its relative insensitivity to acute subarachnoid hemorrhage, and its sensitivity to patient motion make it more easily and appropriately performed for assessment of subacute and chronic TBI. MR imaging can also be used as a problem-solving tool in the setting of neurologic deficits unexplained by CT; MR may identify brainstem injury, ischemia/infarction, small cortical contusions, and white matter injury, all of which are relative "blind spots" on CT.

The key MR imaging sequences to perform include: fluid-attenuated inversion recovery (FLAIR) images for nonhemorrhagic TAI and subarachnoid hemorrhage (SAH); gradient-recalled echo (GRE) or susceptibility-weighted imaging (SWI) for hemorrhagic TAI and blood products in general; and diffusion-weighted imaging (DWI) for ischemia/infarction and TAI. These sequences are now discussed, followed by a brief discussion of more advanced MR imaging techniques.

FLAIR is a T2-weighted inversion recovery sequence that suppresses the T2 bright signal from cerebrospinal fluid (CSF), thus improving lesion conspicuity in the periventricular regions and cerebral cortex. FLAIR is far more sensitive than conventional T2-weighted images to cortical contusions, TAI, and SAH (Figs. 3–6).[25]

GRE T2*-weighted imaging is sensitive to the presence of blood breakdown products: deoxyhemoglobin, intracellular (not extracellular) methemoglobin, ferritin, and hemosiderin. These blood products results in areas of signal loss due to alteration of the local magnetic susceptibility in the tissue (Fig. 7). Because hemosiderin can persist indefinitely, GRE T2*-weighted imaging is recommended for the evaluation of remote TBI[26] as well as for acute and subacute TBI. Small foci of hemosiderin can sometimes

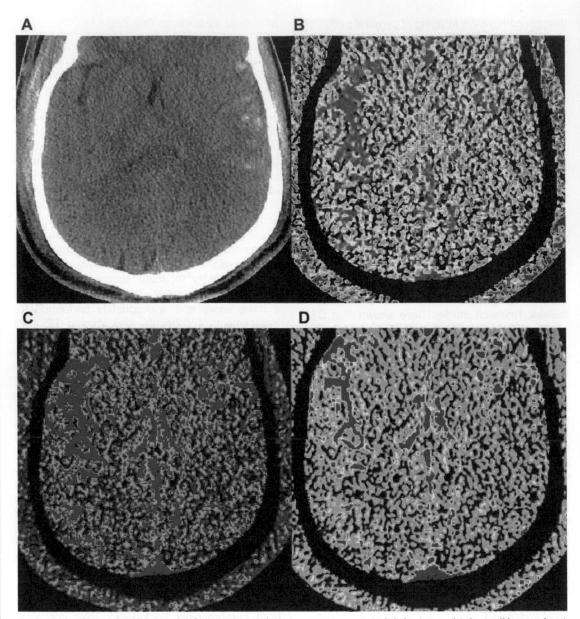

Fig. 1. **CT perfusion (CTP) in cerebral contusion**. Admission noncontrast CT (*A*) depicts multiple small hemorrhagic foci in the left temporal lobe with the so-called "salt and pepper" appearance of an acute contusion. Minimal edema (ie, "pepper") is noted at this hyperacute stage. Mild sulcal effacement is consistent with cerebral hyperemia (dysautoregulation). CTP shows high MTT (*B*), low CBF (*C*), and low CBV (*D*) values. This zone of abnormal perfusion progressed on follow-up imaging into a larger parenchymal lesion. Recent studies have shown that CTP depicts the full extent of cerebral contusions earlier and more accurately than conventional noncontrast CT. Note how the perfusion defect is larger than the area seen on CT, and as stated, this lesion progressed on follow-up (not shown).

be resorbed over time, however, so the lack of evidence of blood products on GRE does not exclude prior TBI.[27]

Limitations of GRE images include geometric distortion, chemical-shift artifacts, and susceptibility artifacts at bone-air-brain interfaces (especially over the frontal and ethmoidal sinuses and mastoid air cells) that obscure the anatomy of the orbitofrontal and inferior temporal lobes, both areas that are typically injured in TBI (Fig. 8). The choice of echo time (TE) affects GRE artifacts and performance: whereas a short TE reduces susceptibility effects at the tissue-air boundaries, a longer TE sequence (which

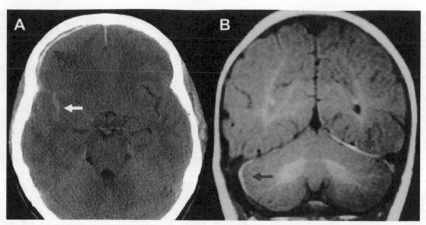

Fig. 2. **"Smear" subdural hematoma (SDH).** (*A*) Axial CT image demonstrates a thin right frontal SDH with minimal mass effect (*red arrow*). Also note subtle SAH within the right Sylvian fissure (*white arrow*). (*B*) Coronal T1-weighted image in a different patient shows thin left tentorial and right infratentorial SDHs (*arrows*); the corresponding CT scan in this case was negative.

maximizes lesion-to-tissue contrast) more sensitively detects TAI lesions. Fortunately, these geometric distortions and susceptibility effects can be mitigated so some extent by parallel imaging and fast image acquisition methods.[28]

SWI can be likened to a supercharged GRE sequence and is the most sensitive sequence for identifying hemorrhage, especially petechial hemorrhage. SWI amplifies susceptibility effects by combining both magnitude and phase information from a high-resolution, fully velocity compensated 3-dimensional (3D) T2*-weighted gradient-echo sequence.[29] Conventional GRE T2*-weighted MR imaging relies only on the magnitude images and ignores the phase images, the latter of which contain valuable information regarding tissue susceptibility differences. SWI is 3 to 6 times more sensitive than GRE T2*-weighted imaging in detecting hemorrhagic TAI.[30–33] In addition, a recent study by Wu and colleagues[33] showed that it is also fairly sensitive to acute SAH as well as subacute and chronic SAH.

DWI is one of the imaging sequences of choice for acute TAI and ischemia/infarction,

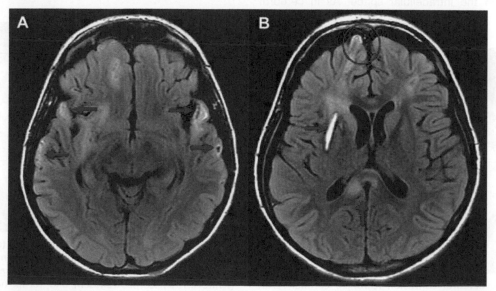

Fig. 3. **FLAIR imaging in cortical contusions (chronic).** (*A*) Axial image demonstrates multiple areas of T2 hyperintensity within the gyral crests of the temporal lobes bilaterally, consistent with old cortical contusions (*arrows*). (*B*) Slightly higher image in the same patient reveals concomitant splenial TAI (*vertical arrow*), hemorrhagic putaminal TAI (*horizontal arrow*), and a contusion of the right superior frontal gyrus (*circle*).

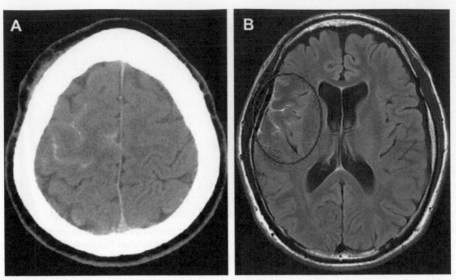

Fig. 4. **Traumatic subarachnoid hemorrhage (SAH).** (*A*) Axial CT shows linear high attenuation within the right frontal convexity sulci consistent with acute blood in the subarachnoid space. This patient also has a small right frontal subgaleal hematoma. (*B*) FLAIR imaging in a different patient with posttraumatic SAH demonstrates increased signal in the right Sylvian fissure (*circle*).

but it is also helpful in identifying cerebral contusions.[34,35] In the central nervous system, the diffusion of water is impeded by tissue structures such as cell membranes, myelin sheaths, intracellular microtubules, and associated proteins. Because living cells and tissues are composed of multiple subcompartments where the magnitude and direction of diffusion vary, diffusion is faster in the extracellular space than in the intracellular space. As in cerebral

infarction, acute TAI lesions also show increased signal (reduced diffusion) on DWI with a corresponding reduction in apparent diffusion coefficient (ADC). DWI generally reveals more lesions than fast spin-echo T2-weighted and GRE T2*-weighted images in patients imaged within 48 hours of injury (**Fig. 9**). Chronic TAI lesions are either invisible or show decreased signal (facilitated diffusion) on DWI.

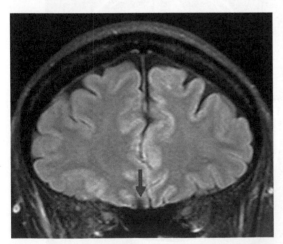

Fig. 5. **Cerebral contusion (chronic).** Coronal FLAIR image in a patient with posttraumatic anosmia demonstrates very subtle T2 hypointensity within the right gyrus rectus (*arrow*), consistent with old hemorrhage.

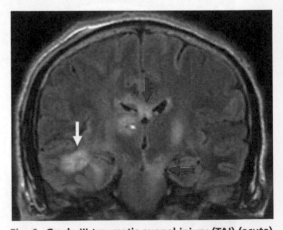

Fig. 6. **Grade III traumatic axonal injury (TAI) (acute).** Coronal FLAIR image reveals multiple abnormal T2-hyperintense foci involving the right temporal stem (*white arrow*), corpus callosum and fornix (*vertical red arrow*), left midbrain (*horizontal red arrow*), and bilateral basal ganglia, all of which are consistent with TAI. This patient had suffered severe head injury in a cycling accident.

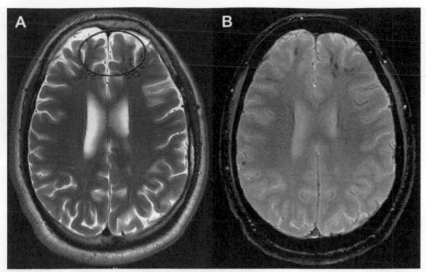

Fig. 7. **Traumatic axonal injury (TAI)**. (*A*) Axial T2-weighted MR shows very subtle hypointense foci within the subcortical white matter of the superior frontal gyrus bilaterally (*circle*). (*B*) The corresponding GRE image more easily demonstrates multiple bilateral subcortical T2 hypointense foci consistent with hemorrhagic TAI.

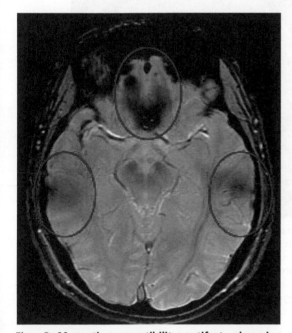

Fig. 8. **Magnetic susceptibility artifact obscuring cortical contusions**. Axial GRE image shows ill-defined hypointense areas in the orbitofrontal and inferior temporal lobes (*circles*). This susceptibility artifact partially obscures regions of the brain that are typically involved by cortical contusion; this is not usually an issue for deep white matter lesions, but it can easily obscure cortical contusions. With the recent advance of parallel imaging technology, however, less spatial distortion and higher signal-to-noise ratio can be achieved in a time-efficient manner to reduce this problem.

Diffusion tensor imaging (DTI) is sensitive to the spatial orientation of water diffusion, and allows for the virtual reconstruction of axonal networks within the brain.[36] DTI has provided important insights into the neurobiological basis for normal development and aging, as well as various disease processes in the central nervous system such as demyelinating disorders, brain tumors, dysmyelination, and TBI. DTI is the study of choice when evaluating the integrity and directionality of white matter fiber tracts, and thus it has been extensively applied as a research tool in the study of TAI.

There are 2 primary indices of DTI: fractional anisotropy (FA) and ADC. FA is an index of water diffusivity in the voxel. FA is low when fibers are not collinear (eg, crossing fibers) or if fibers have been damaged. ADC is an estimate of the average magnitude of water movement in a voxel. Therefore, ADC will increase in the setting of vasogenic edema and when water flows out of capillaries into the interstitial space. ADC decreases with cytotoxic edema and when diffusion is restricted by injured swollen cells. When axons are injured, normal anisotropy decreases because of restricted axoplasmic flow. Several studies have revealed an abnormal decrease in white matter FA when conventional MR imaging was normal.[37–40] A follow-up study in 2 patients with TBI revealed that in some regions with initially reduced FA, the changes were partially or completely corrected 30 days after injury.[40] These results should not necessarily be interpreted as evidence for regeneration of neurons. Instead, a cellular repair mechanism may have corrected the cytoskeletal misalignment before disconnection occurred.

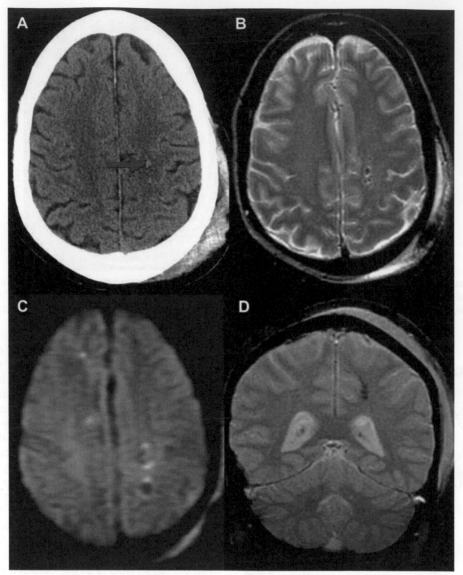

Fig. 9. Grade I TAI (acute). (*A*) Axial CT demonstrates several small subtle hyperdense foci within the posterior left frontal subcortical white matter (*arrow*), compatible with acute hemorrhagic TAI. Extensive ipsilateral scalp soft tissue swelling is also noted. (*B*) Axial T2-weighted MR image reveals corresponding hypointense foci (ie, deoxyhemoglobin) in the same area. (*C*) Axial diffusion-weighted imaging (DWI) demonstrates the previous foci in addition to several additional TAI lesions in the right hemisphere. (*D*) Coronal GRE image shows magnetic susceptibility associated with the lesions, confirming hemorrhagic TAI.

DTI is providing some remarkable insights into TBI, but there appears to be an "irrational exuberance"[41] in the literature, especially for 3D-color tractography (Fig. 10). The sensitivity of fiber-tracking algorithms to many physical and computational variables is still poorly understood, and their behavior in the face of injured tissue even less so. Numerous issues must still be accounted for to reduce false positives and false negatives when interpreting DTI studies. For example, FA and ADC are affected by imaging variables such as field strength and resolution, as well as patient variables including age and preexisting disease. Although single-shot echo-planar imaging (EPI) is fairly immune to extreme variability in phase between applications of diffusion-encoding gradients, it suffers from severe artifacts in the presence of magnetic field inhomogeneities. The significant T2* decay that can occur during long echo trains makes high-resolution acquisitions challenging.

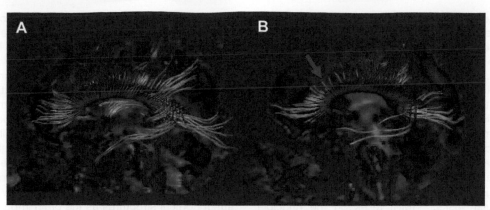

Fig. 10. **Diffusion tensor 3D fiber tractography**. Sagittal tractograms in a normal age-matched patient (*A*) and a TBI patient (*B*) show apparent "pruning" of the frontal white matter fiber tracts (*arrow*), suspicious for TAI. However, it is critical to understand that DTI fiber trajectories do not represent or correspond to actual fibers (given the discrepancy of scale between MR image voxels and axonal fibers, that is quite impossible). While visually seductive, they are nothing more than a mathematical construct that can be used to generate what might be called "pseudoanatomical" displays of hypothetical connections. Indeed, as mentioned in the text, it is likely premature to make this direct diagnosis, as so much remains poorly understood both technically and pathophysiologically.

With the recent advance of parallel imaging technology, less spatial distortion and higher signal-to-noise ratio can be achieved in a time-efficient manner with single-shot EPI. More case-control studies are necessary, however, with age-matched comparisons of DTI results between patients and corresponding control subgroups. Finally, the difficulties of post-processing and the need for statistical analyses to evaluate the effects on FA maps of spatial distortion correction induced by gradient nonlinearity, misregistration, image processing, and variable protocol parameters (b value, number of diffusion-encoding gradient directions, number of excitations, software data analysis package, and so forth) are currently keeping DTI primarily in the research arena.

Magnetization transfer imaging (MTI) takes advantage of the molecular disarrangement of white matter tracts in TAI. MTI exploits the longitudinal (T1) relaxation coupling between bound (hydrated) water protons and free (bulk) water protons. Although classically used to assess demyelination in the setting of multiple sclerosis, MTI may provide a quantitative index of the structural integrity of tissue, and therefore is a potential marker of TAI.[42]

Magnetic resonance spectroscopy (MRS) can reveal posttraumatic neurometabolite abnormalities in the injured brain when conventional neuroimaging is normal.[43,44] The most common brain metabolites that are measured with proton [^{1}H] MRS include *N*-acetylaspartate (NAA), creatinine (Cr), choline (Cho), glutamate (Glu), lactate, and myoinositol. In brief, a reduction of NAA, a marker of axonal and neuronal functional status, has been shown to be a dynamic process after TBI: it remains low in patients with poor recovery and returns to normal in patients with good outcomes. Decreased NAA values represent either neuronal loss or neuronal/mitochondrial dysfunction, because they can recover after the resolution of energy failure.[45,46] Total Cho is considered an indicator of membrane structural integrity, and is typically increased in TBI. Ross and colleagues[47] suggested that elevated Cho levels in white matter may be caused by breakdown products appearing after the shearing of myelin and cellular membranes, and that reduced NAA values result from axonal injury. Changes in Cr, a marker of cell energy metabolism and mitochondrial function, may also be seen. An increased Cr level may be part of a repair mechanism associated with increased mitochondrial function in areas of injury. Perturbations in Glu, the brain's major neurotransmitter, as well as an increase in lactate are also seen following TBI. MRS is not routinely performed in TBI and is usually reserved for experimental studies; this is partially because the data interpretation is complicated by the variability in results depending on the severity of the initial injury, the time after injury that the scan is performed, the types and location of spectral acquisitions, and the outcome measures used to monitor recovery. In addition, results may have been influenced by technical factors involved in the acquisition and processing of MRS data. One cannot account for voxels with spectra that are too distorted or that contain no measurable metabolites because of large amounts of blood products. This latter limitation may cause an underestimation of the overall effect of hemorrhagic damage. Finally, because ratios are often used instead of quantitative metabolite levels, changes in Cr may affect the ratios and may explain why the Cho/Cr ratio is slightly lower in patients with poor outcomes in some regions.

Functional MR imaging (fMRI) indirectly observes the activity of the brain via detection of an alteration in the ratio of cerebral blood deoxyhemoglobin to oxyhemoglobin in response to particular tasks.[48] fMRI relies on the principle that changes in the blood oxygen level dependent (BOLD) signal are caused by changes in CBF, which in turn is thought to be caused by changes in neuronal activity. As neuronal activity increases, blood flow overcompensates such that the local blood oxygenation actually increases. Because deoxyhemoglobin is an endogenous paramagnetic contrast agent, a decrease in its concentration is reflected as an increase in signal intensity on GRE images. This principle has been validated in animal studies, but the fundamental mechanisms underlying the coupling between neuronal activity and blood flow changes have not been elucidated. This aspect is relevant to the topic of TBI because it is possible that abnormalities in fMRI signals could be caused by abnormalities in neuronal activity (as is usually assumed), or by abnormalities in the coupling of neuronal activity to the regulation of CBF (which is rarely assessed).

fMRI can be performed at either 1.5 T or 3 T, but higher field strength is generally preferred. A high-resolution 3D-SPGR (spoiled gradient-recalled acquisition in the steady state), T1-weighted whole brain study is initially obtained. Then, for fMRI data collection, GRE EPI is performed, preferably with parallel imaging. Although "resting state" fMRI can be performed, most fMRI examinations measure the magnetic evoked response to a stimulated task that is subsequently coregistered with the high-resolution MR images.

fMRI research in TBI has centered primarily on the assessment of deficits after mild TBI (Fig. 11), but also offers promise in the understanding of the brain's ability to reorganize after injury. As with the aforementioned advanced MR imaging techniques, however, fMRI has been used in number of research studies of TBI patients but is not yet part of routine clinical care. There is a need for improved standardization of fMRI acquisition and analysis protocols for TBI. A major challenge facing task-related fMR imaging studies is that the changes in BOLD signal are strongly dependent on how well the task is performed, so interpretation of whether fMRI changes are caused by TBI or simply by worse performance is a major issue. Another criticism of fMRI in TBI is the lack of a baseline (pre-trauma) study.

Voxel-based morphometry (VBM) measures the change in volume of the brain and has traditionally been used to assess brain atrophy in Alzheimer disease. Only preliminary research in TBI patients has been performed, but gray matter atrophy has been identified, suggesting that the eventual pathologic end point of TBI is loss of cortical neuronal cell bodies.[49] Two possible mechanisms are thought to be responsible. First, the injury could affect cortical structures as the brain impacts the cranial vault in a coup-contrecoup manner.[39] Second, TAI could cause axonal damage, leading to retrograde degeneration and neuronal somatic loss. Postsynaptic cortical atrophy may also result from diminished anterograde transmission.

Single-photon emission tomography (SPECT) uses the gamma-emitting isotope technetium-99 to image cerebral perfusion. The discovery of significant changes in CBF in patients with TBI makes SPECT a promising tool in evaluating patients with mild TBI.[50–52] Frontal and temporal lobe hypoperfusion is commonly seen in head injury, presumably due to the gliding effect of the brain over the underlying skull. Although this hypoperfusion is generally attributed to the cerebral edema that surrounds the damaged brain and limits CBF, it may also result from vasospasm, direct vascular injury, and/or perfusion changes due to alterations in remote neuronal activity (diaschisis).[53,54] SPECT can show areas of perfusion abnormality following head trauma that are normal on conventional CT and MR imaging.[55] Due to its low spatial resolution, however, SPECT is less sensitive in detecting many smaller lesions that are visible on MR imaging.

Positron emission tomography (PET) uses [^{18}F] 2-fluoro-2-deoxy-D-glucose (^{18}F-FDG) to evaluate cerebral glucose metabolism in vivo. Acutely injured brain cells show increased glucose metabolism following severe TBI because of intracellular ionic perturbation.[56–59] Following the initial hyperglycolysis state, injured brain cells then show a prolonged period of regional hypometabolism. Based on the principle that regional glucose metabolism reflects the neuronal activity of the region, focal hypometabolism indicates an area of neuronal dysfunction. To account for the metabolic reduction, 2 main mechanisms have been proposed: (1) local neuronal loss and (2) decreased neuronal activity as a result of deafferentation. FDG-PET also has an advantage for elucidating focal brain dysfunction compared with the cerebral perfusion information that is

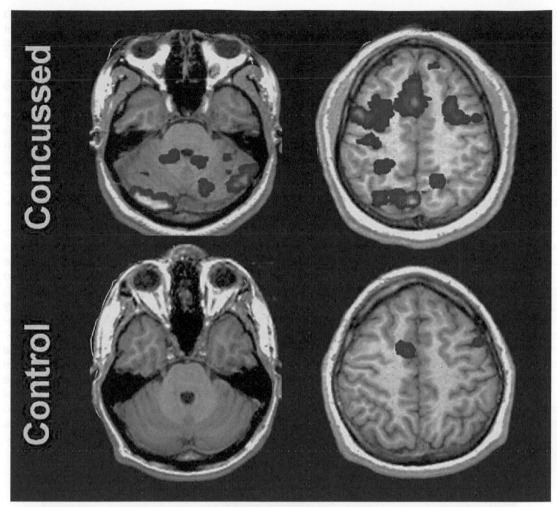

Fig. 11. Functional MR imaging (fMRI) in concussion. Within-subject differences for 2 football players, one who experienced a concussion (*top*) and one who did not (*bottom*). Both players were imaged before the start of the football season. The concussed player was imaged again within a week following his concussion. The second player was imaged again at the end of the season. Colored areas show cortical and subcortical regions where the second imaging session resulted in significantly greater activation than the first. Notice that for the concussed player there is significantly greater activation in numerous brain regions as compared with the nonconcussed player. (*Courtesy* Kelly J. Jantzen).

obtained from SPECT studies. Although a significant number of functional imaging studies in TBI have been performed using perfusion SPECT analysis, metabolic PET technology demonstrates similar overall findings but with increased resolution. Unfortunately, although PET provides information on cerebral metabolism and has shown promise in TBI, it is not widely available, is expensive, and is not regularly reimbursed for the evaluation of TBI.

Magnetoencephalography

Magnetoencephalography (MEG) is a noninvasive functional imaging technique with high temporal resolution (<1 millisecond) and spatial localization accuracy at the cortical level (2–3 mm). Unlike normal spontaneous MEG data, which are dominated by neuronal activity with frequencies above 8 Hz, brain-injured tissue generates abnormal low-frequency delta-wave (1–4 Hz) magnetic signals that can be directly measured and localized using MEG.[60] Abnormal focal slowing can be detected by MEG when other imaging modalities are normal, and MEG appears to be more sensitive than MR imaging and SPECT to TBI.[61] Abnormal MEG delta waves have been observed in subjects without obvious DTI abnormality, indicating that MEG may also be more sensitive than DTI in diagnosing mild TBI.[62] MEG's availability is unfortunately, very limited, with only about 20 whole-head MEG systems in the United States and fewer than 150 systems installed worldwide. This lack of availability will likely relegate MEG to the research arena for the foreseeable future.

THE INJURIES
Extra-Axial Injury

Scalp and skull injury
The scalp is composed of 5 layers: skin; subcutaneous fibro-fatty tissue; galea aponeurotica; loose areolar connective tissue; periosteum.

The subgaleal hematoma is a frequent sequela of head injury resulting from direct impact or shearing of traversing veins. Close examination of the scalp soft tissues should be one of the first steps in interpreting a trauma head CT. Identification of soft tissue injury allows the radiologist to pinpoint the site of impact, or "coup" site, that may be invisible to the clinician because of its small size or obscuration by the patient's hair. Indeed, the presence of a scalp injury may be the only clue to the presence of TBI in a patient presenting with "altered mental status."

The coup site in particular should be carefully inspected for the presence of an underlying skull fracture, as well as for evidence of soft tissue laceration and radiopaque foreign bodies. The 3 main types of skull fractures include linear (most common), depressed, and basilar. Fractures can also be described as comminuted (multiple fragments) or compound (open).

Linear fractures in the axial plane can easily be missed on axial CT slices, but close examination of the "scout" image will often reveal the fracture line (Fig. 12).

Depressed fractures are commonly associated with underlying parenchymal injury (Fig. 13). These fractures are typically explored neurosurgically to evaluate underlying vessels, remove and elevate bone fragments, and diminish the risk of infection.

Basilar skull fractures can be complicated by injury to the petrous and cavernous portions of the internal carotid artery (ICA), the transverse and sigmoid venous sinuses, cranial nerves, and the middle and inner ear structures.

Temporal bone fracture (TBF) classification may be based on the traditional anatomically descriptive system of "longitudinal" versus "transverse" orientation to the long axis of the petrous temporal bone, or the newer more clinically relevant system of "otic capsule sparing" versus "otic capsule involving" fracture.[63] Longitudinal TBF is most common (95%), results from a lateral blow, and is often associated with a fracture extending to

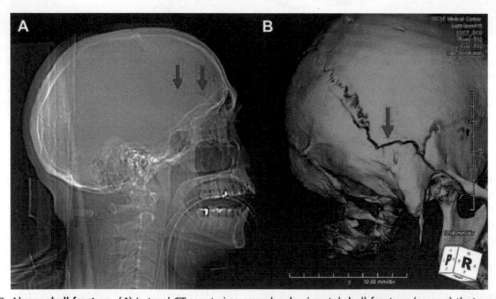

Fig. 12. **Linear skull fracture.** (*A*) Lateral CT scout view reveals a horizontal skull fracture (*arrows*) that was invisible on the corresponding axial images. Fractures that are parallel to the axial imaging plane can be missed if the scout view is not reviewed. The scout view may also reveal clinically unsuspected upper cervical spine and facial fractures. The CT scout image has essentially taken the place of the skull radiograph. (*B*) Oblique 3D volume CT in a different patient demonstrates a linear occipital fracture with diastasis of the lambdoid and occipitomastoid sutures (*arrow*).

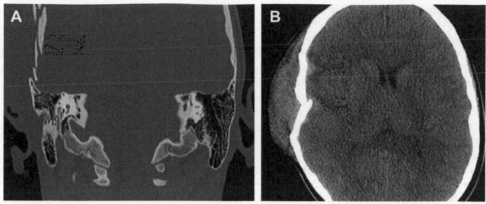

Fig. 13. **"Fracture contusion."** (*A*) Coronal CT displayed in "bone window" shows a depressed and comminuted right frontotemporal skull fracture (*arrow*). (*B*) Axial CT demonstrates subjacent hemorrhagic contusions (*arrows*).

the squamosal portion of the temporal bone. It typically spares the otic capsule but may involve the ossicles, resulting in conductive hearing loss. Transverse TBF is much less common (5%) and results from an occipital impact. Injury to the otic capsule, resulting in sensorineural hearing loss and/or facial nerve injury, is more common with the transverse TBF fracture. Many fractures, however, are actually mixed or obliquely oriented and do not nicely fit into the traditional transverse-longitudinal classification scheme, and so the critical point of interpretation is assessment of which structures have been injured. For suspected CSF leaks, high-resolution CT before and after intrathecal instillation of contrast is often helpful (Fig. 14).

Vascular injury

The subtypes of traumatic cerebrovascular injury can be thought of as a spectrum of injuries to the vessel wall ranging from separation of the intima from the media resulting in dissection, to medial and adventitial perforation resulting in pseudoaneurysm, to complete vascular transection or occlusion. The traumatic arteriovenous fistula (AVF) occurs when laceration of an artery occurs adjacent to a vein, resulting in communication between the 2 systems. The archetypal traumatic AVF is the carotid cavernous fistula (CCF) (Barrow Type A) resulting from a laceration of the ICA with direct communication to the cavernous sinus. Skull base fractures involving the carotid canal should alert the radiologist to a possible CCF

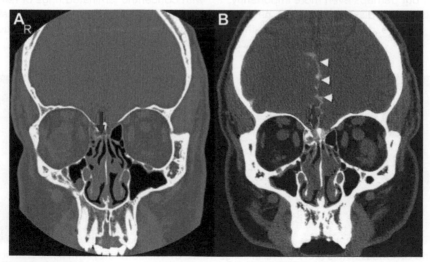

Fig. 14. **Cerebrospinal fluid (CSF) leak.** (*A*) Coronal CT image shows a bony defect of the right cribriform plate and fovea ethmoidalis (*arrow*). (*B*) Coronal CT image from a cisternogram shows leakage of contrast into the right ethmoid sinus through the bony defect (*arrow*). (*From* Le TH, Gean AD. Neuroimaging of traumatic brain injury. Mount Sinai J Med 2009;76:162; with permission.)

(Fig. 15). Symptoms often develop in a delayed fashion, days to weeks after the initial trauma, and therefore these injuries can initially be over-looked. Classic clinical findings of CCF include proptosis, chemosis, and ophthalmoplegia, with vision loss and facial pain variably present. The cross-sectional imaging findings of a CCF include lateral bowing of the cavernous sinus, a dilated superior ophthalmic vein, retrobulbar fat strand-ing, enlarged extraocular muscles, and proptosis. On conventional catheter angiography, there is abnormal early filling of the cavernous sinus during the arterial phase and early venous outflow to the superior ophthalmic vein, inferior petrosal sinus, and/or contralateral cavernous sinus.

A traumatic AVF can also result from laceration of the middle meningeal artery with fistulous communication to the middle meningeal veins. Because the arterial blood is able to drain via the meningeal veins, this type of middle meningeal artery injury rarely leads to the formation of an EDH. Patients are often asymptomatic or present with nonspecific complaints such as a pulsatile scalp mass or pulsatile tinnitus. In addition to these traumatic AVFs that may present acutely, venous thrombosis in the setting of head trauma can lead to formation of indirect, generally lower flow dural AVFs in a delayed fashion.

Dissections of the ICA in the setting of trauma most commonly occur in the distal cervical, petrous, and cavernous portions of the ICA.[64] The distal cervical vertebral artery is also particu-larly prone to dissection in blunt trauma. In a recent study, 35% of patients with a fracture through the carotid canal were shown to have a dissection at angiography, but perhaps even more importantly, 40% patients with a dissection did not have an associated fracture.[65] Twenty to thirty-three percent of patients with dissection are clinically asymptomatic, whereas others may present with delayed cerebral ischemia, neck pain, or Horner syndrome.[66] The diagnosis of dissection can be made with CTA, MR imaging/MR angiography (MRA), or conventional angiography. With recent advances in multidetector CT, CTA has emerged as a promising first-line screening tool for neuro-vascular injury. In addition, because catheter angi-ography only demonstrates the caliber of the patent lumen, MR and CTA can identify a dissected vessel that may appear "normal" on catheter angi-ography. Vascular irregularity, narrowing, or occlu-sion are the most common imaging findings of dissection, but an intimal flap and focal out-pouching of the vessel wall suggesting a traumatic pseudoaneurysm may also be seen. One advan-tage of MR over CTA is the T1-weighted sequence with fat suppression, which can demonstrate a "hyperintense crescent" around the lumen of the dissected vessel, consistent with intramural methemoglobin (Fig. 16).

Pseudoaneurysms are rare in adults but account for 11% of all pediatric aneurysms (Fig. 17). The overall incidence of aneurysms in the pediatric population, however, is lower than in adults. The wall of the pseudoaneurysm is usually an encap-sulated hematoma in communication with the arterial lumen, though on occasion the adventitia may still be intact. Nevertheless, the wall of the pseudoaneurysm provides little support, and hence it has a propensity to rupture. On imaging, the pseudoaneurysm frequently has an irregular contour and a wide neck. Thrombus within the pseudoaneurysm manifests as a rounded mass with concentric laminated rings of heterogeneous density or signal intensity, consistent with thrombus in various stages of evolution. The size

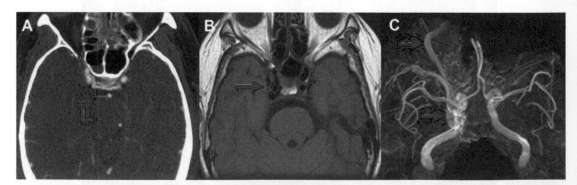

Fig. 15. **Carotid cavernous fistula (CCF).** (A) Axial image from a CTA demonstrates asymmetric enhancement of the right cavernous sinus (arrow). (B) T1-weighted MR image without contrast shows abnormally dilated flow voids within the right cavernous sinus (arrow). (C) Maximum intensity projection (MIP) reconstruction image from an MR angiogram (MRA) demonstrates increased flow-related enhancement (dilated venous channels) within the right cavernous sinus (posterior arrow) and a dilated superior ophthalmic vein (anterior arrow).

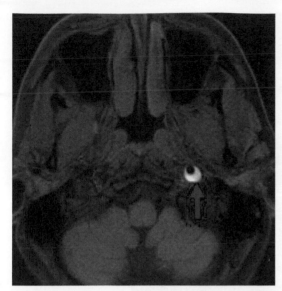

Fig. 16. Internal carotid artery dissection. Axial T1-weighted MR image with fat suppression shows a hyperintense crescent surrounding the left ICA (*arrow*). The high signal represents a subacute (methemoglobin stage) intramural hematoma. Note the preserved flow-void within the artery, underscoring why conventional catheter angiography may be normal in some cases of a vascular dissection.

of a partially thrombosed pseudoaneurysm is often underestimated on conventional angiography because the angiogram only depicts the patent portion of the lesion. In the absence of thrombosis or turbulent flow, the pseudoaneurysm appears as a round area of signal void on both T1- and T2-weighted images. Pulsation within the pseudoaneurysm shows phase artifacts on MR imaging, a helpful imaging clue to the presence of a vascular lesion. Please refer to the chapter by Hetts and English for more information on emergency vascular lesions.

Extra-Axial Hemorrhage

The 4 types of extra-axial hemorrhage include EDH, SDH, SAH, and intraventricular hemorrhage (IVH).

Pneumocephalus (intracranial air) can occur in any of these 4 locations, as well as in the brain parenchyma (pneumatocele). An understanding of normal meningeal anatomy is crucial to understanding the location and imaging appearances of the extra-axial collections. In brief, the 3 meningeal layers include the dura mater, arachnoid mater, and pia mater. The dura is composed of 2 layers: an outer periosteal layer and an inner meningeal layer that forms the dural reflections such as the falx cerebri and tentorium cerebelli.

The underlying arachnoid is superficial to the pia and is attached to it via innumerable arachnoid trabeculations. The pia is the deepest layer of the meninges and completely invests the brain surface, closely following the sulci and gyri.

Epidural hematoma

EDH, seen in 1% to 4% of TBI patients, develops within the potential space located between the outer dural layer and the skull.[67,68] At the moment of impact, the dura may be stripped away from the inner table, and extravasated blood from injured meningeal vessels, diploic veins, or dural sinuses fills the newly created epidural space. Loss of consciousness is frequently immediate, but many patients then experience a "lucid" interval during which time the EDH expands until it becomes large enough to impact on the patient's level of consciousness. Although it is a potential neurosurgical emergency, EDH is generally associated with an excellent prognosis compared with SDH, likely because the EDH is caused by direct rather than shearing forces and hence the injury is more localized.

The source of hemorrhage in an EDH is arterial in 85% of cases, and it most commonly results from fracture of the thin temporal squamosa resulting in laceration of the underlying middle meningeal artery (**Fig. 18**). The vast majority of EDHs occur at the coup site and an underlying fracture is identified in greater than 90% of cases.[32] Venous EDHs are also associated with skull fractures, and typically occur infratentorially or within the anterior aspect of the middle cranial fossa from injury to the transverse/sigmoid sinuses or the sphenoparietal sinus, respectively (**Figs. 19 and 20**).[69]

The imaging appearance of the typical EDH consists of a biconvex, hyperdense, extra-axial collection that does not cross sutures (with an exception at the level of the sagittal suture, as dura does not invest the suture due to the presence of the superior sagittal sinus). The EDH can cross dural reflections such as the falx cerebri and tentorium cerebelli, whereas the SDH is limited by these structures. Previous studies have shown a worse prognosis for lesions with a mixed density ("heterogeneous" EDH) on CT.[70,71] This so-called "swirl sign" (see **Fig. 18**) usually indicates active bleeding, with the hypodense areas representing unclotted blood; these lesions have more of a propensity for further enlargement than EDHs of homogeneous density.

One special scenario to be aware of is the development of a rapidly expanding EDH immediately following a decompressive craniectomy (**Fig. 21**). This development presumably relates to the

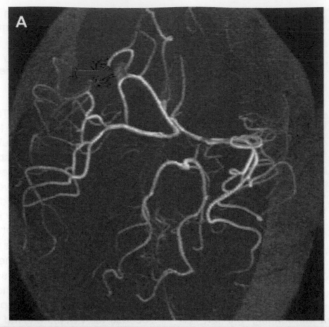

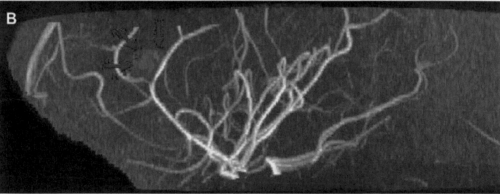

Fig. 17. **Traumatic pseudoaneurysm.** Oblique (*A*) and sagittal (*B*) 3D time-of-flight MIP MRA images demonstrate an ill-defined oval area of flow-related enhancement (*arrows*) protruding from the anterior cerebral artery at the bifurcation of the pericallosal and callosal-marginal branches. The appearance is compatible with a partially thrombosed pseudoaneurysm.

removal of a "tamponade effect" on a small extra-axial collection that is then able to expand once pressure relationships are altered by removal of portions of the cranial vault. An immediate postoperative CT scan may be indicated in these craniectomy patients in whom there is evidence of a skull fracture remote from the planned craniectomy or a small collection remote from the craniectomy that was not considered "surgical" in nature.[72]

The Subdural hematoma

SDH is seen in 10% to 20% of patients with head trauma. It is the traumatic intracranial hemorrhage that most commonly requires operative management, and it has a much higher associated

mortality (50%–85%) than EDH.[73] The SDH occurs between the inner meningeal layer of dura and the arachnoid. The majority of SDHs are caused by traumatic disruption of the bridging cortical veins traversing this space (Fig. 22). Unlike the EDH, the SDH is less often associated with a skull fracture in the adult. The SDH can be seen in both the coup and contrecoup locations, with the contrecoup location being more common. SDH may also be seen in elderly patients or patients with coagulopathy who are at increased risk for a spontaneous SDH or an SDH following minor trauma.

Most SDHs are supratentorial and are located over the cerebral convexities, along the tentorium

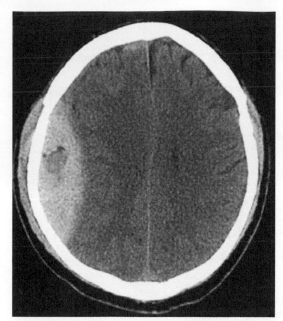

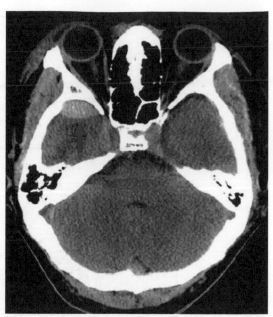

Fig. 18. **EDH "swirl sign."** Noncontrast axial CT shows low attenuation areas within an acute right fronto-parietal EDH. The density within this EDH is secondary to laceration of the middle meningeal artery with mixing of hyperacute unclotted (low attenuation) arterial blood with more dense clotted (high attenuation) blood.

Fig. 20. **Benign anterior temporal EDH ("BAT-EDH").** Axial CT shows a biconvex, homogeneous, high-attenuation extra-axial collection within the anterior aspect of the middle cranial fossa (*arrow*), consistent with a venous EDH due to disruption of the sphenopar-ietal sinus. Note the characteristic ipsilateral periorbital soft tissue swelling. A fracture of the sphenotemporal buttress was also present on the bone window.

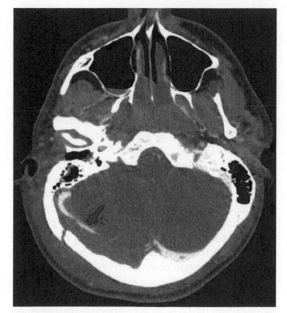

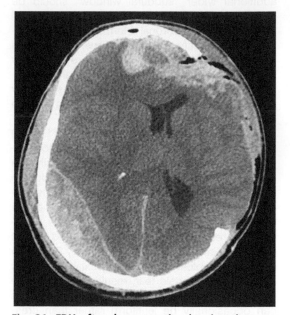

Fig. 19. **Venous EDH.** Contrast-enhanced axial CT shows displacement of the right transverse sinus (*arrow*) from the occiput, thus confirming the epidural location of the collection. Also note the adja-cent occipital skull fracture with overlying scalp swelling.

Fig. 21. **EDH after decompressive hemicraniectomy.** Noncontrast axial CT shows external herniation of the left frontotemporal lobe and a large right parieto-occipital EDH. The EDH developed subsequent to the DCH, likely caused by release of the "tampo-nade effect" by the preoperative elevated intracranial pressure.

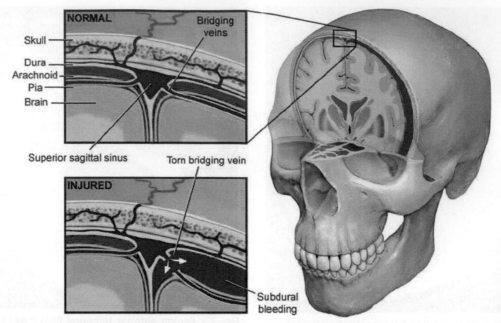

Fig. 22. **Acute SDH**. Schematic drawing showing the most common mechanism of the SDH. Note traumatic disruption of the bridging cortical vein traversing the subdural space. The SDH is located between the inner meningeal layer of dura and the arachnoid.

cerebelli, or along the falx cerebri, in descending order of frequency. Small SDHs may be overlooked on traditional CT "brain windows," and an additional wider "subdural window" should be used in all trauma patients to detect these small SDHs. Reviewing coronal reformations can sometimes help identify these collections. Infratentorial SDHs are rare in adults and are more commonly seen in neonates secondary to perinatal injury.

The SDH can be divided into 3 stages, namely acute, subacute, and chronic, each with its own distinct imaging characteristics.

The CT appearance of an acute SDH (<1 week) consists of a crescentic, hyperdense, holohemispheric, extra-axial collection. Occasionally the acute SDH may be iso- or hypointense due to underlying anemia. It can also be of mixed density in the hyperacute setting because of active bleeding or underlying coagulopathy; the hypodense areas correspond to unclotted blood (Fig. 23). Alternatively, a mixed-density SDH may be due to rebleeding into a preexisting chronic SDH or an arachnoid tear, resulting in admixture of blood with CSF. These "atypical" acute SDHs can occasionally be lentiform rather than crescentic in shape, likely secondary to adhesions in the subdural space.

The subacute SDH (1–3 weeks) gradually decreases in attenuation as the cellular elements are removed. During this subacute period, an isodense phase occurs and the collection can be

difficult to detect on noncontrast CT (Fig. 24). Imaging clues to the presence of an isodense SDH include:

- Medial displacement of the gray-white junction from the inner table ("abnormally thick cortex")
- White matter buckling
- Presence of mass effect manifested by midline shift, compression of the ipsilateral ventricle, or sulcal effacement.

The conspicuous appearance of blood products on MR imaging makes the diagnosis of the subacute SDH fairly straightforward. Of note, the subacute SDH may appear lentiform rather than crescentic in shape, especially in the coronal plane, and thus mimic an EDH. On T1-weighted images, the isointense signal of the acute SDH gradually transitions to hyperintense signal as methemoglobin appears in the subacute phase.

In the absence of recurrent bleeding, the chronic SDH (longer than 3 weeks) appears as a homogeneously hypodense crescentic collection (Fig. 25). If rebleeding occurs, then a bilayered "hematocrit effect" appearance can be seen with the hyperdense acute blood layering dependently. Subdural adhesions and membranes are also common in the chronic setting, producing multiple compartments of different densities. The more uniform hypodense chronic SDH can be confused with a subdural hygroma if it approaches CSF density.

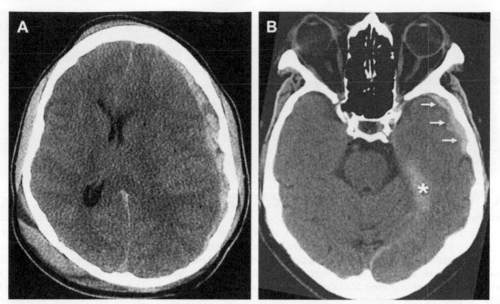

Fig. 23. Acute SDH. (*A*) Axial CT shows a contrecoup left holohemispheric mixed-density extra-axial collection, consistent with an acute SDH. Like the EDH illustrated in Fig. 18, the heterogeneity of the collection is likely due to mixing of actively bleeding unclotted (low attenuation) blood with clotted (high attenuation) blood. The degree of mass effect in this kind of SDH tends to be disproportionate to the size of the collection, suggesting underlying hyperemic swelling. (*B*) Tentorial SDH. Note the ill-defined asymmetric high attenuation layering along the left tentorial incisura (*asterisk*) and a small left temporal SDH (*arrows*).

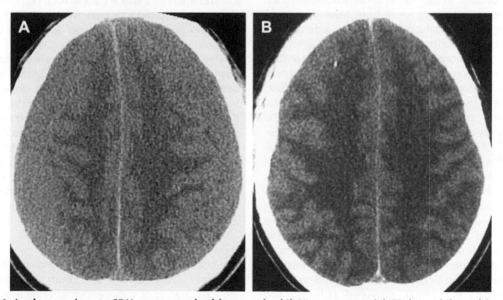

Fig. 24. Isodense subacute SDH versus cerebral hyperemia. (*A*) Noncontrast axial CT shows bilateral isodense SDHs (*asterisk*) that can be difficult to differentiate from the subjacent parenchyma because the collection has the same density as the underlying cortex. Note, however, the displacement of the gray matter ("thick cortex") and the white matter buckling, which serve as important clues in detecting potentially subtle SDHs, especially when they are bilateral. (*B*) Posttraumatic dysautoregulation (hyperemic swelling) on CT shows complete loss of cerebral sulci with preservation of gray-white matter differentiation. Note the absence of white matter buckling.

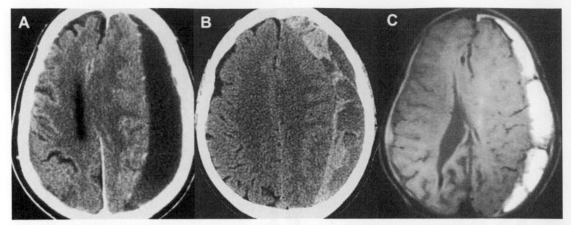

Fig. 25. Chronic SDH. (*A*) "Uncomplicated" SDH. Noncontrast axial CT shows a uniformly hypodense left SDH. Such collections can usually be treated with burr-hole evacuation. (*B*) "Complicated" SDH. Axial CT demonstrates a left holohemispheric SDH with internal septations and mixed density. There is moderate mass effect on the left cerebral hemisphere and mild left-to-right midline shift. (*C*) "Complicated" SDH. Axial T1-weighted MR in a different patient with a chronic SDH shows an extra-axial collection with loculations and mass effect. The hyperintensity is due to the presence of methemoglobin. Such collections usually necessitate evacuation via craniotomy.

A subdural hygroma is a CSF collection caused by a tear in the arachnoid in the setting of trauma. The subdural hygroma presents in a delayed fashion, usually 3 to 30 days after the initial injury, and generally resolves without intervention.

Subarachnoid hemorrhage
SAH occurs in up to 11% of traumatic brain injuries.[74] SAH may result from tearing of small pial or arachnoidal cortical vessels, extension of IVH via the fourth ventricular outlet foramina, or from contiguous extension of an intracerebral contusion/hematoma into the subarachnoid space. Important areas to search for subtle SAH include the interpeduncular cistern, basilar cisterns, contrecoup Sylvian fissure, and the convexity sulci (see **Fig. 4**). Occasionally, "effacement" of the sulci due to the presence of intrasulcal SAH is the only imaging clue to the presence of SAH. Acute SAH is more difficult to detect on conventional T1- and T2-weighted MR imaging than on CT. FLAIR imaging, however, is potentially more sensitive than CT, especially when a volume of at least 1 to 2 mL of blood is present. Note that "abnormal" high signal in the sulci and cisterns of ventilated patients receiving a high inspired oxygen fraction (>0.60) can be observed on FLAIR sequences in normal, uninjured patients, and should not be mistaken for subarachnoid hemorrhage. Communicating hydrocephalus (due to scarring of the arachnoid villi) is thought to be the most common complication of SAH, but traumatic SAH can also cause vasospasm.[75] Subacute SAH is difficult to detect on CT, as the blood is typically

isodense to CSF on CT and is better recognized on MR imaging because of the high sensitivity of the FLAIR sequence to substances that alter the composition of CSF. SAH more than 1 week old is difficult, if not impossible, to detect on CT; chronic SAH is better detected on MR imaging. Chronic blood products, such as hemosiderin in the subarachnoid space ("superficial hemosiderosis"), are best detected on SWI and GRE T2*-weighted images (**Fig. 26**), and appear as areas of decreased signal intensity.

"Pseudo-SAH" is a phenomenon that may be seen in the setting of acute TBI, typically in the setting of diffuse brain swelling and downward transtentorial herniation. The increased density in the subarachnoid space is thought to be caused by contraction of the subarachnoid space and/or engorgement of small pial vessels in conjunction with the "silhouetting" of the subarachnoid space by low-density cerebral edema (**Fig. 27**).[76] It is important not to confuse this with true SAH but rather to recognize it as a generally ominous sign of elevated intracranial pressure.

Intraventricular hemorrhage
IVH occurs in 2.8% of all patients with blunt head trauma.[77] IVH can result from rotationally-induced tearing of subependymal veins along the surface of the ventricles, from contiguous extension of a parenchymal hematoma into the ventricular system, from retrograde flow of SAH into the ventricles, or from a direct penetrating injury. Isolated IVH hemorrhage is rare, as it is usually associated with SAH and contusions. IVH can appear

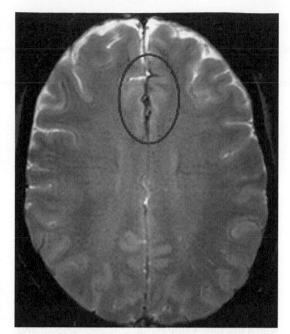

Fig. 26. **Chronic SAH ("superficial hemosiderosis")**. Axial GRE T2*-weighted MR image reveals linear areas of low signal (*vertical arrows*) within the subarachnoid space of the paramedian frontal lobe, consistent with ferritin and hemosiderin deposition related to prior trauma.

as a fluid-fluid level layering dependently within the occipital horns or as a "tumefactive" intraventricular clot (**Fig. 28**). Patients with IVH are at risk for developing noncommunicating hydrocephalus

from obstruction of the aqueduct due to ependymal adhesions and scarring.

Intra-Axial Injury

Cerebral "swelling"

By definition, brain swelling has mass effect that results in effacement of cisterns and sulci and sometimes the ventricle(s). Cerebral swelling may be focal or diffuse. The increase in cerebral volume may be caused by an increase in CBV (hyperemia) or an increase in tissue fluid (cerebral edema). Cerebral edema can be further divided into 2 major types: "vasogenic," due to blood-brain barrier disruption that results in extracellular water accumulation, and "cytotoxic/cellular," due to intracellular water accumulation.[78] A third type, "osmotic" brain edema, is caused by osmotic imbalances between the blood and the brain tissue.

Early on, cerebral hyperemia is seen on imaging as the presence of mass effect with preservation of gray-white matter differentiation (see **Fig. 24**B). Posttraumatic hyperemic swelling is caused by loss of cerebral autoregulation, a complex intrinsic control mechanism that maintains a constant CBF by constantly adjusting the cerebral vascular resistance in response to changing mean arterial pressure. Cerebral "hyperemia" may progress to cerebral "edema." Cytotoxic edema leads to loss of gray-white differentiation due to cell swelling, whereas vasogenic edema is primarily caused by an increase in extracellular water and involves the white matter. Young patients are more

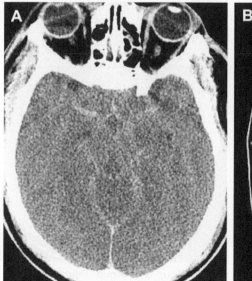
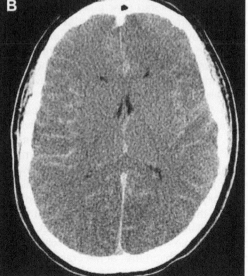

Fig. 27. **Pseudo-SAH**. Axial CT images at the level of the circle of Willis (*A*) and basal ganglia (*B*) show loss of gray-white matter differentiation (including the deep gray nuclei), complete effacement of the cerebral sulci and perimesencephalic cisterns, partial effacement of the ventricles, and linear high attenuation within the subarachnoid space.

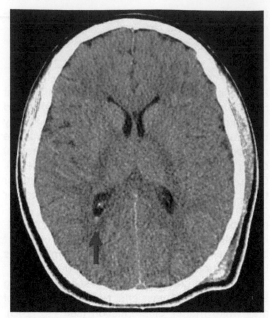

Fig. 28. Acute IVH. Axial CT shows high-density material layering dependently within the occipital horn of the right lateral ventricle (*arrow*), consistent with acute intraventricular blood. Evidence of left occipital scalp trauma is present as well.

susceptible to dysautoregulation in the setting of trauma. In fact, when midline shift or mass effect appears "out of proportion" to the size of an extra-axial collection or intraparenchymal lesion, then underlying cerebral swelling should be suspected. In this situation, a decompressive craniectomy (DC) may be favored over a craniotomy to allow external herniation and avoid secondary injury due to elevated intracranial pressure. The DC is performed in the setting of medically refractory intracranial hypertension to avoid secondary ischemic complications in patients with severe cerebral swelling due to TBI.

Over the last decade, DC has experienced a resurgence, and several studies have shown long-term improvements in functional outcomes.[79–83] Ideally, a bifrontal or wide frontotemporoparietal craniectomy is performed to allow external herniation. If the craniectomy is too small, then externally herniated brain tissue may form acute rather than obtuse angles and result in venous ischemia/infarction of brain tissue at the craniectomy margin. After a DC, CT surveillance frequently shows a "hygroma" at the craniectomy site with gelfilm dura-seal in the middle of the CSF collection. In the chronic setting, the brain tends to develop a concave or "sunken" appearance at the craniectomy site, and paradoxic midline shift may be seen. Early results with CTP

studies have shown reduced CBF in the hemisphere underlying the craniectomy, which improves after replacement of the bone flap.[84]

Cortical contusion

Contusions occur in up to 43% of patients with blunt head injuries.[85] Cortical contusion occurs when the brain surface rubs across the rough inner table of the calvarium, and as such it represents a "brain bruise" of the superficial gray matter. Cortical contusions always involve the gyral crests and may or may not extend into the underlying subcortical white matter. Brain contusions can be classified as fracture contusions, coup contusions, and/or contrecoup contusions. Fracture contusions occur at a site of direct impact, usually beneath a depressed skull fracture (see **Fig. 13**). A coup contusion also occurs at the site of impact, but is caused by a transient inbending of the calvarium, most often due to a blow against the stationary head, and is not necessarily associated with a fracture. Contrecoup contusions occur 180° opposite the site of initial head impact, when the brain is set into motion relative to a stationary calvarium (**Fig. 29**). The classic contrecoup contusion typically results from an occipital impact, and leads to injury of the anterior and inferior orbitofrontal and temporal lobes (**Fig. 30**). "Gliding"

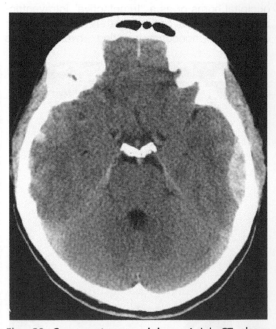

Fig. 29. Coup-contrecoup injury. Axial CT shows a characteristic hyperdense, homogeneous, biconvex left temporal collection (*asterisk*) with overlying scalp soft tissue swelling, consistent with a small EDH at the coup site. A typical mixed-density contrecoup right temporal cortical contusion is also noted.

contusions occur over the parasagittal convexity and are secondary to angular acceleration, with stretching of the parasagittal veins and adjacent cerebrum.

The acute contusion can be very subtle on CT. It may initially appear as a small, round peripheral hemorrhage in one of the common locations already described, and it may be difficult to differentiate from a small extra-axial bleed. As the contusion evolves, however, surrounding vasogenic edema appears, thus confirming the intra-axial location of the hemorrhage. A characteristic "salt and pepper" pattern of mixed areas of hypodensity and hyperdensity becomes more apparent with time. In severe cases the entire temporal lobe may be contused, resulting in the so-called burst lobe. Because of their superficial location, contusions are far more conspicuous on MR than on CT, especially when they involve the gyral crests over the convexity and skull base, where beam-hardening artifact limits CT. On T2-weighted MR imaging, an acute contusion has a central dark signal (deoxyhemoglobin) with surrounding hyperintense edematous cortical tissue. Within a day or two, the subacute contusion develops increased vasogenic edema; in addition, deoxyhemoglobin evolves into intracellular methemoglobin, resulting in T1 hyperintensity (**Fig. 31**). The subacute contusion and hematoma often demonstrate ring enhancement following intravenous contrast administration, and therefore may mimic a brain abscess, infarct, or neoplasm (**Fig. 32**) if prior imaging is not available or a history of trauma is not elicited. The chronic contusion appears as a focal, often wedge-shaped, peripheral area of encephalomalacia, and as such it may mimic an old embolic infarct (see **Fig. 5**). The lesion is often lined with hemosiderin, resulting in the characteristic dark T2 signal intensity seen on GRE and SWI sequences.

Intraparenchymal hematoma

With increasing severity of head injury, the microhemorrhages associated with the cortical contusion may coalesce into a focal intraparenchymal hematoma (IPH). In some cases, therefore, cortical contusion and parenchymal hematoma represent a spectrum of pathophysiology rather than distinct entities. The traumatic IPH may also result from shear-induced hemorrhage due to rupture of small intraparenchymal blood vessels and microcavitation. Like contusion, IPH frequently involves the contrecoup location, especially the orbitofrontal lobes and the temporal lobes. The ICH is usually more well-defined than the cortical contusion and tends to have less surrounding edema. IPH may also occur in the basal ganglia as a result of shear-induced injury to the lenticulostriate vessels. As mentioned, it should be remembered that the subacute hematoma typically shows ring enhancement following intravenous contrast administration and, therefore, may mimic a brain

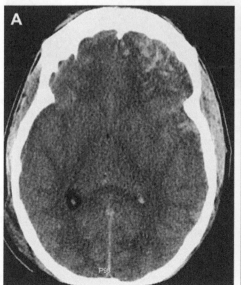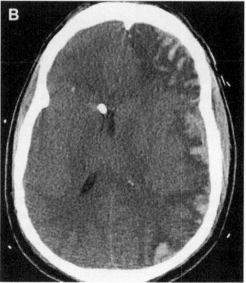

Fig. 30. Contrecoup cortical contusions. (*A*) Admission axial CT shows innumerable ill-defined left frontotemporal hemorrhagic cortical contusions ("salt and pepper" appearance). Right occipital subgaleal soft tissue swelling is noted at the coup site. (*B*) CT examination performed 24 hours later shows evolution and "blossoming" of the contusions with increased surrounding vasogenic edema. A right frontal external ventricular drainage catheter is now present within the right frontal horn.

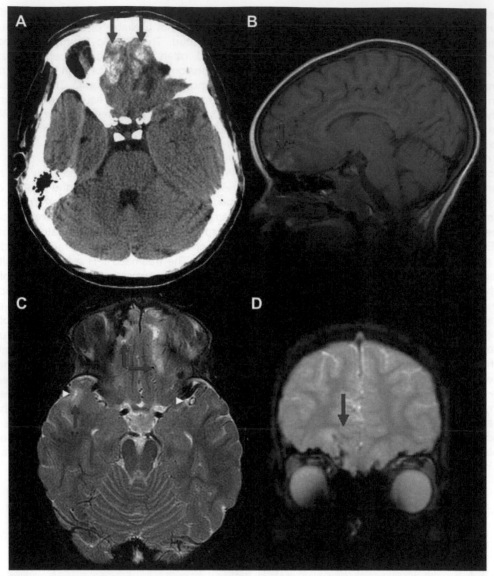

Fig. 31. **Subacute cortical contusions**. (*A*) Axial CT performed 32 hours after injury shows bilateral orbitofrontal hemorrhagic contusions (*arrows*). (*B*) Sagittal T1-weighted MR performed on admission day 4 demonstrates methemoglobin in this area (*arrow*). (*C*) Axial T2-weighted and (*D*) coronal gradient-echo imaging confirm the intracellular methemoglobin content of the contusions (*arrows*).

abscess, infarct, or neoplasm. Rarely, approximately 1 to 4 days following the onset of the initial trauma, delayed intracerebral hematomas can occur in areas that previously demonstrated focal contusions on CT or MR imaging.[86,87] These delayed hematomas tend to occur in multiple lobar locations and are associated with a poor prognosis. The proposed pathogenesis is reperfusion-associated hemorrhage secondary to initial vasospasm with subsequent vasodilation; this leads to initial hypotension with subsequent hypertension, and the injury is often further exacerbated by an underlying coagulopathy. Penetrating injuries (eg, gunshot wounds, sharp objects), of course, can also cause IPH in addition to EDH, SAH, and SDH.

Traumatic axonal injury
The mechanism of TAI is shear-strain deformation, that is, a change in shape of the brain without a change in volume. On the basis of neuropathologic findings, many investigators now consider "diffuse axonal injury/shearing injury" a misnomer because the injury is frequently not diffuse but

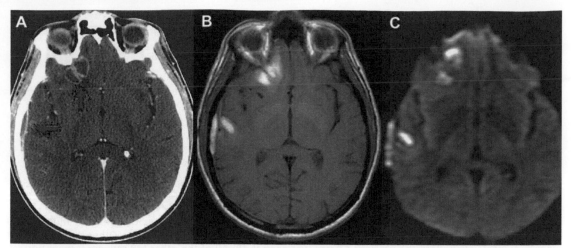

Fig. 32. Subacute contusions/hematoma. (*A*) Axial contrast-enhanced CT shows ring-enhancing lesions in the right anterior-inferior frontal lobe (*vertical arrow*). A peripherally enhancing right temporal extra-axial collection is also present (*horizontal arrow*). The enhancement is related to breakdown of the blood-brain barrier. (*B*) Axial T1-weighted MR image shows T1 shortening consistent with methemoglobin within subacute hemorrhage associated with the contusions and also the extra-axial collection. (*C*) Axial DWI shows hyperintensity within these subacute contusions and the extra-axial collection. It is important to remember that blood products can demonstrate high signal on DWI, mimicking "true" reduced diffusion. It is also important not to confuse this ring-enhancing appearance with neoplasm or infection. The biggest clue is the classic inferior frontal and temporal location, and the associated extra-axial collection; these findings prompted a search for soft tissue and bony injury, which revealed a fracture of the right temporal squamosa.

rather multifocal, and also because it is caused by tensile strain (not shear). Hence, the term TAI has been suggested to be more appropriate and is used here.

TAI typically results from a rotational deceleration/acceleration force that exceeds the elastic limit for the axon. Pathologically, there is an initial misalignment of the cytoskeleton and change in the axolemmal permeability that depends on the severity of the injury. The first evidence of TAI is believed to be focal neurofilament misalignment, which becomes striking within the first 6 hours after injury.[88] This misalignment leads to impaired axoplasmic transport and local accumulation of organelles. The effect continues for several hours after injury, causing local swelling and expansion of the axonal cylinder. Over time, disconnection of the axon occurs at 30 to 60 hours after injury, with eventual fiber loss (Wallerian degeneration).

Because of differences in tissue density and rigidity, as well as relative fixation of certain parts of the brain relative to the rigid calvarium, the deep and superficial regions of the brain may not move at the same rate or in the same direction; this results in strain distributed across axons, causing axonal stretching, swelling, and/or rupture. Initially it was thought that neuronal injury was limited to the acute and subacute phases after the event, followed by a short period of retrograde

and antegrade Wallerian degeneration, which can also be identified as early as 5 days. Newer studies, however, have demonstrated delayed progressive neuronal loss and atrophy[89] occurring days to weeks following the event.

The most common locations of TAI include the lobar gray-white matter junction, the corpus callosum,[90] and the dorsolateral midbrain. These 3 locations comprise the classic "shear injury triad." Other affected areas include the fornices, capsules, periventricular white matter, and superior cerebellar peduncles. The clinical manifestations of TAI depend on the severity of the injury, and can vary from mild postconcussive symptoms to coma.[91,92] The identification of TAI-related white matter lesions is critical, as they are thought to be responsible for the majority of TBI cognitive deficits. Unfortunately, TAI is often underdiagnosed with conventional imaging techniques, hence its description as the "stealth" pathology of TBI.

Patients with a discrepancy between their clinical status and their CT findings should undergo MR imaging, given its increased sensitivity to white matter and brainstem injury[93,94] and hence its far greater sensitivity in diagnosing TAI. On CT and MR imaging, the location of TAI tends to correlate with the severity of the trauma. Specifically, mild TAI (grade I) involves only the gray-white junction

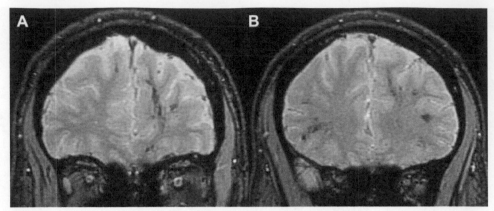

Fig. 33. Grade I TAI (chronic). (*A*) Coronal multiplanar gradient-recalled images demonstrate multiple T2-hyperintense foci involving the subcortical white matter of the frontal lobes bilaterally. Other than subtle left superior frontal volume loss, the patient's CT scan was normal. (*B*) All of the other MR sequences were normal, thus underscoring the role of GRE (and SWI) images in the identification of acute and chronic hemorrhagic TAI.

of the lobar white matter, commonly the parasagittal regions of the frontal lobes, and periventricular regions of the temporal lobes (see **Figs. 7** and **9**; **Fig. 33**). Patients with moderate TAI (Grade II) have lesions involving the corpus callosum, particularly the posterior body and splenium, in addition to the lobar white matter. In severe TAI (Grade III), the dorsolateral midbrain, in addition to the lobar white matter and corpus callosum, is involved (see **Fig. 6**).

In addition to TAI, primary brainstem injury can also occur from a direct contusion of the midbrain against the tentorial incisura. The distinction between a contusion and TAI may be important for long-term prognosis, as outcome from brainstem axonal injury is less favorable. Secondary brainstem injuries include:

- "Duret" hemorrhage (occurring in the setting of abrupt downward herniation)
- Compression of the midbrain by uncal herniation with a contralateral "Kernohan notch"
- Focal primary contusion to the brainstem due to impact with the ipsilateral tentorium
- Ischemic injury.

The most useful routine MR sequences for TBI/TAI include FLAIR, GRE, and DWI sequences. As mentioned, GRE is highly sensitive to small hemorrhagic lesions, but is limited in TAI because the majority of TAI lesions are actually nonhemorrhagic. FLAIR improves the sensitivity to nonhemorrhagic TAI, especially in the coronal and sagittal planes, which best detect injury to the corpus callosum and fornices. DWI may show reduced ADC in the setting of acute TAI, reflecting cytotoxic edema and cellular swelling. Though currently experimental, DTI, with or without 3D-color tractography, has provided insight into TAI, as discussed earlier. Specifically, the greater the proportion of damaged and/or distorted axons in the voxel, the lower the FA. In the more chronic stages, fiber disruption occurs, resulting in lower fiber density (causing decreased FA) and atrophy of white matter tissue on anatomic imaging. It should be noted that microscopically, one typically observes damaged, distorted fibers interspersed among normal appearing fibers; this intermixing of normal and abnormal axons is also represented in a single voxel because of partial volume effects. In summary, decreased FA in association with decreased longitudinal water diffusivity is consistent with impaired axonal transportation and loss of white matter integrity.

Subcortical gray matter injury
Injury to the thalami and basal ganglia is a rare manifestation of TBI, reportedly accounting for about 5% of parenchymal traumatic lesions. In the authors' experience, these lesions are more common in pediatric TBI than in adult TBI. On CT, these lesions may present as small hemorrhages in the basal ganglia, postulated to be secondary to disruption of small perforating blood vessels (see **Figs. 3** and **6**). The lesions are generally associated with a low initial GCS score.[42]

SUMMARY

Despite tremendous technological advances over the last 2 decades, noncontrast CT remains the primary initial imaging modality for acute TBI; concomitant CTA is often performed acutely for cases of suspected vascular injury. Conventional MR imaging is performed subsequently to better evaluate the extent of injury in patients who are not recovering as expected, and to fully characterize the extent of injury. Advanced imaging techniques such as fMR imaging, MRS, MEG, PET, and SPECT are all being investigated in patients with TBI with the hope of more accurately capturing the true burden of disease. These advanced imaging techniques show promise, as they are confirming the heterogeneous and dynamic nature of TBI, but they are largely confined to the research arena. It may turn out that the complementary use of combined advanced MR imaging techniques (eg, DTI + MEG or MRS + DTI)[60,95] is the best way to detect subtle neuronal injuries that cannot be detected by conventional MR imaging or CT techniques. Most of the data available at present are from small case series or case reports, and there are numerous logistic hurdles to overcome before they are "ready for prime time" in routine clinical practice. In addition, the financial burden of combining different neuroimaging techniques in today's cost-conscious, evidence-based climate is a real issue. Therefore, while there are numerous promising imaging biomarkers for TBI on the horizon, they require further study to fully determine their clinical utility in day-to-day practice. Further improvement in the neuroradiological evaluation of TBI should refine our current imaging approach and enhance our understanding of the pathophysiological manifestations (and therefore, treatment) of this epidemic disease. Until these advanced modalities become routine, however, the assessment of TBI will continue to rest on routine noncontrast head CT scans, supplemented, as discussed in this article, with vascular and MR imaging as appropriate.

REFERENCES

1. Marion D. Evidenced-based guidelines for traumatic brain injuries. Prog Neurol Surg 2006;19:171–96.
2. Finkelstein EA, Corso PC, Miller TR, et al. Incidence and economic burden of injuries in the United States, 2000. New York: Oxford University Press; 2006.
3. Corrigan J, Selassie A, Orman (Langlois) J. The epidemiology of traumatic brain injury. J Head Trauma Rehabil 2010;25:72–80.
4. Keenan HT, Bratton SL. Epidemiology and outcomes of pediatric traumatic brain injury. Dev Neurosci 2006;28:256–63.
5. Hyder AA, Wunderlich CA, Puvanachandra P, et al. The impact of traumatic brain injuries: a global perspective. NeuroRehabilitation 2007;22:341–53.
6. Teasdale G, Jennett B. Assessment of coma and impaired consciousness. A practical scale. Lancet 1974;2:81–4.
7. Saatman K, Duhaime C, Bullock R, et al. Classification of traumatic brain injury for targeted therapies. J Neurotrauma 2008;25:719–38.
8. Bazarian JJ, McClung J, Shah MN, et al. Mild traumatic brain injury in the United States, 1998–2000. Brain Inj 2005;19:85–91.
9. Lee H, Wintermark M, Gean AD, et al. Focal lesions in acute mild traumatic brain injury and neurocognitive outcome: CT versus 3T MRI. J Neurotrauma 2008;25:1049–56.
10. Ruff R. Two decades of advances in understanding of mild traumatic brain injury. J Head Trauma Rehabil 2004;20:5–18.
11. Kurca E, Sivak S, Kucera P. Impaired cognitive functions in mild traumatic brain injury patients with normal and pathologic magnetic resonance imaging. Neuroradiology 2006;48:661–9.
12. Stiver SI, Manley GT. Prehospital management of traumatic brain injury. Neurosurg Focus 2008;25:E5.
13. Bergsneider M, Hovda DA, McArthur DL, et al. Metabolic recovery following human traumatic brain injury based on FDG-PET: time course and relationship to neurological disability. J Head Trauma Rehabil 2001;16(2):135–48.
14. Davis PC. Head trauma. AJNR Am J Neuroradiol 2007;28:1619–21.
15. Provenzale J. CT and MR imaging of acute cranial trauma. Emerg Radiol 2007;14:1–12.
16. Stein SC, Burnett MG, Glick HA. Indications for CT scanning in mild traumatic brain injury: a cost-effectiveness study. J Trauma 2006;61:558–66.
17. Haydel MJ, Preston CA, Mills TJ, et al. Indications for computed tomography in patients with minor head injury. N Engl J Med 2000;343:100–5.
18. Stiell IG, Wells GA, Vandemheen K, et al. The Canadian CT head rule for patients with minor head injury. Lancet 2001;357:1391–6.
19. Haydel M. Clinical decision instruments for CT scanning in minor head injury. JAMA 2005;294(12):1551–3.
20. Enterline DS, Kapoor G. A practical approach to CT angiography of the neck and brain. Tech Vasc Interv Radiol 2006;9(4):192–204.
21. Wintermark M, van Melle G, Schnyder P, et al. Admission perfusion CT: prognostic value in patients with severe head trauma. Radiology 2004;232:211–20.
22. Wintermark M, Chiolero R, Van Melle G, et al. Cerebral vascular autoregulation assessed by perfusion-CT in severe head trauma patients. J Neuroradiol 2006;33:27–37.
23. Soustiel JF, Mahamid E, Goldsher D, et al. Perfusion-CT for early assessment of traumatic cerebral contusions. Neuroradiology 2008;50:189–96.
24. Garnett MR, Blamire AM, Corkill RG, et al. Abnormal cerebral blood volume in regions of contused and normal appearing brain following traumatic brain

injury using perfusion magnetic resonance imaging. J Neurotrauma 2001;18(6):585—93.

25. Woodcock RJ Jr, Short J, Do HM, et al. Imaging of acute subarachnoid hemorrhage with a fluid-attenuated inversion recovery sequence in an animal model: comparison with non-contrast-enhanced CT. AJNR Am J Neuroradiol 2001;22: 1698—703.

26. Yanagawa Y, Tsushima Y, Tokumaru A, et al. A quantitative analysis of head injury using T2-weighted gradient-echo imaging. J Trauma 2000; 49:272—7.

27. Messori A, Polonara G, Mabiglia C, et al. Is haemosiderin visible indefinitely on gradient-echo MRI following traumatic intracerebral haemorrhage? Neuroradiology 2003;45(12):881—6.

28. Schmiedeskamp H, Newbould RD, Pisani LJ, et al. Improvements in parallel imaging accelerated functional MRI using multiecho echo-planar imaging. Magn Reson Med 2010;63(4):959—69.

29. Haacke EM, Xu Y, Cheng YC, et al. Susceptibility weighted imaging (SWI). Magn Reson Med 2004; 52:612—8.

30. Babikian T, Freier MC, Tong KA, et al. Susceptibility weighted imaging: neuropsychologic outcome and pediatric head injury. Pediatr Neurol 2005;33: 184—94.

31. Tong KA, Ashwal S, Holshouser BA, et al. Diffuse axonal injury in children: clinical correlation with hemorrhagic lesions. Ann Neurol 2004;56:36—50.

32. Tong KA, Ashwal S, Holshouser BA, et al. Hemorrhagic shearing lesions in children and adolescents with posttraumatic diffuse axonal injury: improved detection and initial results. Radiology 2003;227: 332—9.

33. Wu Z, Li S, Lei J, et al. Evaluation of traumatic subarachnoid hemorrhage using susceptibility weighted imaging comparing with CT. J Magn Reson Imaging.

34. Liu AY, Maldjian JA, Bagley LJ, et al. Traumatic brain injury: diffusion-weighted MR imaging findings. AJNR Am J Neuroradiol 1999;20:1636—41.

35. Huisman TA, Sorensen AG, Hergan K, et al. Diffusion-weighted imaging for the evaluation of diffuse axonal injury in closed head injury. J Comput Assist Tomogr 2003;27:5—11.

36. Mori S, van Zijl PC. Fiber tracking: principles and strategies—A technical review. NMR Biomed 2002; 15:468—80.

37. Shimony JS, McKinstry RC, Akbudak E, et al. Quantitative diffusion-tensor anisotropy brain MR imaging: normative human data and anatomic analysis. Radiology 1999;212:770—84.

38. Niogi SN, Mukherjee P, Ghajar J, et al. Extent of microstructural white matter injury in postconcussive syndrome correlates with impaired cognitive reaction time: a 3T diffusion tensor imaging study of

mild traumatic brain injury. AJNR Am J Neuroradiol 2008;29:967—73.

39. Le TH, Mukherjee P, Henry RG, et al. Diffusion tensor imaging with three-dimensional fiber tractography of traumatic axonal shearing injury: an imaging correlate for the posterior callosal "disconnection" syndrome: case report. Neurosurgery 2005;56:189.

40. Arfanakis K, Haughton VM, Carew JD, et al. Diffusion tensor MR imaging in diffuse axonal injury. AJNR Am J Neuroradiol 2002;23:794—802.

41. Field AS. Diffusion tensor imaging at the crossroads: fiber tracking meets tissue characterization in brain tumors. AJNR Am J Neuroradiol 2005;26(9):2183—6.

42. Sinson G, Bagley LJ, Cecil KM, et al. Magnetization transfer imaging and proton MR spectroscopy in the evaluation of axonal injury: correlation with clinical outcome after traumatic brain injury. AJNR Am J Neuroradiol 2001;22:143—51.

43. Gasparovic C, Yeo R, Mannell M, et al. Neurometabolite concentrations in gray and white matter in mild traumatic brain injury: an ^{1}H-Magnetic Resonance Spectroscopy Study. J Neurotrauma 2009; 26(10):1635—43.

44. Holshouser BA, Tong KA, Ashwal S, et al. Proton MR spectroscopic imaging depicts diffuse axonal injury in children with traumatic brain injury. AJNR Am J Neuroradiol 2005;26:1276—85.

45. Danielsen ER, Christensen PB, Arlien-Soborg P, et al. Axonal recovery after severe traumatic brain injury demonstrated in vivo by 1H MR spectroscopy. Neuroradiology 2003;45:722—4.

46. Ross BD, Ernst T, Kreis R, et al. 1H MRS in acute traumatic brain injury. J Magn Reson Imaging 1998;8:829—40.

47. Govind V, Gold S, Kaliannan K. Whole-brain proton MR spectroscopic imaging of mild-to-moderate traumatic brain injury and correlation with neuropsychological deficits. J Neurotrauma 2010;27:483—96.

48. Logothetis NK, Pauls J, Augath M, et al. Neurophysiological investigation of the basis of the fMRI signal. Nature 2001;412(6843):150—7.

49. Cohen BA, Inglese M, Rusinek H. Proton MR spectroscopy and MRI-volumetry in mild traumatic brain injury. AJNR Am J Neuroradiol 2007;28:907—13.

50. Gowda NK, Agrawal D, Bal C, et al. Technetium Tc-99m ethyl cysteinate dimer brain single-photon emission ct in mild traumatic brain injury: a prospective study. AJNR Am J Neuroradiol 2006;27: 447—51.

51. Hofman PA, Stapert SZ, Kroonenburgh MJ, et al. MR imaging, single photon emission CT, and neurocognitive performance after mild traumatic brain injury. AJNR Am J Neuroradiol 2001;22:441—9.

52. Stamatakis ME, Wilson JT, Hadley DM, et al. SPECT imaging in head injury interpreted with statistical parametric mapping. J Nucl Med 2002; 43:470—00.

53. Fontaine A, Azouvi P, Remy P, et al. Functional anatomy of neuropsychological deficits after severe traumatic brain injury. Neurology 1999;53:1963–8.

54. McAllister TW, Sparling MB, Flashman LA, et al. Neuroimaging findings in mild traumatic brain injury. J Clin Exp Neuropsychol 2001;23:775–91.

55. Kinuya K, Kakuda K, Nobata K, et al. Role of brain perfusion single-photon emission tomography in traumatic head injury. Nucl Med Commun 2004; 25(4):333–7.

56. Ruff RM, Crouch JA, Tröster AI, et al. Selected cases of poor outcome following a minor brain trauma: comparing neuropsychological and positron emission tomography assessment. Brain Inj 1994;8:297–308.

57. Newberg AB, Alavi A. Neuroimaging in patients with head injury. Semin Nucl Med 2003;33:136–47.

58. Nakashima T, Nakayama N, Miwa K. Focal brain glucose hypometabolism in patients with neuropsychologic deficits after diffuse axonal injury. AJNR Am J Neuroradiol 2007;28:236–42.

59. Gross H, Kling A, Henry G, et al. Local cerebral glucose metabolism in patients with long-term behavioral and cognitive deficits following mild traumatic brain injury. J Neuropsychiatry Clin Neurosci 1996;8:324–34.

60. Lewine JD, Davis JT, Bigler ED, et al. Objective documentation of traumatic brain injury subsequent to mild head trauma: multimodal brain imaging with MEG, SPECT, and MRI. J Head Trauma Rehabil 2007;22(3):141–55.

61. Lewine JD, Davis JT, Sloan JH, et al. Neuromagnetic assessment of pathophysiologic brain activity induced by minor head trauma. AJNR Am J Neuroradiol 1999;20(5):857–66.

62. Huang MX, Theilmann RJ, Robb A, et al. Integrated imaging approach with MEG and DTI to detect mild traumatic brain injury in military and civilian patients. J Neurotrauma 2009;26(8):1213–26.

63. Little SC, Kesser BW. Radiographic classification of temporal bone fractures: clinical predictability using a new system. Arch Otolaryngol Head Neck Surg 2006;132:1300–4.

64. Provenzale JM. Dissection of the internal carotid and vertebral arteries: imaging features. AJR Am J Roentgenol 1995;165:1099–104.

65. York G, Barboriak D, Petrella J, et al. Association of internal carotid artery injury with carotid canal fractures in patients with head trauma. AJR Am J Roentgenol 2005;184:1672–8.

66. Krings T, Geibprasert S, Lasjaunias PL. Cerebrovascular trauma. Eur Radiol 2008;18:1531–45.

67. Young RJ, Destian S. Imaging of traumatic intracranial hemorrhage. Neuroimaging Clin N Am 2002;12: 189–204.

68. Zimmerman RA, Bilaniuk LT. Computed tomographic staging of traumatic epidural bleeding. Radiology 1982;144:809–12.

69. Gean AD, Fischbein NJ, Purcell DD, et al. The benign anterior temporal epidural hematoma (BAT_EDH): an indolent lesion with a characteristic imaging appearance. Radiology, in press.

70. Subramanian SK, Roszler MH, Gaudy B, et al. Significance of computed tomography mixed density in traumatic extra-axial hemorrhage. Neurol Res 2002;24:125–8.

71. Pruthi N, Balasubramaniam A, Chandramouli BA, et al. Mixed-density extradural hematomas on computed tomography-prognostic significance. Surg Neurol 2009;71:202–6.

72. Su TM, Lee TH, Chen WF, et al. Contralateral acute epidural hematoma after decompressive surgery of acute subdural hematoma: clinical features and outcome. J Trauma 2008;65:1298–302.

73. Gutman MB, Moulton RJ, Sullivan I, et al. Risk factors predicting operable intracranial hematomas in head injury. J Neurosurg 1992;77:9–14.

74. Greene KA, Marciano FF, Johnson BA, et al. Impact of traumatic subarachnoid hemorrhage on outcome in nonpenetrating head injury. Part I: a proposed computerized tomography grading scale. J Neurosurg 1995;83:445–52.

75. Martin NA, Doberstein C, Alexander M, et al. Post-traumatic cerebral arterial spasm. J Neurotrauma 1995;12:897–901.

76. Given CA 2nd, Burdette JH, Elster AD, et al. Pseudo-subarachnoid hemorrhage: a potential imaging pitfall associated with diffuse cerebral edema. AJNR Am J Neuroradiol 2003;24:254–6.

77. LeRoux PD, Haglund MM, Newell DW, et al. Intraventricular hemorrhage in blunt head trauma: an analysis of 43 cases. Neurosurgery 1992;31: 678–84 [discussion: 684–5].

78. Unterberg AW, Stover J, Kress B, et al. Edema and brain trauma. Neuroscience 2004;129:1021–9.

79. Polin RS, Shaffrey ME, Bogaev CA, et al. Decompressive bifrontal craniectomy in the treatment of severe refractory posttraumatic cerebral edema. Neurosurgery 1997;41:84–92 [discussion: 92–4].

80. Guerra WK, Gaab MR, Dietz H, et al. Surgical decompression for traumatic brain swelling: indications and results. J Neurosurg 1999;90:187–96.

81. Guerra WK, Piek J, Gaab MR. Decompressive craniectomy to treat intracranial hypertension in head injury patients. Intensive Care Med 1999;25: 1327–9.

82. Kunze E, Meixensberger J, Janka M, et al. Decompressive craniectomy in patients with uncontrollable intracranial hypertension. Acta Neurochir Suppl 1998;71:16–8.

83. Albanese J, Leone M, Alliez JR, et al. Decompressive craniectomy for severe traumatic brain injury: evaluation of the effects at one year. Crit Care Med 2003;31:2535–8.

84. Stiver SI, Wintermark M, Manley GT. Reversible monoparesis following decompressive hemicraniectomy for traumatic brain injury. J Neurosurg 2008; 109:245–54.

85. Gentry LR, Godersky JC, Thompson B. MR imaging of head trauma: review of the distribution and radiopathologic features of traumatic lesions. AJR Am J Roentgenol 1988;150:663–72.

86. Lipper MH, Kishore PR, Girevendulis AK, et al. Delayed intracranial hematoma in patients with severe head injury. Radiology 1979;133(3 Pt 1):645–9.

87. Nanassis K, Frowein RA, Karimi A, et al. Delayed post-traumatic intracerebral bleeding. Delayed post-traumatic apoplexy: "Spatapoplexie". Neurosurg Rev 1989;12(Suppl 1):243–51.

88. Povlishock JT. Pathophysiology of neural injury: therapeutic opportunities and challenges. Clin Neurosurg 2000;46:113–26.

89. Hammoud DA, Wasserman BA. Diffuse axonal injuries: pathophysiology and imaging. Neuroimaging Clin N Am 2002;12:205–16.

90. Chang MC, Jang SH. Corpus callosum injury in patients with diffuse axonal injury: a diffusion tensor imaging study. NeuroRehabilitation 2010;26(4):339–45.

91. Rutgers DR, Toulgoat F, Cazejust J, et al. White matter abnormalities in mild traumatic brain injury: a diffusion tensor imaging study. AJNR Am J Neuroradiol 2008;29:514–9.

92. Mittl RL, Grossman RI, Hiehle JF, et al. Prevalence of MR evidence of diffuse axonal injury in patients with mild head injury and normal head CT findings. AJNR Am J Neuroradiol 1994;15:1583–9.

93. Gentry LR, Thompson B, Godersky JC. Trauma to the corpus callosum: MR features. AJNR Am J Neuroradiol 1988;9:1129–38.

94. Gentry LR, Godersky JC, Thompson B, et al. Prospective comparative study of intermediate-field MR and CT in the evaluation of closed head trauma. AJR Am J Roentgenol 1988;150:673–82.

95. Kou Z, Wu Z, Tong KA, et al. The role of advanced MR imaging findings as biomarkers of traumatic brain injury. J Head Trauma Rehabil 2010;25(4):267–82.

Central Nervous System Infection

Ashley H. Aiken

KEYWORDS

- CNS infections • Meningitis • Abscess • Encephalitis
- Subdural empyema

Infections of the brain and its linings pose a growing, worldwide health problem. Widespread immigration, the emergence of multidrug-resistant strains, and HIV infection have all served to change the face of the diagnosis and imaging of central nervous system (CNS) infections.

The radiologist plays a crucial role in identifying and narrowing the differential diagnosis of CNS infection. This article aims to outline a practical imaging approach, which begins with recognizing 1 of 5 basic imaging patterns: (1) extra-axial lesion, (2) ring-enhancing lesion, (3) temporal lobe lesion, (4) basal ganglia lesion, and (5) white matter abnormality.

Within these broad imaging categories, a thorough understanding of the characteristic imaging features of specific pathogens and clinical history, including patient immune status and geographic location, are essential to narrow the differential considerations and propose a more specific diagnosis.

Neuroimaging also plays a pivotal role in diagnosing and monitoring the therapeutic response in opportunistic infections in the setting of HIV. This subset of infections will also be discussed within the context of the 5 basic imaging patterns.

IMAGING MODALITIES

CT is often the first imaging study for the evaluation of suspected CNS infection because of its widespread availability and rapid assessment of complications such as hydrocephalus, mass effect/herniation, and hemorrhage. CT is critical in the emergency room setting to identify these neurosurgical emergencies. However, MRI is the study of choice for further characterization of CNS infection, and it is more sensitive for the identification of leptomeningitis, empyema, ventriculitis, and complications, such as cerebral infarction. The most important MR sequences in this setting include the following:

- Diffusion-weighted imaging (DWI)
- Fluid attenuated inversion recovery (FLAIR)
- T2-weighted (T2W)
- T1-weighted post-gadolinium (GAD)
- Magnetic resonance spectroscopy (MRS).

Diffusion-weighted imaging (DWI) plays an important role in differentiating a pyogenic abscess from other ring-enhancing lesions. Pyogenic abscesses classically have reduced diffusion ("light bulb bright diffusion"), which is thought to reflect the high viscosity of inflammatory cells. However, reduced diffusion is not specific to pyogenic abscess, and it may be present in other ring-enhancing lesions, including hypercellular tumor, subacute hematomas, and nonpyogenic infections.[1–9] DWI is also useful in detecting and characterizing extra-axial collections, as subdural empyemas typically have reduced diffusion.[7]

Fluid attenuated inversion recovery (FLAIR) imaging uses an inversion recovery pulse after an inversion time to nullify the high signal of cerebrospinal fluid (CSF). FLAIR is sensitive in detecting leptomeningeal disease because elevated protein in the subarachnoid space (SAS) causes a decrease in T1 relaxation time and resultant hyperintensity. In spite of the high sensitivity of FLAIR images in the detection of abnormal SAS

Division of Neuroradiology, Emory University Hospital, 1364 Clifton Road, Suite BG 26, Atlanta, GA 30322, USA
E-mail address: Ashley.aiken@emoryhealthcare.org

Neuroimag Clin N Am 20 (2010) 557–580
doi:10.1016/j.nic.2010.07.011

hyperintensity, this finding is not specific for lepto-meningitis; it may also be encountered with lepto-meningeal tumor, subarachnoid hemorrhage, supplemental O_2 administration, and severe arterial occlusive disease with slow flow in leptomeningeal collaterals.

T2-weighted (T2W) imaging is most helpful for evaluation the core signal intensity of ring-enhancing lesions, and to define the extent of surrounding vasogenic edema. T1-weighted post-gadolinium (GAD) imaging is critical to evaluate the enhancement characteristics of infectious etiologies. Specific patterns are discussed in the section on imaging patterns to follow.

Magnetic resonance spectroscopy (MRS) shows increases in lactate (1.3 ppm), acetate (1.92 ppm), and succinate (2.4 ppm) in pyogenic abscesses, presumably from the enhanced glycolysis and fermentation of the organism. Amino acids, including valine and leucine (0.9 ppm), are also known to be the end products of proteolysis by enzymes released by neutrophils in pus. Detection of resonance peaks from acetate, succinate, and such amino acids as valine and leucine is suggestive of abscess, as they have not been reported in proton MR spectra of brain tumors.[10–12]

IMAGING PATTERNS
Extra-axial

With this imaging pattern, it is key to search the paranasal sinuses, middle ear, and mastoid air cells for a source. It is also very important to look for complications including brain abscess, dural sinus thrombosis, infarction, and hydrocephalus.

Epidural empyema

An epidural abscess and/or empyema most commonly extends from the paranasal sinuses, especially the frontal sinus. Extension may be via direct bony erosion or retrograde flow via valveless bridging veins. Other etiologies include recent surgery, trauma, and mastoiditis. This purulent collection localizes outside the dura, which protects the underlying brain parenchyma. Therefore, patients with an epidural empyema tend to have a more benign, insidious course than those with a subdural empyema. Patients often complain only of a fever and headache.

On imaging, epidural abscesses are lentiform in shape, tacked down at the sutures, but they can cross the midline, unlike subdural collections (Fig. 1). The MR signal characteristics include T1 hypointensity, which is brighter than pure CSF given its proteinaceous content and inflammatory debris, and T2 hyperintensity, approaching CSF intensity. On post-GAD images, there is profound enhancement of the inflamed dura, often more than seen in subdural empyemas. Another important imaging feature of epidural empyemas is the relatively normal appearance of the underlying brain parenchyma in contrast to subdural empyemas.[13] Empyemas classically have reduced diffusion. However, the DWI signal characteristics can be more complex in epidural as opposed to subdural empyemas. Because epidural empyemas tend to have a more prolonged course, portions of the lesion may become less viscous, allowing for mixed intensity on DWI.[7] Please refer to "Acute Neuro-Interventional Therapies," elsewhere in this issue, for additional imaging information.

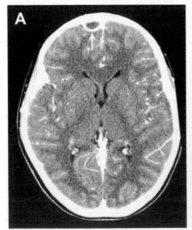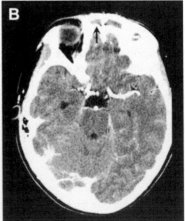

Fig. 1. **Frontal sinusitis and epidural abscess.** 11-year-old boy with severe headache. (*A*) Axial contrast-enhanced CT shows a right frontal peripherally enhancing lentiform collection (*arrow*), compatible with epidural abscess. (*B*) An inferior axial CT slice shows contiguous bilateral frontal sinus opacification (*arrow*).

Key Imaging Features: Epidural Empyema

- Lentiform collection
- Reduced diffusion
- Look for source in paranasal sinuses or mastoid air cells.

Subdural empyema

The source of most subdural empyemas is also sinusitis or mastoiditis, with frontal sinusitis accounting for most cases. Other etiologies include prior trauma with a superinfected subdural hematoma, postcraniotomy, or a complication of meningitis. Patients may present with fever, headache, seizures, and focal neurologic deficits. The subdural empyema is a medical emergency and usually requires neurosurgical intervention.

Neuroimaging plays a key role in early diagnosis and characterization. CT is often used acutely because of its speed and widespread availability. It is most useful in defining the extent and degree of mass effect and herniation; however, small subdural empyemas can be missed on CT, especially when located along the inner table of the skull.[14] MRI is helpful in diagnosing and differentiating a subdural empyema from other subdural collections, including a subdural effusion, chronic subdural hematoma, and a subdural hygroma that may mimic an empyema on CT (Fig. 2). Subdural empyemas have similar T1 and T2 signal characteristics to epidural empyemas, and classically show reduced diffusion, identified as high signal on DWI and low signal on the apparent diffusion coefficient (ADC) map.

Key Imaging Features: Subdural Empyema

- Reduced diffusion
- Look for source in paranasal sinuses or mastoid air cells

Leptomeningitis

Meningitis refers to acute or chronic inflammation of the pia-arachnoid layers and the adjacent CSF. It may be viral, bacterial, or fungal. The diagnosis usually is based on clinical history, physical examination, and CSF analysis, with imaging playing a limited role. The clinical presentation is often characteristic, with fever, headache, neck stiffness, vomiting, and photophobia being most common.

Imaging is most useful to evaluate the complications of meningitis, including vascular thrombosis, infarctions, brain abscess, ventriculitis, hydrocephalus, and extra-axial empyemas. Post-GAD and FLAIR sequences are most sensitive for detecting abnormal meningeal enhancement and SAS disease, respectively.[15] DWI is particularly helpful in the identification of complications, such as infarction or subdural empyema. Acute bacterial or viral meningitis typically shows enhancement over the cerebrum and interhemispheric fissure, whereas chronic tuberculous or fungal meningitis classically shows enhancement in the basal cisterns (Fig. 3).

Tuberculous meningitis, the most common presentation of neurotuberculosis, occurs predominately in young children and adolescents. It usually presents as a long-standing insidious process with exuberant inflammation of the basilar meninges and an obliterative vasculopathy of the basal penetrating vessels. Most infarcts are thus seen in the basal ganglia and internal capsule (see Fig. 3C).[16] The common imaging triad consists of basal meningeal enhancement, hydrocephalus, and cerebral infarction.[17] Leptomeningeal enhancement is not specific for infectious meningitis, and can also be seen with carcinomatous meningitis, sarcoidosis, or chemical meningitis.

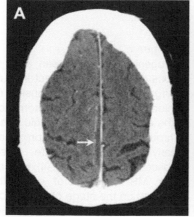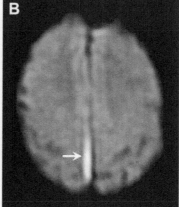

Fig. 2. Meningitis with subdural empyema. 56-year-old female with meningitis and new left leg shaking. (*A*) Axial contrast-enhanced CT shows a right parafalcine subdural collection (*arrow*). (*B*) DWI shows reduced diffusion compatible with subdural empyema (*arrow*).

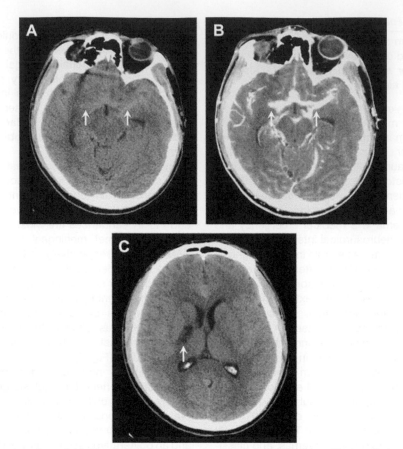

Fig. 3. Coccidiomycosis and basilar meningitis. 23-year-old migrant worker with headache and left upper extremity weakness. (*A*) Noncontrast CT shows hyperdensity in the basilar cisterns (*arrows*). (*B*) Contrast-enhanced CT shows abnormal enhancement of the basilar meninges (*arrows*). (*C*) Noncontrast CT at the level of the basal ganglia shows an infarct in the posterior limb of the right internal capsule (*arrow*), thus explaining the patient's clinical presentation. Perforating artery infarctions are a potential complication of basilar meningitis secondary to the associated inflammatory arteriopathy.

Key Imaging Features: Leptomeningitis

- SAS hyperintensity on FLAIR
- Leptomeningeal enhancement
- Look for hydrocephalus and infarctions as complications.

Ring-enhancing Lesions

This imaging pattern is the classic mimicker, and there is a long list of differential considerations. Frequently, the primary differential can be narrowed to infection versus neoplasm; however, close attention to the imaging features is critical to recognize nonoperative ring-enhancing lesions such as tumefactive demyelination, subacute infarct, and subacute hematoma. The imaging characteristics that favor infection over neoplasm include a thin, smooth, ring-enhancement, "daughter cysts," a thinner ring of enhancement

toward the ventricular surface, and, of course, the "light bulb bright DWI" of a pyogenic abscess.

Pyogenic abscess

Pyogenic abscesses can arise from hematogenous dissemination, direct inoculation (trauma or surgery), contiguous extension (paranasal sinus, middle ear, mastoids), or complicating meningitis. The evolution of a pyogenic abscess progresses through 4 stages over approximately 2 weeks: (1) early cerebritis, (2) late cerebritis, (3) early abscess/capsule, and (4) late abscess/capsule. The MRI features of cerebritis and abscess depend on the stage of this infectious process.

In the early cerebritis stage, ill-defined T1 hypo-intensity and T2 hyperintensity are noted, with mottled heterogeneous enhancement. As the infection matures, the necrotic debris accumulates centrally and the body attempts to isolate the infection with a collagenous capsule. Centrally, the abscess cavity is T1 hypointense (but slightly higher than CSF) and T2 hyperintense (Fig. 4). The abscess capsule is iso- or slightly hyperintense on T1-weighted images and markedly hypointense on T2-weighted imaging; this is thought to be secondary to paramagnetic hemoglobin degradation products or free radicals in macrophages. On post-GAD images, a thin, smooth ring is characteristic, in contrast to necrotic tumors, which typically have a thick nodular ring enhancement (Fig. 5). Another important feature of a brain abscess is its tendency to "grow toward the white matter," resulting in an oval configuration with a thicker enhancing capsule toward the more well-vascularized cortex. The thinner capsule abutting the white matter helps explain the propensity for intraventricular rupture and subsequent ventriculitis. Imaging features of ventriculitis/ependymitis include enhancement of the ventricular wall and reduced diffusion (Fig. 6). Ventriculitis is rarely isolated and usually occurs in the setting of abscess rupture, meningitis, or shunting and increases mortality to 80%.

DWI is extremely useful in identifying a brain abscess. As mentioned previously, the pyogenic brain abscess typically has "light bulb bright"

diffusion signal intensity with corresponding low ADC values. Although some tumors can have low ADC values because of hypercellularity, the necrotic or cystic portions are usually less cellular and therefore do not show the same reduced diffusion.[1,2,4,6,9]

Key Imaging Features: Pyogenic Abscess

- "Light bulb bright" DWI
- Central T2 hyperintensity
- T2 hypointense capsule.

Tuberculoma

A global increase in the incidence of tuberculosis (TB) can be attributed to increased immigration, AIDS, and multidrug-resistant strains. CNS infection with *Mycobacterium tuberculosis* can present as either of the following:

- Diffuse form (eg, basal exudative leptomeningitis, as discussed previously)
- Localized form (eg, tuberculoma, abscess, or cerebritis).

The most common parenchymal form of CNS TB is tuberculous granuloma (tuberculoma). In some countries, TB represents up to 10% to 30% of all focal intracranial masses.

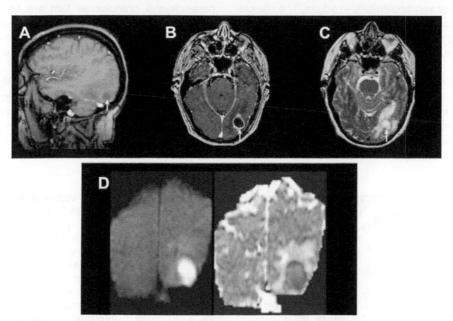

Fig. 4. **Pyogenic abscess.** 65-year-old woman with fever and vision loss. (*A*) Sagittal T1-weighted image shows the typical central T1 hypointensity (*arrow*). A T1 hyperintense rim can be seen in some cases. (*B*) Axial post-GAD T1-weighted image shows thin, smooth, ring enhancement that is typical for infection (*arrow*). Also, small daughter cysts are shown anteriorly and posteriorly. (*C*) Axial T2-weighted image shows the typical T2 hypointense rim, central T2 hyperintensity, and marked surrounding vasogenic edema, characteristic of the pyogenic brain abscess (*arrow*). (*D*) Axial DWI shows "light bulb" bright diffusion and hypointensity on the ADC map, consistent with true reduced diffusion.

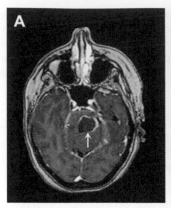
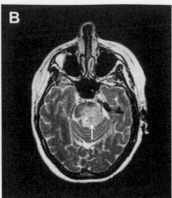
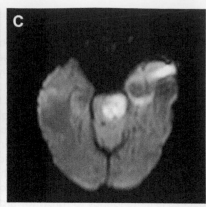

Fig. 5. Brainstem pyogenic abscess mimicking glioblastoma multiforme (GBM). 53-year-old man presented for preoperative evaluation for presumed GBM, without signs and symptoms of infection. (*A*) Axial post-GAD T1-weighted image shows thin, smooth enhancement of the pontine lesion (*arrow*), findings that are more suggestive of infection than neoplasm. (*B*) Axial T2-weighted image reveals ill-defined T2 hyperintensity (*arrow*) rather than the more typical discrete T2 hyperintensity; this finding suggests an earlier stage of infection. (*C*) Axial DWI and ADC map show reduced diffusion. Although GBMs may be hypercellular and show reduced diffusion, the combination of reduced diffusion and thin ring enhancement are key to the diagnosis of an abscess.

Parenchymal TB is more common in HIV-infected patients, can be solitary or multiple, and can occur with or without meningitis.[18] There is hematogenous spread in cases of known pulmonary TB.

Tuberculomas occur at the corticomedullary junction and are more common infratentorially in children and supratentorially in adults. The clinical presentation is often related to the space-occupying mass effect (ie, seizures, focal neurologic signs, headache, papilledema) rather than to the infection.

The MRI features depend on whether the granuloma is noncaseating, solid-caseating, or cystic-caseating. Noncaseating granulomas are T2 hypointense and solidly enhancing. Caseating granulomas have smooth ring enhancement. Solid caseating granulomas have characteristic T2 hypointensity (**Fig. 7**), whereas cystic-caseating granulomas have central T2 hyperintensity similar to pyogenic abscess. The dark T2 signal is thought to be caused by free radicals, and the solid caseation signal is attributed to cellular density.[17,19] Finally, the tuberculous abscess is a rare complication developing from parenchymal granulomas that are teeming with tubercle bacilli. Similar to cystic-caseating granulomas, these lesions show central T2 hyperintensity and even reduced diffusion, which can therefore mimic pyogenic abscess.[17,20] Some investigators suggest that MRS may help differentiate tubercular abscess from pyogenic abscess. Specifically, identification of the amino acids acetate and succinate are found in pyogenic abscesses, but lipid peaks are found in tubercular abscesses.[20]

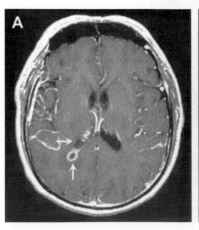
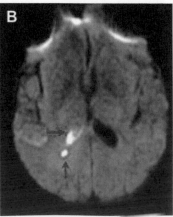

Fig. 6. Ventriculitis. 65-year-old man with fever after shunt placement. (*A*) Axial post-GAD T1-weighted image shows a ring-enhancing abscess adjacent to the atrium of the right lateral ventricle (*vertical arrow*). Note also subtle subependymal enhancement and higher signal intensity in the ventricle indicating ventriculitis (*horizontal arrow*). (*B*) Axial DWI at the same level demonstrates *reduced diffusion* in both the abscess (*vertical arrow*) and the debris within the ventricle (*horizontal arrow*).

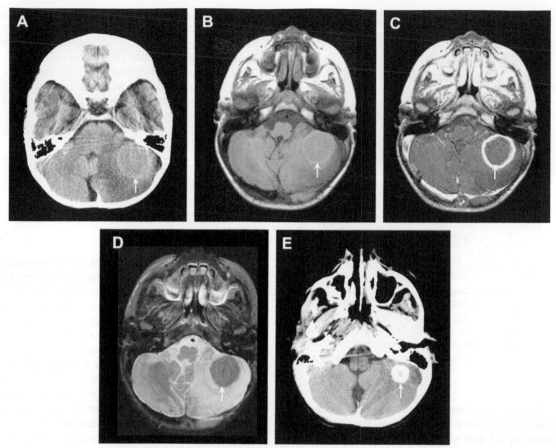

Fig. 7. Caseating tuberculoma. 3-year-old boy with fever, lethargy, and abnormal chest x-ray. (*A*) Axial noncontrast CT shows a round, slightly hyperdense mass with surrounding vasogenic edema located in the left cerebellar hemisphere (*arrow*). Note that the slight hyperdensity would be atypical for pyogenic abscess. (*B*) Axial noncontrast T1-weighted image reveals a thin hyperintense rim around the mass (*arrow*). (*C*) Axial post-GAD T1-weighted image shows smooth ring-enhancement (*arrow*), which favors infection over neoplasm. (*D*) Axial T2-weighted image shows uniform T2 hypointensity (*arrow*), which suggests an atypical infection rather than pyogenic infection. (*E*) Axial CT image obtained 1 year after treatment demonstrates dense calcification that is sometimes termed a "brain stone" (*arrow*).

Key Imaging Feature: Tuberculoma

- Central T2 hypointensity in noncaseating and solid caseating tuberculomas, ± reduced diffusion.

Neurocysticercosis

Neurocysticercosis, caused by the pork tapeworm *Taenia solium,* is the most common parasitic infection of the CNS in immunocompetent individuals. Endemic in Latin America and parts of Asia, India, Africa, and Eastern Europe, it is the most common cause of seizures in young patients in developing countries with poor hygiene. Neurocysticercosis may involve the brain parenchyma, the subarachnoid space, and the ventricles. [21–23]

CT and MRI findings in parenchymal neurocysticercosis depend on the stage of development of the parasite. Four stages have been categorized[24,25]: (1) viable/vesicular, (2) colloidal, (3) nodular-granular, and (4) calcified.

In the first, vesicular, stage, small cysts follow CSF density on CT and CSF intensity on MRI, and show little to no enhancement or edema. Most of these lesions have a "cyst with a dot" appearance representing an eccentric scolex (Fig. 8).

Colloidal lesions develop ring enhancement and surrounding edema as the parasite degenerates and triggers the host immune response. MRI characteristics in the second colloidal phase include central T1 hypointensity, central T2 hyperintensity, ring-enhancement, and *increased* diffusion (Fig. 9).

During the nodular-granular phase, the cyst wall thickens, the cyst involutes, and the surrounding edema decreases.

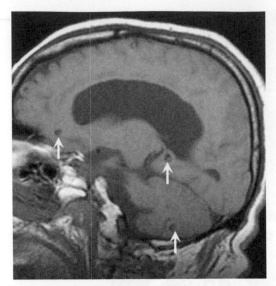

Fig. 8. Vesicular stage of neurocysticercosis. 40-year-old man with seizures. Sagittal T1-weighted image demonstrates multiple lesions that have a "cyst with a dot" appearance (*arrows*). This is a classic finding in vesicular neurocysticercosis where the "dot" represents the scolex. Note the *absence* of mass effect and edema.

Finally, the lesion mineralizes in the calcified stage and appears as small parenchymal calcifications on CT and small areas of susceptibility on MR gradient sequences (see Fig. 9D, E).

The colloidal stage mimics other ring-enhancing lesions. In these cases, DWI may be helpful to differentiate a cysticercosis cyst from a pyogenic abscess because cysticercal cysts are dark.[23] Also, ADC values are higher in neurocysticercosis than in TB granulomas.[26]

Subarachnoid lesions may be small in the cortical sulci, but are often large and "grapelike" when located in the basilar cisterns or Sylvian fissures. In the past, the term "racemose" referred to this form in which the scolex was not thought to develop; however, it is now known that the scolex may be present, yet undergoes degeneration, such that the term "racemose" has fallen into disuse.[23] Ruptured subarachnoid lesions may produce a basilar meningitis and lead to vasculitis and lacunar infarction.[23] Ventricular cysticerci are usually isodense to CSF on CT and isointense to CSF on T2-weighted MR imaging, thus making them difficult to detect. Intraventricular cysticercosis occurs in approximately 20% of cases and is most often located in the aqueduct of Sylvius or fourth ventricle.[13] Frequently, the accompanying hydrocephalus is detected before the obstructing cyst is identified. Therefore, FLAIR is a critical sequence to localize intraventricular

cysts, because the cysts will appear hyperintense to CSF and become more conspicuous (Fig. 10). Cysts can migrate within the ventricular system (the "ventricular migration sign") and cause intermittent obstructive hydrocephalus.[27] Treatment includes antiparasitic medications such as oral albendazole, steroids for edema, and antiseizure medications in selected cases.[23]

Key Imaging Features: Neurocysticercosis

- Central T2 hyperintensity
- Dark DWI (*increased* diffusion)
- Scolex
- Additional calcifications.

Aspergillosis

Invasive CNS aspergillosis is rare, but is seen with increased frequency in immunosuppressed patients, particularly after bone marrow transplantation (BMT).[28] Because humans are infected by inhaling spores, the lungs and paranasal sinuses are the main sites of infection. Cerebral involvement may also result from hematogenous spread from the lungs or direct invasion from the sinuses. Invasive CNS aspergillosis has high morbidity and mortality, but case reports do note survival with early, aggressive antifungal therapy and surgical resection.[29,30] As clinical and laboratory features do not always confirm the diagnosis, neuroimaging plays a key role.[31]

Imaging patterns depend on lesion age and immunologic status of the patient. The angioinvasive nature of the fungus helps explain the CT and MR imaging features of these cortical and subcortical septic infarctions. Aspergillosis also has a unique affinity for perforating arteries that supply the basal ganglia, thalami, and corpus callosum.[32] In severely immunocompromised patients, the lesions appear as poorly defined areas of CT hypodensity or T2 hyperintensity on MRI, without significant mass effect, surrounding edema, or enhancement owing to the lack of a host immune response. In more immunocompetent patients, or as the immune function recovers after BMT, subtle peripheral or ring enhancement may be seen with surrounding vasogenic edema (Fig. 11).[28] Another important clue to the diagnosis is the presence of hemorrhage within these septic infarcts (seen as T1 hyperintensity, T2 hypointensity, and abnormal magnetic susceptibility on gradient sequences). In addition, pyogenic abscesses typically have a *smooth* outer wall, whereas fungal abscesses tend to have a *crenated* wall with intracavitary projections.[20] Although early septic infarcts may show reduced diffusion, Luthra and colleagues[20] found reduced diffusion only in

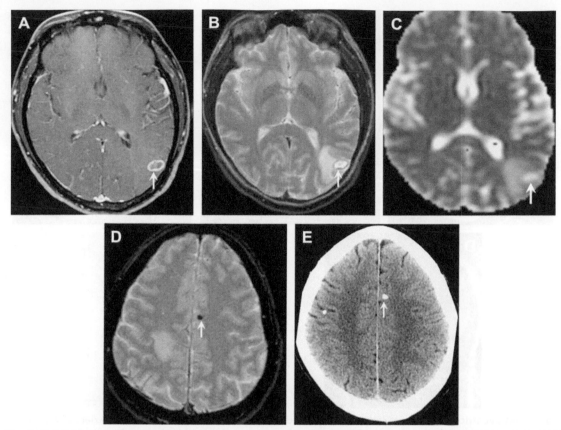

Fig. 9. Colloidal stage and nodular calcified stage of neurocysticercosis. 39-year-old man with new seizure. (*A*) Axial post-GAD T1-weighted image shows a ring-enhancing lesion (*arrow*) with a thin, smooth ring favoring infection. An eccentric, internal "dot" should always raise the possibility of neurocysticercosis. (*B*) Axial T2-weighted image also shows this eccentric "dot" (*arrow*). The central T2 hyperintensity and T2 hypointense rim can mimic pyogenic infection, but DWI should help distinguish. (*C*) Axial ADC map demonstrates *increased* rather than reduced diffusion (*arrow*), suggesting atypical infection rather than pyogenic infection. (*D*) Axial gradient-echo image demonstrates a focus of susceptibility (*arrow*). (*E*) Axial CT shows that the abnormal focus of susceptibility corresponds to calcification (*arrow*). Note the lack of edema and mass effect. Such calcifications are an important clue to the diagnosis of neurocysticercosis which represents the late calcified stage that easily seen on CT.

the wall and projections of the fungal abscess, whereas the core did not show reduced diffusion, distinguishing it from pyogenic and tubercular abscesses.

Key Imaging Features: Aspergillosis

- Angioinvasion with hemorrhage (T2 hypointensity + susceptibility)
- Septic infarcts with minimal mass effect and minimal to no enhancement
- Ring C+ only as immune function recovers
- Mycotic aneurysms.

Toxoplasmosis

Toxoplasmosis is caused by the parasite *Toxoplasma gondii* and is the most common mass lesion in patients with AIDS. Fortunately, the number of cases has declined significantly within the past decade because of the advent of highly active antiretroviral therapy (HAART).[33,34] *T gondii* is an obligate intracellular protozoan that exists in 3 forms: oocysts, tachyzoites, and bradyzoites. Tachyzoites are the rapidly multiplying form and they convert to bradyzoites or tissue cysts when they localize to the CNS.[34] Toxoplasmosis is a ubiquitous organism with titers as high as 70% in the normal adult population. The primary form of transmission is ingestion of undercooked meat, but also blood transfusions, contaminated needles, and contact with cat feces can result in the infection.[35] HIV-infected patients become most susceptible to toxoplasmosis when their CD4 counts are less than 100 cells/μL. The most common presenting symptom is headache, but fever, altered mental status, and focal deficits are also seen.[36]

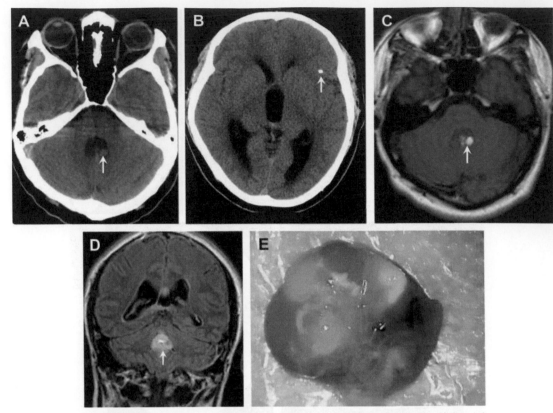

Fig. 10. Intraventricular neurocysticercosis. 30-year-old man with increasing headache. (*A*) Axial noncontrast CT shows enlargement of the fourth ventricle and a round eccentric nodule within the fourth ventricle (*arrow*). Note that the nodule appears too small to obstruct the fourth ventricle. (*B*) Axial CT at a higher level reveals enlargement of the lateral and third ventricles compatible with hydrocephalus. A clue to the etiology of the fourth ventricular lesion is the focal calcification in the left inferior frontal lobe (*arrow*). (*C*) Axial noncontrast T1-weighted image shows an atypical appearance consisting of intrinsic T1 hyperintensity in a neurocysticercosis cyst, secondary to proteinaceous debris (*arrow*). (*D*) Coronal FLAIR image shows that the cyst actually fills the *entire* fourth ventricle (*arrow*), explaining the obstructive hydrocephalus. This case illustrates why FLAIR can be helpful for identifying intraventricular cysts, as they can be difficult to see on CT and on T2-weighted images because they often follow CSF density and intensity, respectively. (*E*) Gross pathologic specimen revealing the proteinaceous components of this cyst.

On noncontrast CT, lesions are usually multiple, hypodense, and located in the basal ganglia, thalami, and corticomedullary junction.[37] The lesions frequently calcify after treatment. On MRI, the T2 signal characteristics can be variable, ranging from T2 hyperintense to T2 iso- or even hypointense.[38] On T1-weighted images, the lesions are hypointense, but intrinsic T1 shortening has been described in a few cases, thought to represent hemorrhage.[39] Smooth, ring enhancement is typically seen on post-GAD images, but smaller lesions may have more nodular enhancement. An imaging finding highly suggestive of toxoplasmosis is the "asymmetric target sign," which consists of a small eccentric nodule of enhancement along the enhancing wall, thought to represent infolding of the cyst wall (**Fig. 12**).[35] This sign is specific, but not sensitive (seen in ~30% cases).[34] Recently, a similar target sign has been described on FLAIR and T2-weighted imaging that consists of 3 layers: T2 hypointense core alternating with an intermediate zone of T2 hyperintensity and a T2 hypointense rim.[40] Although DWI signal can be variable in toxoplasmosis, most investigators have found that most lesions have *increased* diffusion on DWI.[8,41]

In the HIV-infected patient, the major differential consideration for multiple ring-enhancing lesions is primary CNS lymphoma. Imaging features that favor lymphoma include subependymal spread, reduced diffusion owing to hypercellularity, and corpus callosum involvement. Most patients are treated empirically for toxoplasmosis with

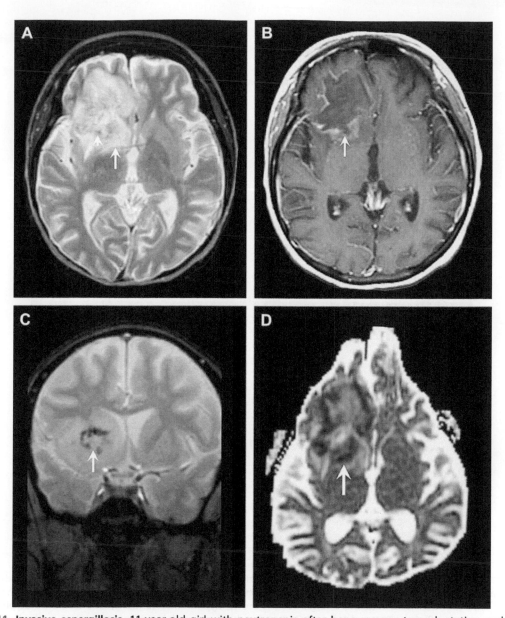

Fig. 11. Invasive aspergillosis. 11-year-old girl with neutropenia after bone marrow transplantation and new fevers. (*A*) Axial T2-weighted image shows a large, predominately T2 hyperintense lesion that involves most of the right inferior frontal lobe, putamen, and caudate head (*large arrow*). Note the small amount of mass effect given the size of the lesion. Also, note the small T2-hypointense areas within this lesion (*short arrow*). (*B*) Axial post-GAD T1-weighted image shows mild peripheral ring enhancement (*arrow*). Again, there is little to no mass effect. (*C*) Coronal gradient-echo image demonstrates susceptibility within this mass (*arrow*), consistent with hemorrhage. *Minimal enhancement, minimal mass effect, and hemorrhage are all clues* to diagnosis of invasive aspergillosis in this neutropenic patient. (*D*) Axial ADC map demonstrates reduced diffusion along the margins of the lesion (*arrow*), but no centrally reduced diffusion that is typical for pyogenic infection.

pyrimethamine and sulfadiazine for a duration of 6 weeks.[42] Radiographic improvement should occur in most (>90%) patients by 14 days.[36] If a follow-up MRI does not show improvement after empiric therapy, thallium-201 brain single-photon emission computed tomography (SPECT) or fluoro-deoxyglucose positron emission tomography (FDG PET) may be useful. Both studies classically show increased uptake only in lymphoma, but have variable sensitivities. Other useful MR techniques include DWI, MRS, and MR perfusion. Lymphoma tends to have reduced diffusion because of its hypercellularity, whereas toxoplasmosis tends to show facilitated diffusion. MRS in

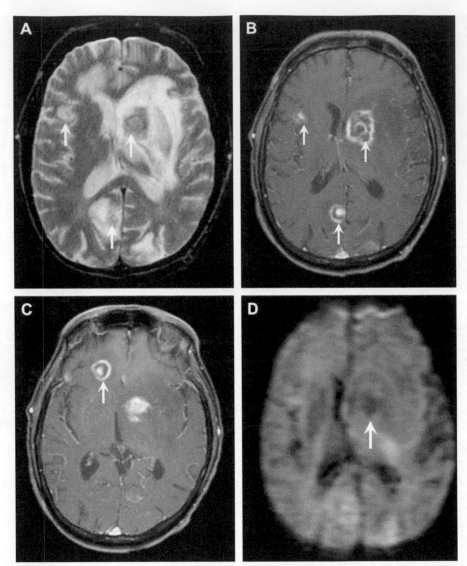

Fig. 12. Toxoplasmosis. 41-year-old HIV-positive man with new right-sided weakness. (*A*) Axial T2 image shows 3 dominant lesions with surrounding vasogenic edema: left caudate head, right parahippocampal gyrus, and right frontal lobe (*arrows*). Note that the 2 larger lesions are *T2 hypointense centrally*; this would be atypical for pyogenic abscess. (*B*) Axial T1-weighted post-GAD image shows ring enhancement (*arrows*). Note the "eccentric target sign," which is shown best in the right parahippocampal lesion. Although this sign is not sensitive, it is fairly specific for toxoplasmosis. (*C*) An additional axial T1-weighted post-GAD image shows another lesion in the right inferior frontal lobe, which also demonstrates the "eccentric target sign" (*arrow*). (*D*) Axial DWI shows no evidence of reduced diffusion within the left basal ganglia lesion (*arrow*).

lymphoma shows marked elevation of choline owing to hypercellularity and membrane turnover. In contrast, MRS in toxoplasmosis confirms the infectious origin with elevated lactate and lipid peaks. On MR perfusion, because lymphoma is a hypervascular neoplastic process, there is elevated relative cerebral blood volume (rCBV), whereas toxoplasmosis shows decreased rCBV.[43] In persistently equivocal cases, a biopsy is usually the next course of action.

Key Imaging Feature: Toxoplasmosis

- Asymmetric or eccentric target sign in the setting of an HIV patient with multiple ring-enhancing lesions.

Acute disseminated encephalomyelitis
Acute disseminated encephalomyelitis (ADEM) is a monophasic inflammatory demyelinating disorder associated with a recent infection or vaccination.[44] Infection or vaccination is thought

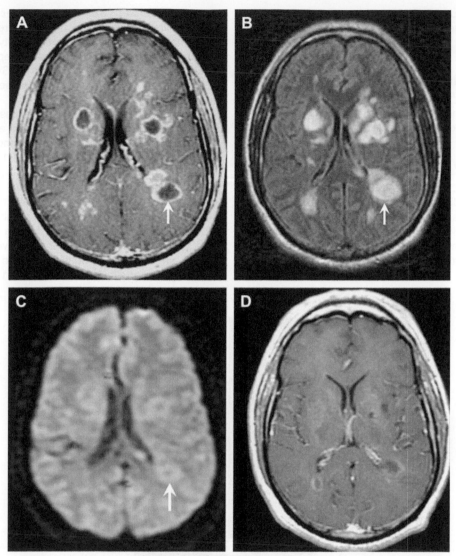

Fig. 13. Acute disseminated encephalomyelitis (ADEM). 43-year-old man with acute altered mental status. (*A*) Axial T1-weighted post-GAD image shows multiple ring-enhancing lesions along with additional smaller nodules of enhancement. (*B*) Axial FLAIR image shows T2 hyperintensity within these lesions; however, there is little to no surrounding vasogenic edema or mass effect. This is a clue that the lesion is a demyelinating process rather than tumor or infection. (*C*) Axial DWI shows no reduced diffusion, also mitigating against pyogenic infection. (*D*) Axial T1-weighted post-GAD image obtained 1 week following steroid treatment shows marked interval improvement with near resolution of many of the lesions.

to trigger an autoimmune attack, possibly via "molecular mimicry." Patients usually present with nonspecific symptoms, including headache, vomiting, fever, and lethargy. Children are affected more often than adults. On MR imaging, multifocal T2 hyperintense lesions are typically seen in the subcortical white matter, thalami, and basal ganglia, but lesions may be tumefactive and mimic other ring-enhancing infections and tumors (Fig. 13).[44,45] Therefore, it is crucial for the radiologist to consider tumefactive demyelination with all

ring-enhancing lesions because of the drastically different management. Specifically, ADEM is treated medically with intravenous high-dose steroids and surgery should be avoided. Nonresponsive patients can also be treated with plasma exchange or immunoglobulins.

The imaging features most suggestive of tumefactive demyelinating lesions include large lesions with little to no mass effect, minimal edema, incomplete ring of enhancement at the "leading edge" of demyelination on the white matter side of the lesion, central dilated veins within the lesion, and decreased perfusion (rCBV).[46–48]

Key Imaging Features: Acute Disseminated Encephalomyelitis

- Minimal mass effect
- Incomplete "leading edge" enhancement.

Temporal Lobe

When this imaging pattern is encountered, the primary diagnostic consideration should always be herpes encephalitis in the infectious category. Noninfectious considerations, including middle cerebral artery (MCA) infarct, glioma, and limbic encephalitis, are discussed briefly in the following sections.

Herpes encephalitis and other viral encephalitis

Encephalitis refers to a diffuse parenchymal inflammation seen as T2 hyperintensity on MR imaging. The most common viral encephalitides include herpes simplex viruses (HSV-1 and HSV-2), herpes zoster, arboviruses, and enteroviruses.[13]

HSV-1 is responsible for 95% of herpes encephalitides and occurs primarily in adults and older children. This devastating necrotizing encephalitis results from reactivation of latent HSV-1 infection within the trigeminal (or gasserian) ganglion, and is the most common cause of fatal sporadic encephalitis.[49] The infection spreads intracranially along meningeal branches of the trigeminal nerve, thus explaining the predilection for the temporal lobe. Patients typically present with fever, headaches, seizures, and focal neurologic deficits. The high mortality rate of HSV-1 herpes

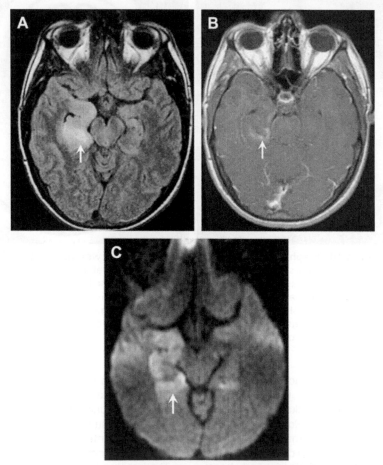

Fig. 14. **Herpes encephalitis.** 26-year-old man with new seizure and fever. (*A*) Axial FLAIR image demonstrates right medial temporal lobe enlargement and hyperintensity (*arrow*). (*B*) Axial T1-weighted post-GAD image shows slight linear enhancement posteriorly (*arrow*). Note that enhancement in HSV is variable and dependent on the time after onset. (*C*) Axial DWI shows reduced diffusion (*arrow*) and confirms involvement of the left medial temporal lobe.

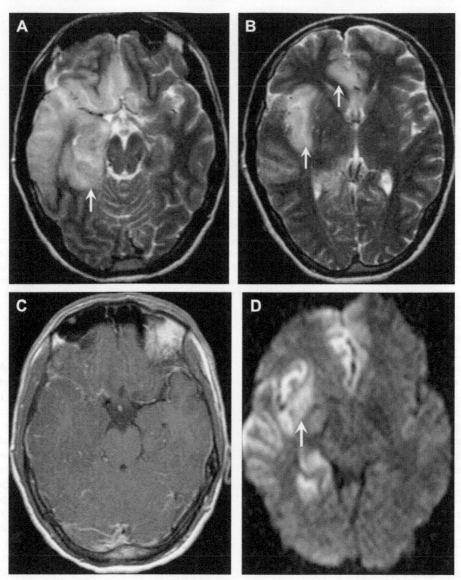

Fig. 15. Herpes encephalitis (typical distribution). 44-year-old woman with mental status changes. (*A, B*) Axial T2-weighted images at 2 different levels show bilateral, asymmetric involvement of the right temporal lobe, insula, and cingulate gyrus (*arrows*). (*C*) Axial T1-weighted post-GAD image shows little to no enhancement. (*D*) Axial DWI demonstrates reduced diffusion.

encephalitis, approaching 70% without treatment, and the availability of effective antiviral drugs, make early diagnosis key. Because polymerase chain reaction (PCR) is not 100% sensitive, early recognition of MR imaging findings can be critical.

The spectrum of imaging findings reflects the edema, hemorrhage, and necrosis seen pathologically. CT can be normal or show ill-defined areas of hypodensity in the medial temporal lobes and/or inferior frontal lobes. MRI better characterizes the extent of injury and classically shows bilateral, but asymmetric, involvement of the limbic system. Cortical swelling with T2 hyperintensity

and T1 hypointensity are seen in the medial temporal lobe, insular cortex, cingulate gyrus, and inferior frontal lobe (Figs. 14 and 15). The pons may also be involved, likely from retrograde transmission along the cisternal segment of the trigeminal nerve.[49] Petechial hemorrhages can manifest as T1 shortening or abnormal susceptibility on gradient-echo sequences. T1 shortening can also be seen in a gyriform configuration owing to cortical hemorrhage.[50] Enhancement is variable, may be patchy or gyral, and generally develops later in the infection (after the T2 abnormality). Areas of reduced diffusion have been

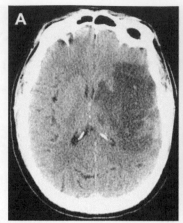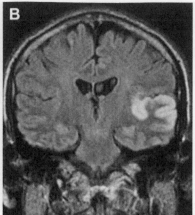

Fig. 16. Middle cerebral artery infarction (contrast with HSV). (*A*) Axial CT shows hypodensity involving the left basal ganglia and temporal lobe. Note that involvement of the basal ganglia is atypical for HSV and this distribution suggests a large left MCA infarct involving the M1 segment and lenticulostriate vessels. (*B*) Coronal FLAIR in a different patient shows hyperintensity in the lateral temporal lobe with relative sparing of the medial temporal lobe, suggesting MCA infarction rather than HSV. HSV usually involves the medial temporal lobe first.

shown to be one of the earliest findings[51,52]; however, DWI can be variable. Some investigators report more severe, nonresponsive cases to have reduced diffusion, whereas cases with a good response to treatment and more favorable outcome show resolution of reduced diffusion, or even increased diffusion at the onset.[53,54]

The primary differential considerations for abnormalities of the temporal lobe include MCA infarct, infiltrating gliomas, and limbic encephalitis. The basal ganglia are usually spared, and the medial temporal lobe is usually involved before the lateral temporal lobe, in herpes encephalitis, thus helping to differentiate from an acute MCA infarct (**Fig. 16**). The clinical history, including the onset and chronicity of symptoms, should help differentiate infarct from infiltrating tumor.

Key Imaging Feature: Herpes Encephalitis and Other Viral Encephalitis

- HSV-1 should be the diagnosis of choice in ANY patient with fever and signal abnormality in the medial temporal lobe until proven otherwise.

Basal Ganglia Lesions

Primary differential considerations for bilateral basal ganglia abnormalities include infection, toxic-metabolic etiologies, venous ischemia, hypoxic-ischemic injury, and neoplasm. It is critical to know the patient's history and specifically his or her immune status.

Cryptococcus

Cryptococcus neoformans is the most common CNS fungal infection in patients with AIDS and the third most common cause of CNS infection in AIDS, after HIV encephalopathy and toxoplasmosis.[34] It typically manifests as a chronic basilar meningitis or meningoencephalitis with minimal inflammation.[13] *C neoformans* is a ubiquitous yeastlike fungus found in soil contaminated by bird excreta. Patients are most vulnerable to *Cryptococcus* when their CD4 counts drop below 100 cells/μL. The diagnosis of CNS cryptococcosis can be made on the basis of a series of microbiologic investigations, including CSF culture and positive identification of the yeast with India ink staining; elevations in cryptococcal antigen latex agglutination titers in CSF and blood; and positive results with blood culture.

The most common imaging finding for cryptococcal meningitis, albeit nonspecific, is communicating or noncommunicating hydrocephalus.[55] Cryptococcus tends to spread along the perivascular (Virchow-Robin) spaces resulting in "gelatinous pseudocysts." These appear as multiple, nonenhancing, rounded, T2 hyperintense, T1 hypointense lesions in the basal ganglia (**Fig. 17**). Other imaging findings include meningeal enhancement and ring-enhancing granulomas ("cryptococcomas") with a predilection for the choroid plexus. Immunocompromised patients are less likely to have hydrocephalus or enhancing parenchymal lesions and are more likely to have gelatinous pseudocysts on imaging. Patients are treated with antifungal agents such as fluconazole or amphotericin B.

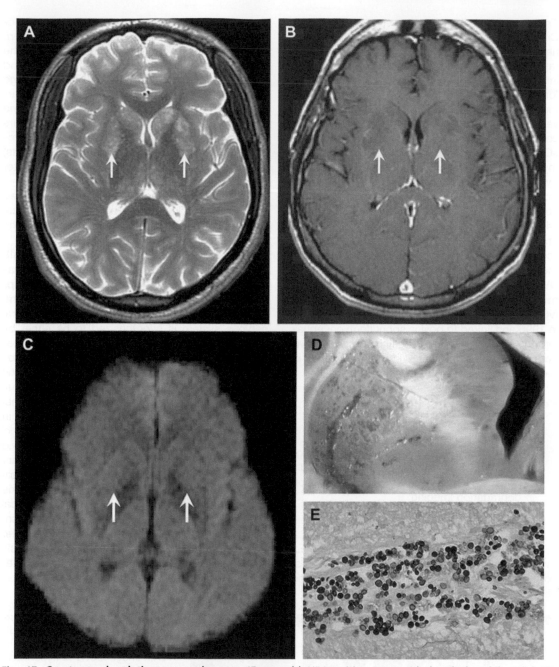

Fig. 17. **Cryptococcal gelatinous pseudocysts.** 47-year-old HIV-positive man with headache. (*A*) Axial T2-weighted image shows innumerable tiny T2 hyperintense foci within the caudate head, lentiform nuclei, and thalamus, bilaterally (*arrows*). (*B*) Axial T1-weighted post-GAD image shows *no enhancement*, thus excluding other entities found in the basal ganglia such as toxoplasmosis and lymphoma. (*C*) Axial DWI shows *no reduced diffusion*, thus excluding acute and/or subacute ischemic injury. (*D*) Coronal gross specimen at the level of the right frontal horn demonstrates mucinous material filling the putaminal perivascular spaces. (*E*) Histology slide shows positive India ink staining.

Key Imaging Features: Cryptococcus

- Nonenhancing T2 hyperintense lesions in the basal ganglia
- *Increased* diffusion.

Toxoplasmosis: Toxoplasmosis is a key differential consideration for ring-enhancing lesions in the basal ganglia in the HIV-infected patient. It was discussed previously in the section on ring-enhancing lesions.

Creutzfeldt-Jakob disease

Creutzfeldt-Jakob disease (CJD) is a rare fatal neurodegenerative disease characterized by rapidly progressive dementia. It is caused by an infectious protein known as a prion. Four different forms of CJD are known: the sporadic type (sCJD), the genetic type, the iatrogenic type, and the variant type (vCJD). The sporadic form is most common (85%).[56] Clinical diagnosis of probable sCJD includes at least 2 of 4 clinical features: myoclonus, visual or cerebellar disturbances, pyramidal/extrapyramidal dysfunction or akinetic mutism, and periodic sharp and slow wave complexes on EEG. The analysis of CSF for the 14-3-3 neuronal protein is also helpful.[56,57] The characteristic MR imaging features include "cortical ribboning" (ribbonlike hyperintensity in the gyri of the cerebral cortex on FLAIR and DWI), and hyperintensity of the caudate and putamen on FLAIR and DWI (Fig. 18). Variant CJD (vCJD) was first reported in the United Kingdom in 1996 and linked to bovine spongiform encephalopathy.[58] The classic imaging finding is the "pulvinar sign," seen as bright DWI and FLAIR signal in the pulvinar nucleus of the thalamus.

Key Imaging Features: CJD

- Bright DWI in putamen and caudate
- "Cortical ribboning"
- DWI is the most useful sequence to diagnose and follow these patients, especially because these patients are prone to motion degradation imaging.

White Matter Lesions

Lyme disease

Lyme disease is seen worldwide, but is the most common vector-borne disease in the United States. It is a tick-transmitted multisystem infection caused by the spirochete *Borrelia burgdorferi*. The incidence peaks in the summer months in the coastal northeast states, also Michigan and Minnesota.[59,60] The disease has 3 stages. Stage 1 occurs 3 to 32 days after the tick bite, with a characteristic targetlike rash, known as erythema migrans, and flulike symptoms. Stage 2 occurs after several weeks to months, consisting of neurologic (15% patients) and cardiac (8% patients) involvement.[59,61] Stage 3 can occur years later as chronic arthritis and neurologic symptoms. The diagnosis of Lyme disease should be based on a history of tick exposure, epidemiology, clinical signs and symptoms at different stages of the disease, and the use of serologic tests.

Lyme neuroborreliosis (LNB) may present with peripheral or central nervous system manifestations, including peripheral neuropathy, myelopathy, encephalitis, lymphocytic meningitis, and cranial nerve palsies. Involvement of the central nervous system is hypothesized to be either by retrograde spread via peripheral nerves or hematogenous spread, leading to a meningoencephalitis. Although the reported rate of abnormal MR findings in LNB varies from 17% to 43%, the most common imaging pattern is nonspecific abnormal white matter T2 prolongation, predominately in the frontal subcortical white matter (Fig. 19).[61–63] The distribution of brain involvement, including the callososeptal interface, may mimic a primary demyelinating disease such as multiple sclerosis (MS). When the characteristic clinical prodrome and exposure history are lacking, the multifocal clinical findings on neurologic examination, positive oligoclonal bands, and white matter patterns on MR imaging may confuse the diagnosis with MS. Patients may also present with leptomeningeal and cranial nerve enhancement, which is

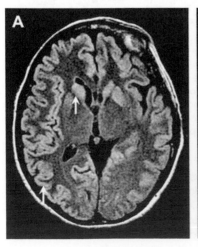
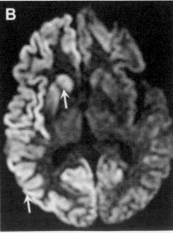

Fig. 18. Creutzfeldt Jacob disease. 60-year-old woman with rapidly progressive dementia. (*A*) Axial FLAIR image shows T2 hyperintensity in the caudate heads (*top arrow*) and putamina bilaterally. Note also abnormal hyperintensity of the cerebral cortex, greater on the right than left, consistent with so-called "cortical ribboning" (*bottom arrow*). (*B*) Axial DWI shows reduced diffusion in these same areas, predominately on the right.

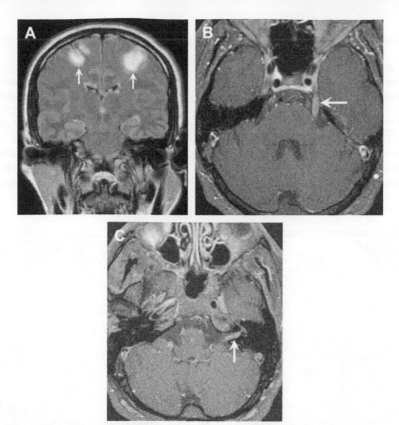

Fig. 19. **Neuroborreliosis (Lyme disease).** 19-year-old man with multiple cranial neuropathies. (*A*) Coronal FLAIR image shows bilateral T2 hyperintensity in the frontal white matter with extension to the cortex (*arrows*). No significant mass effect is noted. Lyme lesions can often mimic demyelinating disease. (*B, C*) Axial T1-weighted post-GAD images demonstrate enhancement of the left fifth, seventh, and eighth nerves (*arrows*).

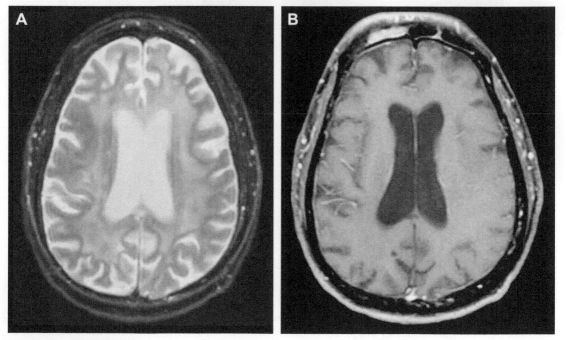

Fig. 20. **HIV encephalopathy.** 43-year-old HIV-positive man with dementia. (*A*) Axial T2-weighted image demonstrates global volume loss and diffuse periventricular white matter T2 hyperintensity. The history of HIV and the *symmetry* of the white matter abnormality are clues to the correct diagnosis of AIDS dementia complex. (*B*) Axial T1-weighted post-GAD image shows *no enhancement*. Note that the areas of T2 hyperintensity are barely visible on this T1-weighted image, ie, the lesions are T1 isointense.

not seen in MS, and is therefore another clue to the correct diagnosis in the setting of nonspecific white matter lesions (see Fig. 19B, C).[61]

Key Imaging Features: White Matter Lesions

- Multiple nonspecific T2 hyperintense lesions in the subcortical white matter
- Leptomeningeal and/or cranial nerve enhancement.

HIV encephalopathy

HIV encephalopathy is a progressive neurodegenerative disease resulting from direct infection of CNS mononuclear cells and microglial cells. Infected cells in the brain ultimately result in microglial activation, diffuse myelin loss, neuronal death, and astroglial proliferation.[64] Patients present with a subcortical dementia and cognitive and behavioral deficits including inattention,

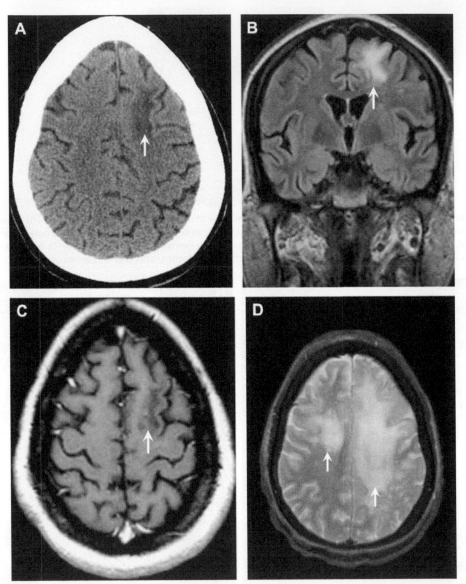

Fig. 21. **Progressive multifocal leukoencephalopathy (PML).** 34-year-old HIV-positive woman with right hand weakness. (*A*) Axial noncontrast CT image shows focal hypodensity within the subcortical white matter of the left superior frontal gyrus (*arrow*). (*B*) Coronal FLAIR image demonstrates corresponding T2 hyperintensity (*arrow*). Note *lack* of mass effect and involvement of subcortical U-fibers. (*C*) Axial T1-weighted post-GAD image shows no enhancement (*arrow*). Note the T1 hypointensity in contrast to the T1 isointense signal seen in the previous case of HIV encephalopathy (see Fig. 20B). (*D*) Three-month follow-up axial T2-weighted image in the same patient demonstrates rapid progression (*arrows*).

indifference and psychomotor slowing (AIDS Dementia Complex).

The imaging features of HIV encephalopathy include diffuse cerebral atrophy and *symmetric* T2 hyperintensity in the periventricular and deep white matter (Fig. 20). There is *no* mass effect or contrast enhancement. The symmetric white matter involvement helps to distinguish it from progressive multifocal leukoencephalopathy (PML), which tends to be asymmetric and involve subcortical U-fibers. HAART may not prevent HIV encephalopathy, but it can decrease the severity. Some studies have even shown that diffuse white matter abnormalities seen on brain MRI can exhibit partial resolution after HAART.[65]

Key Imaging Features: HIV Encephalopathy

- Diffuse cerebral atrophy
- Symmetric periventricular white matter T2 hyperintensity that is barely visible on T1-weighted images.

Progressive multifocal leukoencephalopathy

Progressive multifocal leukoencephalopathy (PML) is a progressive demyelinating disease caused by a DNA papovavirus, the John Cunningham virus (JC virus), which directly infects the myelin-producing oligodendrocytes. Although PML can be seen in many immunocompromised states, the greatest risk occurs in HIV-infected patients with CD4 counts ranging from 50 to 100 cells/μL. Other patients with impaired T-cell function, including patients with long-standing hematological disorders and immunosuppression after organ transplantation, are also at risk. Patients present with progressive neurologic decline. PCR testing of the CSF for the JC virus assists in making the diagnosis with approximately 96% specificity.[34]

The typical MR imaging features include asymmetric T2 hyperintensity in the periventricular white matter with involvement of subcortical U-fibers that create a sharp border with the cortex (Fig. 21). Remarkably, the lesions are particularly hypointense on T1-weighted images. The involved areas may be single or multiple, unilateral or bilateral, but classically asymmetric with frequent involvement of the parieto-occipital areas. There is usually no enhancement or mass effect. These typical imaging features are seen in 90% of cases.[66] Atypical patterns can occur, however, including faint peripheral enhancement, mass effect, and even focal hemorrhage. Some investigators have described contrast enhancement as a positive development, heralding an inflammatory reaction and elimination of the JC virus, but it can also be seen with immune reconstitution

syndrome exacerbating PML.[67] Reduced diffusion has been described in the early phases of the disease at the leading edge of active demyelination, and may be a poor prognostic sign indicating a phase of disease progression.[67–69]

The primary differential consideration is HIV encephalopathy, which can be distinguished from PML by its more symmetric white matter involvement, less intense T2 hyperintensity, lack of subcortical U-fiber involvement, and barely visible lesions on the T1-weighted sequence.

Key Imaging Features: Progressive Multifocal Encephalopathy

- Asymmetric white matter T2 hyperintensity
- Subcortical U-fibers involved
- T1 hypointense
- Typically no enhancement or mass effect.

PML and immune reconstitution inflammatory syndrome

Immune reconstitution following the initiation of combined antiretroviral therapy (HAART) may lead to activation of an inflammatory response to detectable or latent JC virus. Partial restoration of specific immunity may paradoxically lead to a worsening of a number of preexisting infections including PML, CMV, or *Cryptococcus*. Immune

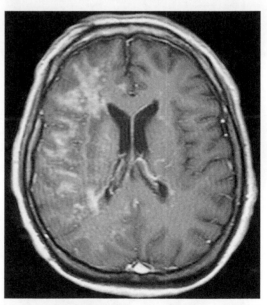

Fig. 22. **Immune reconstitution syndrome (IRIS) in PML.** 39-year-old HIV-positive man with acute worsening after initiation of HAART therapy. Axial T1-weighted post-GAD image shows extensive linear and nodular enhancement in this patient with PML. The enhancement is somewhat atypical for PML and should thus raise the possibility of lymphoma or immune reconstitution.

reconstitution inflammatory syndrome (IRIS) usually occurs in the initial months after beginning HAART, ranging from 1 week to 26 months in one study.[70] Patients with IRIS demonstrate paradoxic deterioration in their clinical status when their CD4 counts rise and viral replication appears to be under control. This often leads to a confusing clinical and radiographic picture. The neuroimaging features may vary depending on the underlying infection and timing of HAART therapy. Atypical imaging features may be encountered, such as mass effect and enhancement in PML lesions, which can mimic lymphoma (Fig. 22).

CMV encephalitis

CMV is a common herpes virus that does not cause clinical disease in immunocompetent

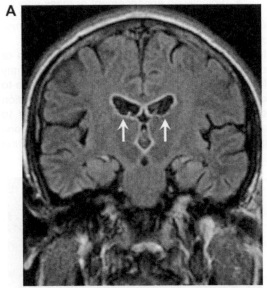

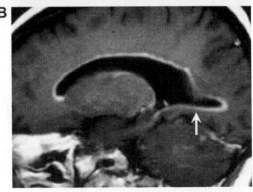

Fig. 23. **Cytomegalovirus ventriculitis.** 28-year-old HIV-positive woman with headache. (*A*) Coronal FLAIR image demonstrates a thin rim of T2 hyperintensity surrounding the frontal horns and third ventricle (*arrows*). (*B*) Parasagittal T1-weighted post-GAD image shows abnormal subependymal enhancement (*arrow*).

patients, but can reactivate in the setting of immunosuppression. CMV infection usually occurs in patients with HIV when the CD4+ count falls less than 50 cells/μL. Although CNS involvement typically takes the form of a meningoencephalitis or ventriculitis, it can also present as myelitis, polyradiculitis, and retinitis. Therefore, CMV retinitis, which is seen in 25% of AIDS patients, may provide a clue to the diagnosis. Patients present with acute onset encephalitis and the diagnosis can be confirmed by positive CMVpp65 antigen.[71] CMV infection may progress to death within days. Patients are currently treated with gangcyclovir and foscarnet.

CMV involves the gray matter and ventricular ependyma to a greater degree than the white matter, thus distinguishing it from other encephalitides in patients with AIDS, such as HIV or PML.[13] Although imaging of CMV has low sensitivity and specificity, MRI is the method of choice. The most characteristic imaging finding is the presence of thin subependymal FLAIR hyperintensity and contrast enhancement (Fig. 23). CMV infection may also have a centrifugal spread from the ventricular system, with focal or diffuse increased T2 signal involving the gray matter or white matter.[13]

Key Imaging Feature: CMV Encephalitis

- Pencil-thin T2 hyperintensity surrounding the ventricles on FLAIR imaging with subependymal enhancement.

REFERENCES

1. Chiang IC, Hsieh TJ, Chiu ML, et al. Distinction between pyogenic brain abscess and necrotic brain tumour using 3-tesla MR spectroscopy, diffusion and perfusion imaging. Br J Radiol 2009;82(982): 813–20.
2. Desprechins B, Stadnik T, Koerts G, et al. Use of diffusion-weighted MR imaging in differential diagnosis between intracerebral necrotic tumors and cerebral abscesses. AJNR Am J Neuroradiol 1999; 20(7):1252–7.
3. Ferreira NP, Otta GM, do Amaral LL, et al. Imaging aspects of pyogenic infections of the central nervous system. Top Magn Reson Imaging 2005; 16(2):145–54.
4. Guo AC, Provenzale JM, Cruz LC Jr, et al. Cerebral abscesses: investigation using apparent diffusion coefficient maps. Neuroradiology 2001;43(5): 370–4.
5. Lai PH, Ho JT, Chen WL, et al. Brain abscess and necrotic brain tumor: discrimination with proton MR spectroscopy and diffusion-weighted imaging. AJNR Am J Neuroradiol 2002;23(8):1369–77.

6. Reddy JS, Mishra AM, Behari S, et al. The role of diffusion-weighted imaging in the differential diagnosis of intracranial cystic mass lesions: a report of 147 lesions. Surg Neurol 2006;66(3):246—50 [discussion: 250—1].

7. Tsuchiya K, Osawa A, Katase S, et al. Diffusion-weighted MRI of subdural and epidural empyemas. Neuroradiology 2003;45(4):220—3.

8. Camacho DL, Smith JK, Castillo M. Differentiation of toxoplasmosis and lymphoma in AIDS patients by using apparent diffusion coefficients. AJNR Am J Neuroradiol 2003;24(4):633—7.

9. Castillo M. Imaging brain abscesses with diffusion-weighted and other sequences. AJNR Am J Neuroradiol 1999;20(7):1193—4.

10. Burtscher IM, Holtas S. In vivo proton MR spectroscopy of untreated and treated brain abscesses. AJNR Am J Neuroradiol 1999;20(6):1049—53.

11. Chang KH, Song IC, Kim SH, et al. In vivo single-voxel proton MR spectroscopy in intracranial cystic masses. AJNR Am J Neuroradiol 1998;19(3):401—5.

12. Lai PH, Li KT, Hsu SS, et al. Pyogenic brain abscess: findings from in vivo 1.5-T and 11.7-T in vitro proton MR spectroscopy. AJNR Am J Neuroradiol 2005;26(2):279—88.

13. Karampekios S, Hesselink J. Cerebral infections. Eur Radiol 2005;15(3):485—93.

14. Nathoo N, Nadvi SS, van Dellen JR, et al. Intracranial subdural empyemas in the era of computed tomography: a review of 699 cases. Neurosurgery 1999;44(3):529—35 [discussion: 535—6].

15. Singer MB, Atlas SW, Drayer BP. Subarachnoid space disease: diagnosis with fluid-attenuated inversion-recovery MR imaging and comparison with gadolinium-enhanced spin-echo MR imaging—blinded reader study. Radiology 1998;208(2):417—22.

16. Gupta RK, Gupta S, Singh D, et al. MR imaging and angiography in tuberculous meningitis. Neuroradiology 1994;36(2):87—92.

17. Bernaerts A, Vanhoenacker FM, Parizel PM, et al. Tuberculosis of the central nervous system: overview of neuroradiological findings. Eur Radiol 2003;13(8):1876—90.

18. Garcia-Monco JC. Central nervous system tuberculosis. Neurol Clin 1999;17(4):737—59.

19. Jinkins JR, Gupta R, Chang KH, et al. MR imaging of central nervous system tuberculosis. Radiol Clin North Am 1995;33(4):771—86.

20. Luthra G, Parihar A, Nath K, et al. Comparative evaluation of fungal, tubercular, and pyogenic brain abscesses with conventional and diffusion MR imaging and proton MR spectroscopy. AJNR Am J Neuroradiol 2007;28(7):1332—8.

21. Del Brutto OH, Sotelo J. Neurocysticercosis: an update. Rev Infect Dis 1988;10(6):1075—87.

22. Garcia HH, Del Brutto OH. Imaging findings in neurocysticercosis. Acta Trop 2003;87(1):71—8.

23. Castillo M. Imaging of neurocysticercosis. Semin Roentgenol 2004;39(4):465—73.

24. Escobar A, Aruffo C, Cruz-Sanchez F, et al. [Neuropathologic findings in neurocysticercosis]. Arch Neurobiol (Madr) 1985;48(3):151—6 [in Spanish].

25. Carpio A, Placencia M, Santillan F, et al. A proposal for classification of neurocysticercosis. Can J Neurol Sci 1994;21(1):43—7.

26. Gupta RK, Prakash M, Mishra AM, et al. Role of diffusion weighted imaging in differentiation of intracranial tuberculoma and tuberculous abscess from cysticercus granulomas—a report of more than 100 lesions. Eur J Radiol 2005;55(3):384—92.

27. Rangel-Guerra RA, Herrera J, Elizondo G, et al. Neurocysticercosis. Arch Neurol 1988;45(5):492.

28. Guermazi A, Gluckman E, Tabti B, et al. Invasive central nervous system aspergillosis in bone marrow transplantation recipients: an overview. Eur Radiol 2003;13(2):377—88.

29. Schwartz S, Milatovic D, Thiel E. Successful treatment of cerebral aspergillosis with a novel triazole (voriconazole) in a patient with acute leukaemia. Br J Haematol 1997;97(3):663—5.

30. Khoury H, Adkins D, Miller G, et al. Resolution of invasive central nervous system aspergillosis in a transplant recipient. Bone Marrow Transplant 1997;20(2):179—80.

31. DeLone DR, Goldstein RA, Petermann G, et al. Disseminated aspergillosis involving the brain: distribution and imaging characteristics. AJNR Am J Neuroradiol 1999;20(9):1597—604.

32. Foerster BR, Thurnher MM, Malani PN, et al. Intracranial infections: clinical and imaging characteristics. Acta Radiol 2007;48(8):875—93.

33. Levy RM, Mills CM, Posin JP, et al. The efficacy and clinical impact of brain imaging in neurologically symptomatic AIDS patients: a prospective CT/MRI study. J Acquir Immune Defic Syndr 1990;3(5):461—71.

34. Smith AB, Smirniotopoulos JG, Rushing EJ. From the archives of the AFIP: central nervous system infections associated with human immunodeficiency virus infection: radiologic-pathologic correlation. Radiographics 2008;28(7):2033—58.

35. Ramsey RG, Geremia GK. CNS complications of AIDS: CT and MR findings. AJR Am J Roentgenol 1988;151(3):449—54.

36. Porter SB, Sande MA. Toxoplasmosis of the central nervous system in the acquired immunodeficiency syndrome. N Engl J Med 1992;327(23):1643—8.

37. Navia BA, Petito CK, Gold JW, et al. Cerebral toxoplasmosis complicating the acquired immune deficiency syndrome: clinical and neuropathological findings in 27 patients. Ann Neurol 1986;19(3):224—38.

38. Brightbill TC, Post MJ, Hensley GT, et al. MR of Toxoplasma encephalitis: signal characteristics on T2-weighted images and pathologic correlation. J Comput Assist Tomogr 1996;20(3):417—22.

39. Trenkwalder P, Trenkwalder C, Feiden W, et al. Toxoplasmosis with early intracerebral hemorrhage in a patient with the acquired immunodeficiency syndrome. Neurology 1992;42(2):436–8.

40. Masamed R, Meleis A, Lee EW, et al. Cerebral toxoplasmosis: case review and description of a new imaging sign. Clin Radiol 2009;64(5):560–3.

41. Batra A, Tripathi RP, Gorthi SP. Magnetic resonance evaluation of cerebral toxoplasmosis in patients with the acquired immunodeficiency syndrome. Acta Radiol 2004;45(2):212–21.

42. Nath A, Sinai AP. Cerebral toxoplasmosis. Curr Treat Options Neurol 2003;5(1):3–12.

43. Ernst TM, Chang L, Witt MD, et al. Cerebral toxoplasmosis and lymphoma in AIDS: perfusion MR imaging experience in 13 patients. Radiology 1998;208(3):663–9.

44. Menge T, Hemmer B, Nessler S, et al. Acute disseminated encephalomyelitis: an update. Arch Neurol 2005;62(11):1673–80.

45. Canellas AR, Gols AR, Izquierdo JR, et al. Idiopathic inflammatory-demyelinating diseases of the central nervous system. Neuroradiology 2007;49(5): 393–409.

46. Given CA 2nd, Stevens BS, Lee C. The MRI appearance of tumefactive demyelinating lesions. AJR Am J Roentgenol 2004;182(1):195–9.

47. Cha S, Pierce S, Knopp EA, et al. Dynamic contrast-enhanced T2*-weighted MR imaging of tumefactive demyelinating lesions. AJNR Am J Neuroradiol 2001;22(6):1109–16.

48. Masdeu JC, Moreira J, Trasi S, et al. The open ring. A new imaging sign in demyelinating disease. J Neuroimaging 1996;6(2):104–7.

49. Tien RD, Felsberg GJ, Osumi AK. Herpesvirus infections of the CNS: MR findings. AJR Am J Roentgenol 1993;161(1):167–76.

50. Baskin HJ, Hedlund G. Neuroimaging of herpesvirus infections in children. Pediatr Radiol 2007;37(10): 949–63.

51. Heiner L, Demaerel P. Diffusion-weighted MR imaging findings in a patient with herpes simplex encephalitis. Eur J Radiol 2003;45(3):195–8.

52. Kuker W, Nagele T, Schmidt F, et al. Diffusion-weighted MRI in herpes simplex encephalitis: a report of three cases. Neuroradiology 2004;46(2):122–5.

53. Duckworth JL, Hawley JS, Riedy G, et al. Magnetic resonance restricted diffusion resolution correlates with clinical improvement and response to treatment in herpes simplex encephalitis. Neurocrit Care 2005; 3(3):251–3.

54. Sener RN. Herpes simplex encephalitis: diffusion MR imaging findings. Comput Med Imaging Graph 2001;25(5):391–7.

55. Takasu A, Taneda M, Otuki H, et al. Gd-DTPA-enhanced MR imaging of cryptococcal meningoencephalitis. Neuroradiology 1991;33(5):443–6.

56. Tschampa HJ, Zerr I, Urbach H. Radiological assessment of Creutzfeldt-Jakob disease. Eur Radiol 2007;17(5):1200–11.

57. Zerr I, Pocchiari M, Collins S, et al. Analysis of EEG and CSF 14-3-3 proteins as aids to the diagnosis of Creutzfeldt-Jakob disease. Neurology 2000;55(6): 811–5.

58. Will RG, Ironside JW, Zeidler M, et al. A new variant of Creutzfeldt-Jakob disease in the UK. Lancet 1996;347(9006):921–5.

59. Hildenbrand P, Craven DE, Jones R, et al. Lyme neuroborreliosis: manifestations of a rapidly emerging zoonosis. AJNR Am J Neuroradiol 2009;30(6): 1079–87.

60. Lyme disease—United States, 2003–2005. MMWR Morb Mortal Wkly Rep 2007;56(23):573–6.

61. Agarwal R, Sze G. Neuro-lyme disease: MR imaging findings. Radiology 2009;253(1):167–73.

62. Rafto SE, Milton WJ, Galetta SL, et al. Biopsy-confirmed CNS Lyme disease: MR appearance at 1.5 T. AJNR Am J Neuroradiol 1990;11(3):482–4.

63. Fernandez RE, Rothberg M, Ferencz G, et al. Lyme disease of the CNS: MR imaging findings in 14 cases. AJNR Am J Neuroradiol 1990;11(3):479–81.

64. Archibald SL, Masliah E, Fennema-Notestine C, et al. Correlation of in vivo neuroimaging abnormalities with postmortem human immunodeficiency virus encephalitis and dendritic loss. Arch Neurol 2004;61 (3):369–76.

65. Thurnher MM, Schindler EG, Thurnher SA, et al. Highly active antiretroviral therapy for patients with AIDS dementia complex: effect on MR imaging findings and clinical course. AJNR Am J Neuroradiol 2000;21(4):670–8.

66. Sarrazin JL, Soulie D, Derosier C, et al. [MRI aspects of progressive multifocal leukoencephalopathy]. J Neuroradiol 1995;22(3):172–9 [in French].

67. Kuker W, Mader I, Nagele T, et al. Progressive multifocal leukoencephalopathy: value of diffusion-weighted and contrast-enhanced magnetic resonance imaging for diagnosis and treatment control. Eur J Neurol 2006;13(8):819–26.

68. Mader I, Herrlinger U, Klose U, et al. Progressive multifocal leukoencephalopathy: analysis of lesion development with diffusion-weighted MRI. Neuroradiology 2003;45(10):717–21.

69. Ohta K, Obara K, Sakauchi M, et al. Lesion extension detected by diffusion-weighted magnetic resonance imaging in progressive multifocal leukoencephalopathy. J Neurol 2001;248(9):809–11.

70. Tan K, Roda R, Ostrow L, et al. PML-IRIS in patients with HIV infection: clinical manifestations and treatment with steroids. Neurology 2009;72(17): 1458–64.

71. Kastrup O, Wanke I, Maschke M. Neuroimaging of infections of the central nervous system. Semin Neurol 2008;28(4):511–22.

Maxillofacial (Midface) Fractures

Jane J. Kim[a],* and Kevin Huoh[b]

KEYWORDS

- Maxillofacial fractures • Midface trauma • Orbit
- Zygomaticomaxillary complex • Naso-orbito-ethmoid
- Le Fort • Facial buttress

Maxillofacial fractures are most commonly caused by traffic accidents, assaults, falls, and sports-related injuries. Studies on the epidemiology and characterization of facial trauma have shown that the specific etiology and incidence of fracture types vary extensively by geographic location.[1,2] Even within the same geographic region, radiologists may encounter different types of facial trauma, depending on their individual practice setting (eg, level 1 trauma center, community hospital, outpatient clinic, or academic center). Regardless of practice type, nasal and orbital fractures are common, and radiologists should be familiar with the imaging findings of these injuries and other common maxillofacial fractures that are relevant to clinical management.

Maxillofacial trauma can be broadly divided into fractures involving the (1) upper face, including the frontal bone and supraorbital rim; (2) midface, including nasal, orbital, maxillary, and zygomatic injuries, in addition to more complex fracture patterns, such as Le Fort fractures; and (3) lower face, including the mandible. Midface fractures are the most common injuries, accounting for approximately 70% of all maxillofacial fractures, according to one large review, followed by mandible fractures (25%) and frontal or supraorbital fractures (5%).[3] Given their high incidence in craniofacial trauma, midface fractures are the focus of this content.

BASIC APPROACH TO FACIAL FRACTURES

The plastic, oral-maxillofacial, or otolaryngologist/head and neck surgeon examining a patient with a facial fracture is broadly interested in two things: form and function. Does the fracture cause a significant cosmetic deformity that requires repair (form)? And, does the fracture pattern cause injury to an adjacent anatomic structure that disrupts normal function and creates symptoms for the patient (function)?

In conjunction with a clinical examination, thin-section noncontrast CT is the best imaging modality to answer these questions. Imaging review should include studying the thin-section axial source images in both bone and soft tissue algorithm as well as coronal and sagittal multiplanar reformations. The reformatted images are particularly useful for assessing fractures oriented in the axial plane, such as orbital floor fractures and Le Fort 1, or floating palate, fractures, which are best appreciated in the coronal plane. Additional 3-D reformations of facial fractures provide a big-picture, overall rendering of facial skeletal alignment that is more difficult to appreciate on the axial images, and this greatly aids surgeons in evaluating cosmetic deformity. The impact of the fracture on facial width, height, and projection is more easily assessed on 3-D than 2-D imaging, and obtaining 3-D reformations in all patients with facial fractures is routine at the authors' institution.

Although addressing the issues of form and function with respect to facial fractures is important, radiologists should also carefully review soft tissue windows for signs of injury to the brain or globe. Intracranial hemorrhage or globe injury necessitates immediate neurosurgical or ophthalmologic consultation and may alter the

[a] Department of Radiology and Biomedical Imaging at University of California, San Francisco, San Francisco General Hospital, 1001 Potrero Avenue, Box 1325, San Francisco, CA 94143, USA
[b] Department of Otolaryngology - Head and Neck Surgery at University of California, San Francisco, 2233 Post Street, 3rd Floor, Box 1225, San Francisco, CA 94143, USA
* Corresponding author.
E-mail address: jane.kim@radiology.ucsf.edu

Neuroimag Clin N Am 20 (2010) 581–596
doi:10.1016/j.nic.2010.07.005
1052-5149/10/$ – see front matter © 2010 Elsevier Inc. All rights reserved.

timing of surgery. Many maxillofacial surgeons have experienced evaluating bony structures on CT for purposes of planning their operative approach, but they may not be familiar with the imaging manifestations of intracranial and orbital soft tissue injury.

NASAL AND NASAL-SEPTAL COMPLEX FRACTURES

Nasal and nasal-septal complex fractures are the most common of all facial fractures because the prominent, central position of the nose renders it susceptible to injury and the thin nasal bones require less force to fracture than other facial bones. The paired nasal bones articulate with each other in the midline at the top of the nose as well as with the frontal bone and the frontal process of the maxilla (Fig. 1). The nasal septum is comprised of a cartilaginous portion anteriorly and bony portion posteriorly, with the perpendicular plate of the ethmoid making up the superior portion of the bony septum and the vomer making up the inferior portion.

The perichondrium that lines the cartilaginous nasal septum provides nutrients and oxygen to the nasal septum, which has no other source of blood supply. If a septal hematoma develops between the perichondrium and septal cartilage, stripping the latter of its blood supply, the septal cartilage may undergo necrosis with resultant infection and/or saddle nose deformity. For this reason, septal hematomas must be recognized and evacuated promptly. This is an uncommon entity that is more common in children. It is usually diagnosed clinically, with no role for imaging to the authors' knowledge.

In the context of nasal fractures, imaging can provide an accurate description of the fracture, such as whether or not it is unilateral or bilateral, is comminuted, or involves an associated septal fracture (Fig. 2). Imaging may also identify complications, such as fracture extension into the anterior skull base and cribiform plate that may result in anosmia or cerebrospinal fluid leak. Suspicion of a nasal fracture in and of itself is not an indication for facial imaging; imaging is reserved for cases in which other facial fractures are suspected.

Clinical evaluation, not the imaging appearance, remains the mainstay for treatment decisions with respect to nasal fractures. Although there is no clear consensus on the optimal treatment of nasal fractures, patients who sustain a nasal fracture may undergo a trial of closed reduction within 3 hours of injury or within 3 to 10 days post injury. Open treatment of nasal fractures is usually reserved for patients with persistent nasal deformity or nasal obstruction after the acute treatment period

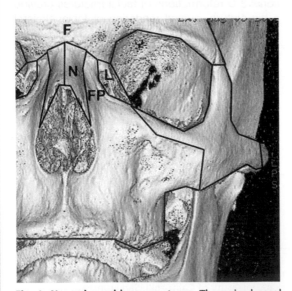

Fig. 1. Normal nasal bone anatomy. The paired nasal bones (N) articulate with each other, the frontal bone (F), and the frontal process of the maxilla (FP). The lacrimal bone (L) is deep to the frontal process of the maxilla.

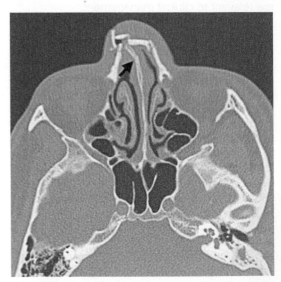

Fig. 2. Nasal-septal complex fracture. There are bilateral comminuted fractures of the nasal bones as well as a fracture of the bony septum (*arrow*). The nasal tip and septum are deviated to the right. It would be reasonable to attempt closed reduction of the nasal bone fractures with the understanding that the patient may need future revision open functional rhinoplasty to correct residual deformity or functional nasal obstruction.

ORBITAL FRACTURES

The superior, inferior, medial, and lateral orbital rims comprise the anteriorly palpable, circumferential bony framework encircling the globe. The corresponding orbital walls project posteriorly and converge toward the orbital apex, rendering the orbit a conical structure. The inferior and medial orbital walls are particularly delicate and vulnerable to fracture after blunt trauma to the eye.

Fractures of the orbit can be characterized as blow-out or blow-in depending on whether or not the fracture fragments extend beyond the orbit into adjacent structures, such as the maxillary or ethmoid sinus (blow-out) or buckle into the orbit (blow-in). Blow-out fractures, particularly of the weak inferior and medial orbital walls, are more common than blow-in injuries, which are rare and are not discussed in this review. Pure blow-out or blow-in fractures involve only the orbital walls and leave the orbital rims intact. Complex orbital injuries, such as the zygomaticomaxillary complex (ZMC), naso-orbito-ethmoidal (NOE), or Le Fort fractures, however, may fracture both the orbital walls and rims.

Blow-out Fractures

Fractures of the orbital floor are more common than fractures of the medial wall (lamina papyracea), and superior blow-out fractures are exceedingly uncommon. There are several important complications of form and function that may follow orbital blow-out fractures, and all of these must be considered at the time of CT interpretation.

The most significant cosmetic complication is the development of enophthalmos due to a fracture that enlarges the volume of the bony orbit, allowing the globe to sink posteriorly (Fig. 3). It is generally thought that enophthalmos greater than 2 mm creates a significant cosmetic deformity, but this can be difficult to determine at the time of acute fracture because the enophthalmos may not develop immediately after trauma and because the examination is impaired by acute periorbital swelling and edema.

There is great clinical interest in using CT features, such as the size of the fracture defect and/or enlargement of orbital volume after injury to predict which patients will develop enophthalmos and thus require surgical repair of their fracture.[4–6] Unfortunately, this is not straightforward given the conical shape of the orbit. The methods used in the literature to estimate the size of fracture defect vary widely and are not easily performed in a busy clinical setting because they require the use of computer-aided algorithms or mathematical calculations. The general surgical recommendation is that large orbital fracture defects (>50% of the orbital floor) should undergo operative repair rather than conservative management because of the high risk of subsequent enophthalmos.[7,8] Surgery is usually undertaken within 2 weeks of the acute trauma, because this allows time for the initial edema and hemorrhage to subside but it is

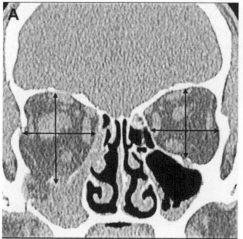 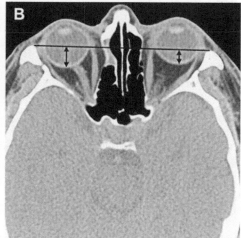

Fig. 3. **Enophthalmos after orbital floor blow-out fracture.** This patient suffered an orbital floor blow-out fracture 2 months before this CT and subsequently developed cosmetically significant enophthalmos. (A) Coronal CT shows an unrepaired right orbital floor blow-out fracture. Note the significant increase in orbital volume on the right as compared with the left. (B) Corresponding axial CT shows enophthalmos with posterior displacement of the right globe as compared with the left (horizontal line drawn between the zygomaticofrontal articulation). This patient underwent subsequent surgical repair.

before significant fibrosis and scarring typically occurs. At the authors' institution, visual estimation rather than a quantitative area calculation of the orbital floor fracture defect on CT generally guides surgical management.

An important functional complication of the blow-out fracture is diplopia caused by entrapment of an extraocular muscle and/or its fascial attachment in the fracture defect. Entrapment is a clinical, not radiologic, diagnosis that is made on forced duction testing. Muscle entrapment may also be difficult to distinguish on clinical examination, however, due to extraocular muscle edema or hemorrhage, which can also limit ocular

motility and cause diplopia. CT can be helpful if there is evidence of muscle or surrounding soft tissue herniation into the fracture defect (Fig. 4). The size and position of the inferior and medial rectus muscles (and their surrounding fat) should always be described in fractures of the orbital floor and medial wall, respectively.

CT may underestimate the extent of muscle entrapment if only a few fibers of the muscle or its fascial attachment to the periorbita are incarcerated or if the fracture defect is very small, as in the case of many trapdoor floor fractures that typically occur in the pediatric population.[9] In this injury, the greater elasticity in the orbital floor

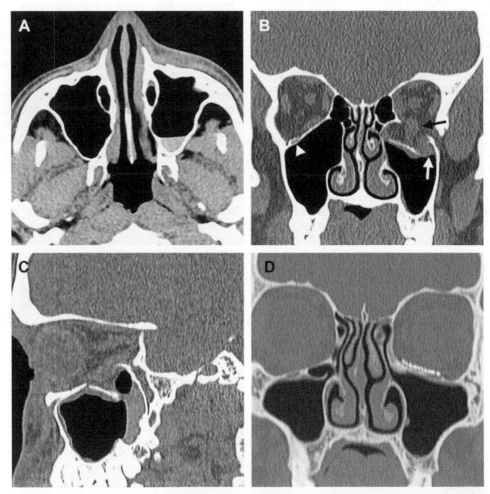

Fig. 4. **Orbital floor blow-out fracture.** (A) Axial noncontrast CT shows hemorrhage layering in the left maxillary sinus, suspicious for orbital fracture. The orbital floor blow-out fracture is best seen in the coronal (B) and sagittal (C) planes and involves more than 50% of the orbital floor on visual approximation. (B) The inferior rectus muscle is enlarged (*black arrow*) and inferiorly displaced with the orbital fat through the fracture defect. Hematoma is also seen in the inferolateral orbit (*white arrow*). Note that the fracture disrupts the infraorbital foramen, which can result in cheek and gum anesthesia (normal contralateral infraorbital foramen designated by white arrowhead for comparison). (D) This fracture was repaired with mesh along the orbital floor.

of young patients is thought to allow the fractured, buckled orbital floor to spring back nearly to its normal position and ensnare orbital contents that are not always readily appreciated on CT. Trapdoor fractures are linear and hinged medially. Careful evaluation of the orbital floor on coronal imaging is important in children with trauma to the orbit, because trapdoor fractures can be subtle and early diagnosis and treatment are critical to good outcome (Fig. 5). Children with trapdoor orbital floor fractures and acute incarceration of the inferior rectus muscle can present as a white-eyed blow-out fracture with few signs of periorbital swelling and bruising, making the clinical diagnosis a difficult one.[10] Early diagnosis is crucial, however, because surgical repair within the first few days of injury is necessary to avoid the oculocardiac reflex and permanent motility restriction resulting from muscle ischemia and necrosis.

Infraorbital anesthesia is another potential functional complication of orbital floor blow-out fractures if the fracture extends through the infraorbital foramen containing the infraorbital nerve (see Fig. 4). Anesthesia of the cheek and upper gum is typically temporary but may last up to 6 months or longer and even permanently in severe cases. Imaging disruption of the infraorbital foramen is not an indication for surgical intervention. Table 1 summarizes the relevant imaging features to describe in cases of orbital blow-out fractures.

BUTTRESS SYSTEM OF THE FACE

The remaining facial fractures discussed in this article involve multiple facial bones. NOE, ZMC, and Le Fort fractures occur at characteristic locations in the facial skeleton. Knowledge of the buttress system of the face is crucial when evaluating these fractures and understanding the approach to repair, because surgery is typically directed toward realigning any displaced components of the facial buttress.

In brief, the buttress system provides structure to the midface and stability against the strong forces associated with mastication. The midface can be conceptualized as a lattice of both vertically and horizontally oriented buttresses, or areas of thicker bone, that support the face. There are three main vertical and three main horizontal buttresses of the midface (Fig. 6). The vertical buttresses, from anteromedial to posterolateral, include the nasomaxillary, zygomaticomaxillary, and pterygomaxillary buttresses. The three horizontal buttresses, from superior to inferior, include the superior orbital rim, inferior orbital rim, and alveolar ridge. The vertical buttresses are stronger than the horizontal ones. NOE fractures disrupt the nasomaxillary buttres; ZMC fractures injure the zygomaticomaxillary buttress; and Le Fort fractures show variable injury to the facial buttresses depending on fracture type, although all three types of Le Fort injuries disrupt the pterygomaxillary buttress. Surgical treatment is aimed at re-establishing

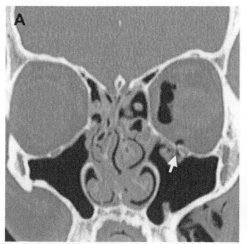 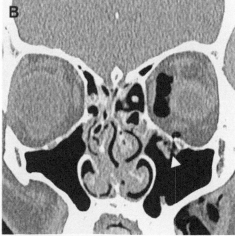

Fig. 5. Trapdoor orbital floor fracture. (A) This orbital floor fracture (*arrow*) requires careful evaluation of the coronal images to appreciate as it is flush with the remainder of the orbital floor. (B) The fracture is hinged medially and has snapped back into place with herniated orbital fat (*arrowhead*) trapped below the fracture defect. Even though the inferior rectus muscle lies above the fracture defect, clinical entrapment and vertical gaze restriction may still be present if the fascial attachment of the muscle to the periorbita is trapped below the fracture defect.

Table 1
Imaging checklist for orbital blow-out fractures

Relevant Imaging Findings to Report	Clinical Significance
Size of fracture defect (>50% of orbital floor?)	Predicts enophthalmos >50% defect is a relative indication for surgery
Grossly abnormal globe position (enophthalmos)	Cosmetically disfiguring Indication for surgical repair
Extraocular muscle or soft tissue herniation	Risk of entrapment and diplopia Entrapment indicates surgical repair
Involvement of infraorbital foramen (for orbital floor fractures)	Risk of cheek, gum anesthesia
Trapdoor fracture in children (for orbital floor fractures)	Easy to miss on imaging (indication for early surgical repair)
Globe injury or orbital hematoma	Risk of blindness (indication for urgent ophthalmologic consult)

normal, anatomic alignment of the main facial buttresses that have been disrupted.

NASO-ORBITO-ETHMOIDAL FRACTURES

NOE injuries are uncommon fractures that involve the orbital rim and nasal bones. They typically result in a telescoped-in appearance of the nose. The skeleton between the orbit and nose is a complex anatomic area reflecting the intersection of multiple bones, including the maxillary, lacrimal, nasal, and frontal bones. NOE fractures involve the inferior orbital rim, medial orbital wall and rim, nasal bones, and ethmoid. The bony nasal septum (perpendicular process of the ethmoid) also frequently collapses with the nasal bones and the normal pyramidal projection of the nose is lost, resulting in a sunken in appearance.

NOE fractures can be disfiguring and result in significant cosmetic deformity if not accurately repaired. Not only is the nose telescoped in but also the normal distance between the eyes (ie, intercanthal distance) may be disrupted. This is because the medial canthal tendon inserts onto the medial orbital rim at the confluence of the lacrimal bone and frontal process of the maxilla, and the medial orbital rim is a central component of the NOE fracture pattern (**Fig. 7**). If the medial canthal tendon is disrupted, or the bone bearing

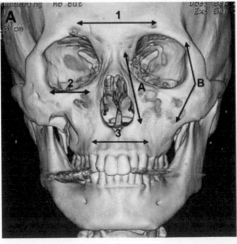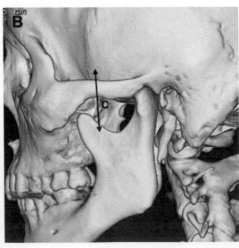

Fig. 6. **Buttress system of the face.** (*A, B*) The buttresses of the midface are areas of thick bone that lend structural support to the face. Three main vertical buttresses, from medial to lateral, include nasomaxillary (A), zygomaticomaxillary (B), and pterygomaxillary (C) buttresses. Three main horizontal buttresses, from superior to inferior, include the superior orbital rim (1), inferior orbital rim (2) and alveolar ridge (3).

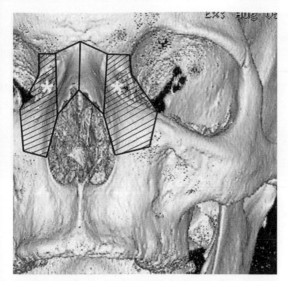

Fig. 7. **Anatomy of the NOE fracture.** The shaded region reflects the area of the medial orbital rim that is disrupted in NOE fractures. The medial canthal tendon inserts onto the medial orbital rim, at the junction of the lacrimal bone and frontal process of the maxilla (*white asterisk* at tendon insertion). The status of this bone, whether or not it is a single segment fracture or comminuted, should always be described.

the tendinous insertion is displaced, the inner corners of the eyes will appear too far apart (telecanthus) and the normal soft tissue contour in the medial canthal area will be lost.

Classification of NOE fractures depends on the status of the central bone fragment of the medial orbital rim onto which the medial canthal tendon inserts. According to Markowitz and colleagues,[11] type I injuries are single-segment fractures of the medial orbital rim without comminution. Type II injuries involve comminution of the medial orbital rim but the tendon remains attached. Type III injuries involve comminution of the bone at the site of tendon attachment or tendon avulsion. CT can determine whether or not the fracture is single segment or comminuted, but the status of the medial canthal tendon and the bone to which it inserts is an intraoperative assessment, not a radiologic one. Radiologic assessment of NOE fractures should specifically describe the status of the medial orbital rim near the lacrimal fossa and whether or not the fracture is single segment or comminuted (Fig. 8). This aids surgical planning for the type of exposure and amount of stabilization that is needed.

Functional complications of NOE fractures include nasolacrimal duct injury and dacrocystitis or dacrocystocele formation. The nasolacrimal duct should be evaluated for fracture extension or disruption. NOE fractures may also extend into the anterior skull base, resulting in cerebrospinal fluid leak, olfactory bulb injury, or frontal lobe contusion. The brain should be evaluated for evidence of hemorrhage in all patients with a NOE fracture. (See Table 2 for a checklist of relevant imaging findings to describe with NOE fractures.)

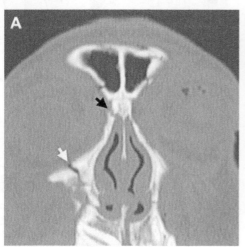
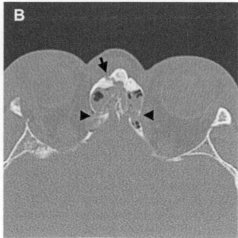

Fig. 8. **NOE fracture.** (*A, B*) There are fractures through the medial orbital rim involving the frontal process of the maxilla (*black arrow*) and (*A*) inferior orbital rim (*white arrow*). This is a single segment NOE fracture because there is no comminution of the central fragment bearing the medial canthal tendon. (*B*) Note fractures through the medial orbital walls and ethmoid air cells bilaterally (*arrowheads*) with concomitant posterior buckling or telescoping of the ethmoid.

Table 2
Imaging checklist for naso-orbito-ethmoidal fractures

Relevant Imaging Findings to Report	Clinical Significance
Single segment versus comminuted fracture of medial orbital rim	Helps surgical planning
Fracture through nasolacrimal duct	Risk of dacrocystitis and dacrocystocele
Anterior skull base fracture extension	Risk of cerebrospinal fluid leak, olfactory disruption, intracranial injury
Frontal lobe contusion	Worse functional outcome (indication for urgent neurosurgical consult)

ZYGOMATICOMAXILLARY COMPLEX FRACTURES

As with all facial fractures, the optimal evaluation of the ZMC fracture requires an accurate understanding of the anatomy and structural supports of the midface. Radiologists are accustomed to describing the individual components through which each fracture line passes (eg, anterior wall of the maxillary sinus or posterior wall of the maxillary sinus). Although this is important, a 3-D conceptual understanding of the ZMC fracture pattern and its relationship to the structural support of the facial skeleton is also important. Because treating surgeons need to restore normal facial contour, they approach ZMC fractures from the standpoint of which key articulations and buttresses have been disrupted and need to be carefully realigned.

The zygoma, which is central to normal malar projection, has four key articulations with the frontal, maxillary, temporal, and sphenoid bones: zygomaticofrontal, zygomaticomaxillary, zygomaticotemporal, and zygomaticosphenoid, respectively (Fig. 9). The classic ZMC fracture disrupts all four articulations and, although frequently known as a tripod fracture, it is more accurately termed a *tetrapod* fracture (Fig. 10). The lateral orbital rim is fractured with injury to the zygomaticofrontal articulation; the inferior orbital rim, orbital floor, and maxillary sinus walls are fractured with injury to the zygomaticomaxillary articulation; the zygomatic arch with the zygomaticotemporal articulation; and the lateral orbital wall with the zygomaticosphenoid articulation (Table 3). The ZMC fracture is actually a spectrum of injuries, and not all four fracture components may be present. The zygomaticofrontal articulation is the strongest of the four articulations and may be the last to fracture.

Cosmetically, malar asymmetry is a significant complication of ZMC fractures (Fig. 11). After the blunt impact that causes the characteristic ZMC fracture pattern and isolates the zygoma from the rest of the facial skeleton, the pull of the masseter muscle, which extends from the zygoma to insert on the ramus of the mandible, can cause an additional rotational deformity of the zygoma and malar depression. Restoring a patient's premorbid facial contour is a chief goal of the surgeon, who pays particular attention to re-establishing accurate alignment across the zygomaticofrontal and zygomaticomaxillary articulations, inferior orbital rim, and lateral orbital wall (zygomaticosphenoid

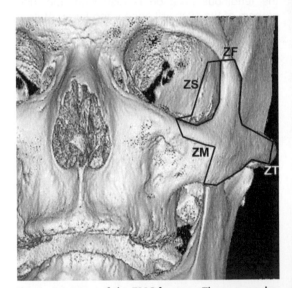

Fig. 9. **Anatomy of the ZMC fracture.** The zygoma has four articulations with other facial bones: zygomaticomaxillary (ZM), zygomaticotemporal (ZT), zygomaticofrontal (ZF), and zygomaticosphenoid (ZS), which makes up the lateral orbital wall. The classic ZMC fracture disrupts all four articulations and is, therefore, a tetrapod fracture, although there is a spectrum of ZMC fractures, and not all four articulations may be disrupted.

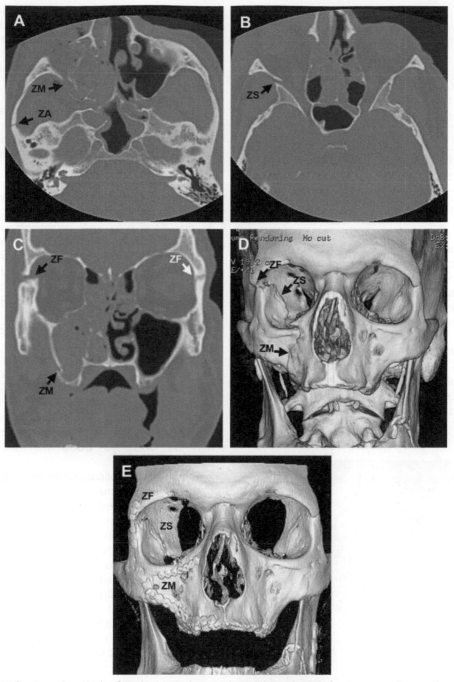

Fig. 10. **ZMC fracture.** (*A–C*) The four key articulations disrupted with ZMC fractures are shown: the zygomatic arch (ZA) and zygomaticosphenoid articulation (ZS) are best seen in the axial plane; the zygomaticofrontal articulation (ZF) in the coronal plane; and the zygomaticomaxillary buttress (ZM) in either axial or coronal plane. The normal contralateral zygomaticofrontal articulation is labeled in white. (*D*) 3-D reformation better depicts the overall relationship of the fracture fragment to the rest of the facial skeleton, showing that the fragment is medially displaced. Medial buckling at the zygomaticosphenoid articulation, which makes up the lateral orbital wall, is well seen on this view. (*E*) 3-D reformation after surgical repair shows that normal facial alignment has been restored by miniplating across the zygomaticofrontal and zygomaticomaxillary articulations, including the inferior orbital rim. Note that plating across these key regions has re-established normal alignment across the zygomaticosphenoid articulation.

Table 3
Zygomaticomaxillary complex or tetrapod fracture

Four key Articulations	Visualized Fracture Lines
Zygomaticofrontal	Lateral orbital rim
Zygomaticomaxillary	Inferior orbital rim; orbital floor; maxillary sinus walls
Zygomaticotemporal	Zygomatic arch
Zygomaticosphenoid	Lateral orbital wall

suture). Fractures that are not displaced do not require surgery.

For fractures that are displaced, the extent of displacement and comminution helps to guide surgical decision making with respect to the type of reduction performed (open versus closed), the type of exposure and incision made, and the extent of fixation required. If a ZMC fracture is significantly displaced and comminuted, open reduction is performed and restoration of alignment is often accomplished by the use of miniplates across select, load-bearing regions. As discussed previously, the zygomaticofrontal and

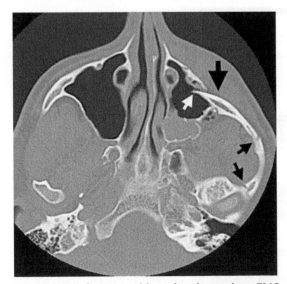

Fig. 11. **ZMC fracture with malar depression.** ZMC fracture with disruption of the zygomatic arch (*small black arrows*) and zygomaticomaxillary articulation (*white arrow*) is associated with significant malar depression (*large black arrow*) as compared with the contralateral side. The zygoma will need to be elevated during surgery to re-establish normal facial contour.

zygomaticomaxillary articulations are part of an important vertical buttress in the midface that bears high physiologic loads due to the forces of mastication.[12] Miniplating is often performed across one or both of these articulations to stabilize and maintain the reduction (see Fig. 10). ZMC fractures that are not comminuted or significantly displaced may be repaired without fixation by closed reduction, although there is considerable controversy regarding the optimal surgical management of various types of ZMC fractures.[13,14]

Enophthalmos is another significant cosmetic complication, given the orbital floor fracture that invariably accompanies the ZMC fracture. As discussed previously, significant depression of the orbital floor with more than 50% involvement of the floor may enlarge the volume of the orbit to such a degree that visually apparent enophthalmos results. Large defects of the orbital floor are an indication for open surgical repair. In addition to the orbital floor fracture, the fracture through the zygomaticosphenoid articulation (lateral orbital wall) may displace laterally, enlarging the orbit and contributing to enophthalmos. In addition to enophthalmos, ZMC fractures may result in a downward sloping of the outer corner of the eye because the lateral canthal ligament inserts approximately 1 cm below the zygomaticofrontal articulation and may be displaced along with the zygoma fracture.

Functional complications of the ZMC fracture can include trismus if the zygomatic arch becomes depressed and strikes the coronoid process onto which the temporalis muscle inserts (Fig. 12). In addition, fractures of the maxilla that are depressed into the sinus or obstruct the maxillary sinus ostium can result in posttraumatic sinusitis. Other functional complications, such as diplopia and infraorbital anesthesia, are due to the orbital fracture component (discussed previously). (See Table 4 for a checklist of relevant imaging findings to describe with ZMC fractures.)

LE FORT FRACTURES

In the early twentieth century, René Le Fort described three predictable types of midface fracture patterns after blunt force injury to cadaver skulls. All three types of Le Fort fractures disrupt the pterygomaxillary buttress. This injury detaches the maxilla from the skull base and results in varying degrees of midface detachment depending on the severity of injury (Fig. 13). In a Le Fort I fracture, also known as the floating

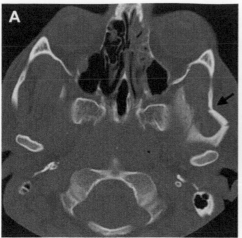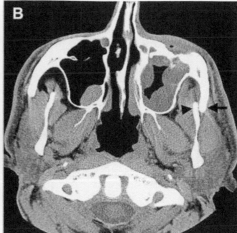

Fig. 12. **ZMC fracture with trismus.** (*A*) This patient with a ZMC fracture and comminuted, depressed zygomatic arch (*arrow*) had trismus. (*B*) The depressed zygomatic arch (*arrow*) impales the temporalis muscle at its insertion on the coronoid process of the mandible (*arrowhead*) and has resulted in trismus, a known functional complication.

palate injury, the fracture occurs in a horizontal plane and detaches the hard palate or maxillary alveolus from the skull base. In a Le Fort II injury, fractures through the medial and inferior orbital rims and zygomaticomaxillary buttress dissociate the central midface from the rest of the skull, allowing the nose and hard palate to move as a unit. A Le Fort III injury is complete midface dissociation.

Pure Le Fort injuries are uncommon because the forces incurred to the face during motor vehicle and other types of accidents are often greater and more complex than taken into consideration by Le Fort. Fractures may occur as a simultaneous

Table 4
Imaging checklist for zygomaticomaxillary complex fractures

Relevant Imaging Findings to Report	Clinical Significance
Displaced versus nondisplaced (malar depression, rotation)	Displaced fracture is indication for surgery
Comminuted versus noncomminuted	Helps surgical planning
Associated skull base or craniofacial fractures	Helps surgical planning
Depression of zygomatic arch contacting coronoid process of mandible	Risk of trismus
Angulation of lateral orbital wall (zygomaticosphenoid suture)	May be overlooked clinically; can cause enophthalmos
Fragments in the maxillary sinus	Risk of sinusitis; sinus obstruction if not surgically repositioned
Extent of orbital floor disruption and change in orbital volume[a]	Large defects result in enophthalmos if not repaired
Extraocular muscle or soft tissue herniation[a]	Indication for surgical repair if there is entrapment
Fracture through infraorbital foramen[a]	Risk of cheek, gum anesthesia
Globe injury or orbital hematoma[a]	Risk of blindness (indication for urgent ophthalmologic consult)
Intracranial hemorrhage	Poorer functional outcome (indication for urgent neurosurgical consult)

[a] Same considerations as for isolated orbital floor blow-out fractures.

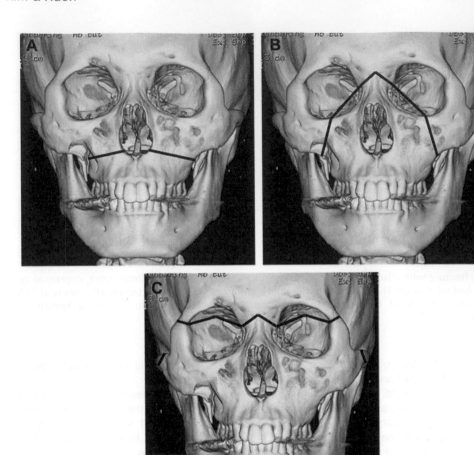

Fig. 13. Le Fort fracture patterns. All three Le Fort fractures disrupt the pterygomaxillary buttress (not pictured), which allows for varying degrees of maxillary separation from the rest of the skull base depending on the specific type of Le Fort fracture. (*A*) Le Fort I fracture is a horizontal fracture through all walls of the maxillary sinus, allowing free movement of the hard palate. (*B*) Le Fort II fracture is a pyramidal fracture that spares the medial wall of the maxillary sinus (unlike Le Fort I) and involves the medial and inferior orbital rim/wall and nasofrontal articulation. This allows for free movement of the nose and hard palate as a unit. (*C*) Le Fort III fracture is complete midface dissociation with fractures through the zygomatic arch, which is unique to this type of Le Fort injury. Fractures are also seen through the medial and lateral orbital wall/rim and nasofrontal articulation, allowing free movement of the entire midface.

combination of Le Fort patterns (eg, both Le Fort I and III injuries), affect only one side of the face (eg, Le Fort I on the right and Le Fort II on the left), or occur in combination with other fracture types, such as ZMC. Despite the difficulties of oversimplification inherent to any classification system, the Le Fort system continues to remain a useful way to approach midface fractures and succinctly communicate complex fracture patterns to other physicians.

To identify a Le Fort fracture pattern on CT, it is useful to look first at the pterygoid plates. As

discussed previously, all Le Fort fractures disrupt the pterygomaxillary buttress and so are associated with fractures of the pterygoid plate. If the pterygoid plates are fractured, the rest of the facial skeleton should be examined for a Le Fort injury.[15]

The Le Fort I fracture is a horizontally oriented fracture line, which is best appreciated on coronal reformatted images as a fracture through all walls of the maxillary sinus. It is this disruption of the maxillary sinus and pterygoid plates that allows free movement of the hard palate (Fig. 14). Unlike Le Fort I injuries, Le Fort II fractures are pyramidal

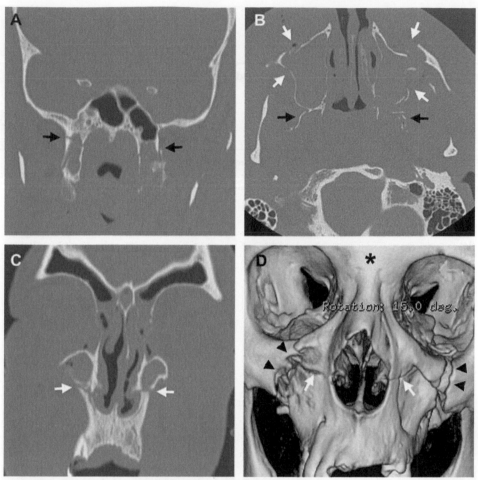

Fig. 14. Bilateral Le Fort I fractures. (*A*) Coronal CT shows fractures through the pterygoid plates bilaterally (*black arrows*), which raise suspicion for Le Fort injury. (*B, C*) All walls of the maxillary sinuses are fractured bilaterally (*white arrows*), consistent with bilateral Le Fort I fractures. Note that the coronal view shows the horizontal nature of this fracture particularly well, with characteristic fractures through the anteromedial walls of both maxillary sinuses, adjacent to the nasal fossa (*white arrows* [*C*]). (*D*) Coronal 3-D reformation again shows the horizontal fracture line (*white arrows*) though the maxillary sinuses above the alveolar ridge that results in the floating palate. Le Fort fractures are often associated with other fractures, and this patient also had bilateral inferior orbital rim fractures through the zygomaticomaxillary buttress (*black arrowheads*) as part of bilateral ZMC fractures (not pictured). Although the inferior orbital rims are fractured, this is not a Le Fort II injury because the medial orbital rims and nasofrontal articulation (*asterisk*) are intact.

in shape and spare the medial wall of the maxillary sinus. Le Fort II fractures disrupt the anterior and posterolateral walls of the maxillary sinus, inferior orbital rim/floor, and medial orbital rim/wall through the nasofrontal articulation or frontal process of the maxilla. Fracture of the inferior orbital rim is unique to Le Fort II injuries as compared with the other types of Le Fort fractures. Le Fort III fractures involve the zygomatic arch. Because this is a distinguishing feature from Le Fort I and II injuries, fractures through the pterygoid plates and zygomatic arch should raise

suspicion for a Le Fort III injury (**Table 5**).[15] Le Fort III fractures disrupt the zygomatic arch, lateral orbital rim (zygomaticofrontal articulation), and lateral orbital wall (zygomaticosphenoid articulation), similar to ZMC fractures. Unlike ZMC injuries, however, Le Fort III fractures spare the inferior orbital rim and instead disrupt the medial orbital rim/wall and nasofrontal articulation. Le Fort III injuries are more extensive than ZMC fractures in that the entire midface, including the nose, maxilla, and zygoma, is freely mobile with respect to the rest of the skull (**Fig. 15**).

Table 5
Le Fort fracture[a]

Injury	Distinguishing Features[b]	Helpful Clues
Le Fort I	All walls of maxillary sinus involved	Best seen in coronal plane
Le Fort II	Inferior orbital rim involved	Spares medial wall of maxillary sinus, unlike Le Fort I
Le Fort III	Zygomatic arch involved	Distinguish from ZMC by medial orbital and pterygoid plate fractures

[a] All Le Fort fracture types are associated with fractures through the pterygoid plates.
[b] *Data from* Rhea JT, Novelline RA. How to simplify the CT diagnosis of Le Fort fractures. AJR Am J Roentgenol 2005;184:1700–5. (Discussion on how to quickly and accurately identify Le Fort fracture patterns.)

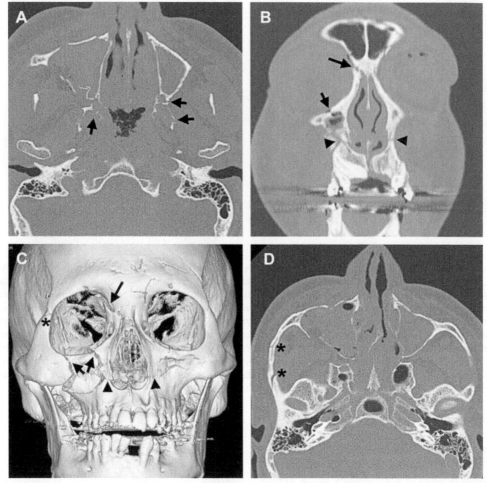

Fig. 15. **Bilateral Le Fort I and right Le Fort II-III fractures.** (*A*) Axial CT scan shows fractures through the pterygoid plates bilaterally (*arrows*), concerning for Le Fort injury. (*B*) Coronal CT shows horizontally oriented fractures through the medial maxillary sinus adjacent to the nasal fossa (*arrowheads*), consistent with Le Fort I fracture as confirmed in other planes. There are additional fractures through the right inferior orbital rim (*short arrow*) and medial right orbit (*long arrow*), through the frontal process of the maxilla, consistent with Le Fort II injury. (*C*) 3-D reformation shows the bilateral horizontally oriented Le Fort I fracture (*arrowheads*) and right Le Fort II fracture with disruption of the inferior orbital rim (*short arrows*) and medial orbit (*long arrow*). There is a non-displaced fracture of the right lateral orbital rim (*). (*D*) Axial CT shows fractures through the right zygomatic arch (*). This was associated with fractures of the lateral orbital wall and rim and consistent with additional Le Fort III injury on the right.

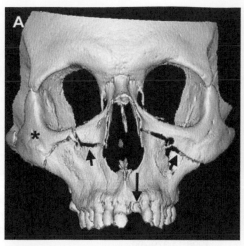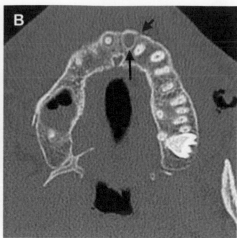

Fig. 16. **Le Fort I fracture and dentoalveolar trauma.** (*A*) 3-D reformation shows bilateral Le Fort I fractures (*short arrows*) resulting in a floating palate. The left central incisor is absent (*long arrow*). Also note an associated ZMC fracture on the right with a freely mobile zygoma (*). (*B*) Axial noncontrast CT shows the empty tooth socket (*long arrow*) and a fracture through the anterior maxillary alveolus as part of a dental avulsion injury (*short arrow*).

Complications of Le Fort fractures include not only significant cosmetic deformity but also serious functional sequelae. The most worrisome acute complication is airway obstruction due to posterior and inferior displacement of the detached midface fracture fragment. Because they result in separation of the maxilla, Le Fort fractures can also cause dental malocclusion. Le Fort fractures, in particular Le Fort I injuries, may also be associated with dentoalveolar trauma because the forceful impact on the maxilla may result in dental avulsion, displacement, loosening, or fracture (**Fig. 16**). Another serious complication

that may be overlooked is blunt cerebrovascular injury. Le Fort II and III fractures are associated with a higher risk of cerebrovascular injury, such as internal carotid artery dissection or pseudoaneurysm and are indications for screening with CT angiography.[16–18] Other functional complications that may result from Le Fort fractures, such as injury to the nasolacrimal duct, infraorbital nerve, and extraocular muscle, depend on whether or not the fracture involves the orbit or other anatomic structures (discussed previously). Finally, it is always important to remember to inspect the brain for associated hemorrhagic injury

Table 6
Imaging checklist for Le Fort fractures

Relevant Imaging Findings to Report	Clinical Significance
Type of Le Fort fracture	Accurate communication among physicians Helps surgical planning
Dentoalveolar trauma	Helps treatment planning
Fracture through nasolacrimal duct	Risk of dacrocystitis and dacrocystocele
Globe injury or orbital hematoma	Risk of blindness (indication for urgent ophthalmologic consult)
Intracranial hemorrhage	Worse functional outcome (indication for urgent neurosurgical consult)
Associated skull base fractures	Helps surgical planning Risk of cerebrospinal fluid leak
Consider screening intracranial CT angiogram for Le Fort II and III fractures	Association with blunt cerebrovascular injury

as well as the skull base (particularly on coronal and sagittal reformatted views) for fractures or defects that may predispose to cerebrospinal fluid leak because of the high incidence of skull base fractures that may occur with Le Fort fractures. (See Table 6 for a checklist of relevant imaging features to describe with Le Fort fractures.)

SUMMARY

Recognizing typical midface fracture injuries and describing the relevant imaging findings are important, and particular attention should be paid to findings that potentially result in significant cosmetic or functional complications. Radiologists should evaluate facial fractures in multiple planes with coronal and sagittal reformats, which are especially helpful for horizontally oriented facial fractures, such as injuries to the orbital floor and the hard palate. 3-D images can also facilitate a broader understanding of the fracture impact on facial width, height, and projection and are useful for an overview of more complex fracture patterns that involve multiple facial bones.

REFERENCES

1. Aksoy E, Unlu E, Sensoz O. A retrospective study on epidemiology and treatment of maxillofacial fractures. J Craniofac Surg 2002;13:772−5.

2. Motamedi MH. An assessment of maxillofacial fractures: a 5-year study of 237 patients. J Oral Maxillofac Surg 2003;61:61−4.

3. Gassner R, Tuli T, Hachl O, et al. Cranio-maxillofacial trauma: a 10 year review of 9,543 cases with 21,067 injuries. J Craniomaxillofac Surg 2003;31:51−61.

4. Ahn HB, Ryu WY, Yoo KW, et al. Prediction of enophthalmos by computer-based volume measurement of orbital fractures in a Korean population. Ophthal Plast Reconstr Surg 2008;24:36−9.

5. Jin HR, Shin SO, Choo MJ, et al. Relationship between the extent of fracture and the degree of enophthalmos in isolated blowout fractures of the medial orbital wall. J Oral Maxillofac Surg 2000;58: 617−20 [discussion: 620−1].

6. Whitehouse RW, Batterbury M, Jackson A, et al. Prediction of enophthalmos by computed tomography after 'blow out' orbital fracture. Br J Ophthalmol 1994; 78:618−20.

7. Burnstine MA. Clinical recommendations for repair of isolated orbital floor fractures: an evidence-based analysis. Ophthalmology 2002;109:1207−10 [discussion: 1210−1; quiz: 1212−3].

8. Hawes MJ, Dortzbach RK. Surgery on orbital floor fractures. Influence of time of repair and fracture size. Ophthalmology 1983;90:1066−70.

9. Parbhu KC, Galler KE, Li C, et al. Underestimation of soft tissue entrapment by computed tomography in orbital floor fractures in the pediatric population. Ophthalmology 2008;115:1620−5.

10. Jordan DR, Allen LH, White J, et al. Intervention within days for some orbital floor fractures: the white-eyed blowout. Ophthal Plast Reconstr Surg 1998;14:379−90.

11. Markowitz BL, Manson PN, Sargent L, et al. Management of the medial canthal tendon in nasoethmoid orbital fractures: the importance of the central fragment in classification and treatment. Plast Reconstr Surg 1991;87:843−53.

12. Linnau KF, Stanley RB Jr, Hallam DK, et al. Imaging of high-energy midfacial trauma: what the surgeon needs to know. Eur J Radiol 2003;48:17−32.

13. Zingg M, Laedrach K, Chen J, et al. Classification and treatment of zygomatic fractures: a review of 1,025 cases. J Oral Maxillofac Surg 1992;50: 778−90.

14. Zachariades N, Mezitis M, Anagnostopoulos D. Changing trends in the treatment of zygomaticomaxillary complex fractures: a 12-year evaluation of methods used. J Oral Maxillofac Surg 1998;56: 1152−6 [discussion: 1156−7].

15. Rhea JT, Novelline RA. How to simplify the CT diagnosis of Le Fort fractures. AJR Am J Roentgenol 2005;184:1700−5.

16. Biffl WL, Moore EE, Offner PJ, et al. Optimizing screening for blunt cerebrovascular injuries. Am J Surg 1999;178:517−22.

17. Cothren CC, Moore EE, Ray Jr CE, et al. Screening for blunt cerebrovascular injuries is cost-effective. Am J Surg 2005;190:845−9.

18. Schneidereit NP, Simons R, Nicolaou S, et al. Utility of screening for blunt vascular neck injuries with computed tomographic angiography. J Trauma 2006;60:209−15 [discussion: 215−6].

Intracranial Hypotension and Intracranial Hypertension

Esther L. Yuh* and William P. Dillon

KEYWORDS

- Intracranial hypotension • Intracranial hypertension
- Pseudotumor cerebri • Intracranial pressure

INTRACRANIAL PRESSURE

Intracranial pressure (ICP) is the pressure within the intracranial space. In the steady state, pressure within the brain parenchyma and intracranial extra-axial spaces are equal. Normal values of ICP are 5 to 15 mm Hg (6–20 cm H_2O) in adults and older children (ages 8 years and older) in the supine position, 1 to 7 mm Hg (1–10 cm H_2O) in younger children, and up to 18 mm Hg (25 cm H_2O) in obese patients.[1,2] ICP increases with Valsalva maneuver, and falls below atmospheric pressure in the standing position. In the lateral decubitus position with lower extremities and neck in neutral position, ICP is approximately equal to intraspinal pressure, and can be estimated by measurement of the cerebrospinal fluid (CSF) opening pressure at lumbar puncture.

Intracranial hypotension is a clinical syndrome in which low CSF volume results in orthostatic headache. Severe cases can result in nausea, vomiting, photophobia, and, rarely, decreased level of consciousness and coma. CSF opening pressures of less than 6 cm H_2O are typical in intracranial hypotension. However, because CSF opening pressure can be within the normal range in spontaneous (or primary) intracranial hypotension (SIH), imaging tests frequently play a key and decisive role in its diagnosis.

Intracranial hypertension occurs in a chronic form known as idiopathic intracranial hypertension (IIH), as well as in a large variety of neurologic and systemic disorders, including intracranial mass, traumatic brain injury, ischemic or hemorrhagic stroke, hydrocephalus, dural sinus thrombosis, dural arteriovenous fistula, and diffuse cerebral edema such as in liver failure. ICP in the range of 20 to 30 mm Hg is considered mildly increased, whereas ICP persistently exceeding 40 mm Hg is severe and life threatening. Symptoms of intracranial hypertension include headache, nausea and vomiting, blurred vision, and in severe cases, altered level of consciousness and death. Direct measurements of CSF pressure through lumbar puncture (in IIH) or invasive ICP monitoring (in acute intracranial hypertension) are essential diagnostic tests. Imaging is used primarily to determine causes of increased ICP, to assess for impending brain herniation, and to evaluate ventricular size.

The Monro-Kellie doctrine[3] describes the relationship among volumes and pressures in the intracranial space, and is relevant to both intracranial hypotension and intracranial hypertension clinical syndromes. It is based on the principle that, within the fixed volume of the intracranial and intraspinal spaces, the total volume of CSF, brain and spinal cord, and intracranial and intraspinal blood volume remains approximately constant. A change in the volume of any one of the compartments is offset by compensatory changes in the other two compartments. For example, in intracranial hypotension, a reduction of CSF volume results in compensatory enlargement of intracranial venous and arterial structures. If expansion of the cerebral vascular volume does not offset the loss of CSF, formation of subdural collections and subdural hematomas may occur. In

Department of Radiology, University of California at San Francisco, 505 Parnassus Avenue, San Francisco, CA 94143-0628, USA
* Corresponding author.
E-mail address: esther.yuh@radiology.ucsf.edu

Neuroimag Clin N Am 20 (2010) 597–617
doi:10.1016/j.nic.2010.07.012

neuroimaging.theclinics.com

intracranial hypertension caused by space-occupying mass lesions, the Monro-Kellie doctrine may be manifested by effacement of cerebral sulci and brain herniation.

INTRACRANIAL HYPOTENSION

In intracranial hypotension, low CSF volume results in orthostatic headache, and, less commonly, nausea, vomiting, photophobia, and, rarely, decreased level of consciousness. Intracranial hypotension results from loss of CSF through a dural defect in the spine, cranial vault, or skull base. SIH refers loosely to cases of intracranial hypotension in which a dural defect is identified and cannot be attributed to a prior procedure or to trauma. Causes of secondary intracranial hypotension include lumbar puncture, cranial or spinal surgery, and head or spine trauma.

CLINICAL PRESENTATION
Symptoms

The most common symptom in intracranial hypotension is orthostatic, or postural, headache. The classic orthostatic headache commences within 15 minutes, but occasionally up to several hours, after assuming a standing or upright sitting position.[4,5] Improvement or resolution typically occurs within 15 to 30 minutes of lying down. Orthostatic headache in SIH is most likely caused by downward displacement of the brain and resulting traction on the richly innervated dura. Orthostatic headaches are generally gradual in onset, and vary in severity from mild to debilitating.[4,6] Over time, the orthostatic feature of the headache may lessen, with a pattern of chronic daily headache ensuing. Very rarely, presentation with a thunderclap headache may mimic acute aneurysmal subarachnoid hemorrhage.[7] Secondary subdural effusions or hematomas may also complicate SIH, leading to constant, nonpostural headaches. Following treatment, rebound increase in ICP with constant headaches may occur.[8,9]

Secondary symptoms often seen in conjunction with the postural headache include posterior neck pain or stiffness, and nausea and vomiting, attributable to meningeal irritation in approximately 50% of patients, sometimes with accompanying photophobia and, less commonly, hypacusia and tinnitus, attributable to either vestibulocochlear nerve traction associated with the sagging brain, or transmission of low CSF pressure to the perilymph.[6] Presence of at least one of these secondary symptoms, in addition to orthostatic headache, is required for the diagnosis of

headache due to SIH in the 2004 International Classification of Headache Disorders (ICHD-2).[5]

Less common symptoms include vertigo, balance disturbance, blurred vision or visual field deficits, diplopia, facial pain or numbness, facial weakness or spasm, and dysgeusia, also attributed to cranial nerve distortion or compression caused by downward displacement of the brain.[6]

Although very uncommon, stupor or coma, rarely progressing to demise from tonsillar herniation and brainstem compression, can be the initial presentation in severe intracranial hypotension.[10–17]

Demographics

SIH occurs more often in women, with a female/male ratio of 3:2. Peak incidence is at approximately 40 years of age, with most cases presenting in the 40- to 60-year age range. However, the condition has been reported in patients as young as 3 years and as old as 86 years.[4] Although the prevalence and incidence of SIH are unknown, one study reported an estimated annual incidence of 5/1000, based on the frequency of this diagnosis in an emergency department setting.[4] The observation that reported incidences of SIH have increased in the past decade implies that the condition is likely still underdiagnosed, because the condition has only recently been recognized.[6]

PATHOPHYSIOLOGY

Most CSF is formed in the ventricular system through active secretion by the choroid plexus. The average CSF volume in adults is approximately 150 mL, and the rate of CSF formation in adults is approximately 500 mL/d.[18,19] The arachnoid granulations (projections of the arachnoid membrane into the venous sinuses) are the major site of CSF absorption.

Post–lumbar puncture headache was described as early as 1899 by Dr August Bier, a pioneer of spinal anesthesia, who stated after undergoing such a procedure himself, "All these symptoms [pressure in the head and dizziness] disappeared as soon as I lay down horizontally, but returned when I arose."[20] In 1938, the German neurologist Georg Schaltenbrand described a condition of low or negative CSF pressure with associated orthostatic headache, and postulated 3 possible causes for the syndrome he termed "essential aliquorrea": low CSF production, high CSF absorption rate, and CSF leakage. Although low ICP caused by impaired CSF production or increased absorption is theoretically possible (the former has been shown in knockout animals lacking normal aquaporin channels[21]), no cases in humans have yet been documented.

The imaging features of intracranial hypotension were first reported in the early 1990s.[22-26] These included demonstrations of subdural collections, sagging of the brain, engorgement of dural sinuses and other intracranial and intraspinal venous structures, enlargement of pituitary gland, and diffuse dural enhancement on magnetic resonance (MR) imaging. These features can be understood as consequences of the Monro-Kellie doctrine,[3] in which the total volume of CSF, brain and spinal cord, and intracranial and intraspinal blood volume remains approximately constant, with a change in any one of the compartments counteracted by compensatory changes in the other two compartments.

Causes

In both spontaneous and secondary types of intracranial hypotension, the cause is generally CSF leakage through a dural defect. Causes of secondary intracranial hypotension include lumbar puncture,[27,28] cranial or spinal surgery,[29] and head or spine trauma. Incidence of post—lumbar puncture headache is reported at 10% to 30%.[27,28]

In SIH, the exact distribution of causes is unclear, but can be inferred from features of the subset of cases in which an actual dural defect or underlying predisposing clinical factor is identified. The following dural defects have been identified during surgical repair:

1. Defects associated with meningeal diverticula, usually along spinal nerve roots within the neural foramina
2. Total absence of the dural covering, often at the level of the exiting nerve roots
3. Frank holes or tears.

In addition to meningeal diverticula, direct mechanical perforation of the dura secondary to degenerative disc-osteophyte is recognized.[30-34] Approximately one-third of patients with SIH also describe a history of recent minor trauma, although the significance of this is not certain.[6]

Even when a direct cause of CSF fistula is found, a predisposing underlying structural weakness of the spinal meninges may be present. As many as two-thirds of patients with a diagnosis of SIH have some clinical features suggestive of an underlying connective tissue disorder, such as Marfan or Ehlers-Danlos syndromes, autosomal dominant polycystic kidney disease, neurofibromatosis type 1, or Lehman syndrome.[4,6] Even in the absence of a confirmed diagnosis of connective tissue disorder, reports have documented an association of SIH with physical examination findings suggestive of connective tissue disorder, including marfanoid body habitus, joint hypermobility, and spontaneous retinal detachment.[4,6]

DIAGNOSIS

The diagnosis of SIH is based on a combination of clinical signs and symptoms, head and spine imaging, and intrathecal pressure measurements.

Diagnostic Criteria for SIH

The ICHD-2 criteria for SIH are the presence of orthostatic headache with at least one item in each of the following two sets of features:

1. Neck stiffness, tinnitus, hypacusia, photophobia, nausea
2. CSF opening pressure less than 6 cm H_2O, observation of CSF leakage on an imaging study, MR imaging features of SIH.

More recently, Schievink and colleagues[35] offered a scheme that incorporates both clinical and imaging criteria. Although its sensitivity and specificity were not established because of a lack of a gold standard, the investigators applied these criteria in the evaluation of 107 consecutive patients with suspected SIH and found that the criteria were satisfied in 94 of the 107 patients (88%).

Imaging Features of Intracranial Hypotension

CT and MR imaging

At least 4 classic imaging features of intracranial hypotension have been described (Fig. 1). Most of these are understood as consequences of the Monro-Kellie doctrine.[3] With loss of CSF from the subarachnoid space, total intracranial blood volume increases to counteract loss of CSF volume. This increase results in enlargement of intracranial venous and arterial structures (see Fig. 1B, E), which manifests as enlargement and rounding of the dural venous sinuses; engorgement of the epidural vertebral venous plexus, often most notable in the upper cervical spine; and enlargement and engorgement of the pituitary gland.

Diffuse dural enhancement (see Fig. 1C, D) results from continued vascular engorgement and transudation of intravascular fluid (and thus intravenously administered gadolinium) into the subdural space, producing a dura that appears boggy. Continued transudation of fluid results in frank subdural collections (see Fig. 1C, D), which further compensate for low CSF volume.

Brain sagging (see Fig. 1A) is one of the most specific MR imaging findings in intracranial

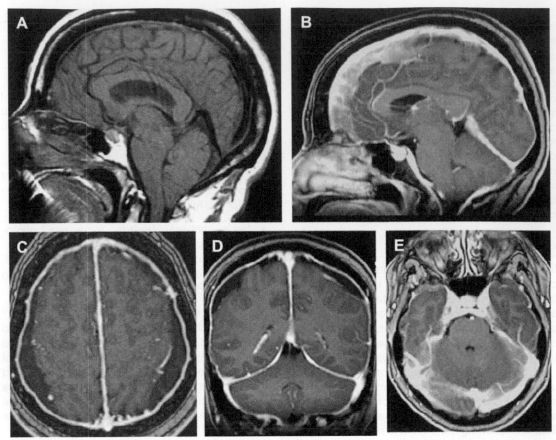

Fig. 1. **MR imaging findings in intracranial hypotension.** (*A*) Brain sagging is manifested as obliteration of the prepontine cistern with varying degrees of flattening of the ventral pons against the clivus, inferior displacement of the floor of the third ventricle, descent of the cerebellar tonsils that can simulate Chiari 1 malformation, and obliteration of the basal cisterns with draping of the optic chiasm over the pituitary gland. (*B, E*) Engorgement of intracranial venous structures. Total intracranial blood volume increases to counteract loss of CSF volume. This manifests as enlargement and rounding of the dural venous sinuses; engorgement of the epidural vertebral venous plexus, often notable along the skull base and in the upper cervical spine; and enlargement of the pituitary gland. (*C, D*) Diffuse smooth dural enhancement and subdural collections. Subdural collections are another compensatory action, believed to result from transudation of intravascular fluid into the subdural space to counteract the decrease in ICP. Diffuse dural enhancement is closely related to the presence of subdural collections, being a result of transudation of fluid and thus intravenously administered gadolinium into the subdural space.

hypotension. Although postulated to be the result, in part, of mass effect from subdural fluid collections, it is more likely the result, at least in part, of decreased buoyancy of the brain caused by the paucity of surrounding CSF. As the brain gains more fluid content and its density increases and more closely matches that of the subarachnoid space CSF, it sinks lower in the fluid column formed by the intracranial and intraspinal subarachnoid space. Brain sagging is manifested on MR imaging as varying degrees of flattening of the ventral pons against the clivus, inferior displacement of the floor of the third ventricle, decreased mamillopontine distance, descent of

the cerebellar tonsils that can simulate Chiari 1 malformation, and obliteration of the basal cisterns with draping of the optic chiasm over the pituitary gland.

Of note, there may be a progression of findings, from initial enlargement of veins, to dural enhancement, to subdural effusions and sagging brain. Thus, the earliest manifestations may be subtle (**Figs. 2** and **3**). These findings are more effectively shown by MR imaging than computed tomography (CT), particularly in early or subtle cases. In addition, up to 20% of patients with clinically apparent SIH reportedly have no abnormal brain MR imaging findings.[4,36]

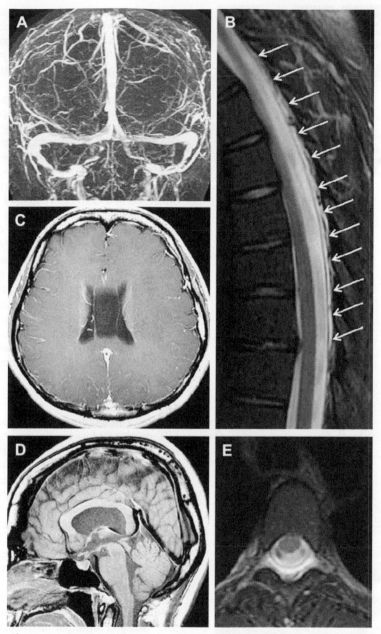

Fig. 2. Isolated dural venous sinus prominence in SIH. 24-year-old woman with a 3-day history of positional headaches. (*A, C, D*) Normal brain MR imaging, with the exception of subtle prominence of the dural venous sinuses. (*B, E*) Subsequent spine MR imaging showed a posterior epidural fluid collection (*arrows*), consistent with spinal CSF leak. Thus, the earliest imaging manifestations of SIH may be subtle, with a progression of findings from initial subtle enlargement of veins, as in this case, to dural enhancement and finally to subdural effusions and sagging brain in untreated severe cases.

CT myelography

CT myelography is the most widely used imaging test to show the site of a suspected CSF leak. After intrathecal administration of iodinated contrast via lumbar puncture, the patient is placed in the Trendelenburg position for approximately 10 minutes. Thin-section axial CT is then performed through the entire spine, and images examined for extrathecal contrast leakage (**Fig. 4**). Most spontaneous CSF leaks are found near the cervicothoracic junction or in the thoracic spine.[37]

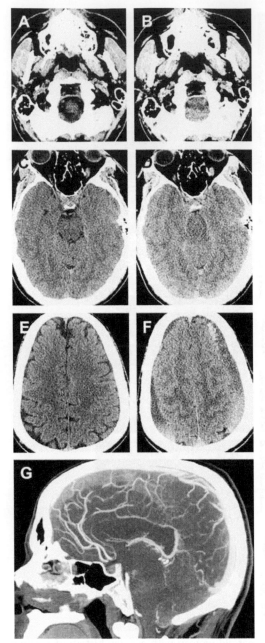

Fig. 3. **Limited sensitivity of CT in early SIH.** 37-year-old man with a 3-month history of progressive headache, which had become severe and debilitating by the time of clinical presentation. (*A, C, E*) Initial noncontrast head CT was normal. Seven weeks later, follow-up head CT (*B, D, F*) and CT angiography (*G*) showed bilateral subdural collections and new downward sagging of the brain, including cerebellar tonsillar herniation. Early MR imaging, in conjunction with the clinical history suggestive of SIH, may have showed subtle early findings leading to an earlier diagnosis. The patient underwent a nontargeted epidural blood patch, followed by a second blood patch targeted to disc-osteophytes at the T5-T6 and T6-T7 levels, with subsequent complete resolution of symptoms.

Although the presence of extradural contrast on initial CT myelography is typically apparent in patients with SIH, subtle or slow leaks may be seen only after additional delayed CT imaging. Although the presence of extradural contrast confirms a leak, the source of the fistula may not be readily apparent because of the quick dispersal of contrast within the epidural space. The use of digital subtraction myelography to identify the site of a rapid CSF leak in the setting of a large cervicothoracic epidural fluid collection has been described.[38] In addition, of note, retrospinal fluid collections at C1-C2 have been reported to be observed in a disproportionately large number of cases of SIH, and should not be mistaken for the site of CSF leakage.[39] These collections have been described in both CT and MR myelography, and most likely represent the egress of extrathecal CSF traveling along the epidural space gutter that allows little impedance to flow of fluid over long distances, and thus represent a false-localizing sign (**Fig. 5**).[40,41] However, others have postulated that this results from transudation of CSF from dilated suboccipital veins (ie, similar in cause to the intracranial subdural collections observed in SIH).

MR myelography

Several investigators have proposed the use of MR myelography, employing injection of intrathecal gadolinium, for the detection of CSF leaks.[42–44] This technique is performed by intrathecal instillation of 0.5 mL or less of gadopentetate dimeglumine diluted with approximately 4 mL of CSF. Axial, coronal, and sagittal fat-suppressed T1-weighted imaging is performed from one to several hours later (see **Fig. 5**). The main advantages of MR imaging include lack of ionizing radiation, increased contrast sensitivity for small subtle leaks, and the possibility of additional delayed imaging, which is generally precluded by CT radiation dose considerations and delayed contrast dispersal with iodinated contrast. The use, in particular, of delayed imaging in MR myelography may increase sensitivity for small or slow CSF leaks, though this hypothesis requires further investigation (**Fig. 6**).

Of note, intrathecal gadolinium administration is not currently approved by the US Food and Drug Administration. A high concentration of gadolinium in the subarachnoid space may cause seizures.[45] In addition, the kinetics of elimination of gadolinium from the CSF space differ than those for intravenously administered gadolinium. In animal studies, gradual enhancement of the brain parenchyma has been observed following intrathecal gadolinium administration, raising concern for the

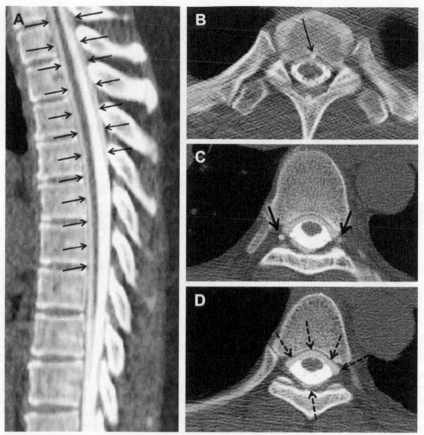

Fig. 4. CT myelography in SIH. 43-year-old woman with a 6-week history of orthostatic headache, photophobia, intermittent nausea, and orthostatic hypacusia. (*A*) Sagittal reformatted CT image and (*B–D*) axial CT images show an extradural CSF collection (*D, arrows*) along the upper and mid thoracic spine (*arrows*). Although no definite focal site of CSF leakage was identified, a dorsal disc-osteophyte at T1-T2 (*B, arrow*) and perineural cysts at multiple spinal levels (*C, arrows*) were suspicious for possible sites of the dural defect.

possibility of acute central nervous system toxicity. However, histologic studies in animals have shown no evidence of injury, and an international registry has reported no significant toxicity with the use of 0.5 to 1 mL of intrathecally administered gadopentetate dimeglumine in humans.[43]

The overall sensitivity of CT and MR myelography for spinal CSF leak is not known. One prospective study successfully showed CSF leaks in 17 of 19 patients, and meningeal diverticula without definite leak in an additional 1 of 19 patients, who satisfied the ICHD-2 criteria for SIH, using CT myelography and heavily T2-weighted MR myelography.[46] Nonetheless, personal observations suggest that a group of patients exists with typical clinical and MR features of SIH in whom no leak can be found, despite CT and MR myelography. These patients typically have numerous perineural cysts, and it

is presumed that one or more of the cysts may be associated with a very slow leak. Other investigators have advocated placing blood patches adjacent to all of the perineural cysts in an effort to stop the presumed leakage. Surgical dural reduction surgery has also been applied to such cases, reducing the volume of the subarachnoid space.[47]

Lumbar Puncture with Opening Pressure Measurement

Normal CSF opening pressure ranges from 1 to 10 cm H_2O in young children, 6 to 20 cm H_2O in adults, and up to 25 cm H_2O in obese patients. To measure CSF opening pressure, the patient should be in the lateral decubitus position with the legs extended and neck in a neutral position. Intracranial hypotension is confirmed with CSF

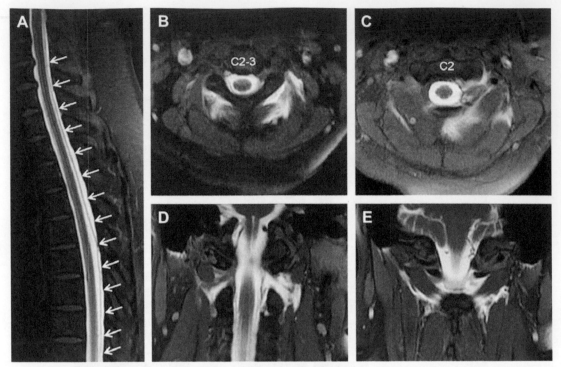

Fig. 5. **MR myelography in SIH.** Sagittal (*A*), axial (*B, C*), and coronal (*D, E*) fat-suppressed T1-weighted images following intrathecal gadolinium administration reveal a dorsal epidural fluid collection compatible with spontaneous CSF leakage (*arrows*). Note the abnormal asymmetric epidural and paraspinal fluid at the left C2-C3 level, a false-localizing sign. After epidural blood patches failed to provide sustained relief of symptoms, the patient underwent surgical repair of dural defect associated with a T3-T4 disc-osteophyte.

opening pressure of less than 6 cm H_2O. CSF pressures can approach zero and can even be slightly less than atmospheric pressure.[4] CSF pressure within the normal range has been documented in some patients with SIH. In such patients, the CSF pressure has presumably fallen but remains within the average normal range.

CSF diagnostic studies in patients with SIH may show normal to increased white blood cell count and a lymphocytic pleocytosis up to 50 cells/mm³. Protein content is normal or increased, sometimes leading to a misdiagnosis of viral meningitis. Xanthochromia is common, and has been postulated to be caused by increased meningeal blood vessel permeability and/or decreased CSF flow in the lumbar subarachnoid space.[4]

TREATMENT

Although recognition of SIH has increased in the past decade because of the increased sensitivity of MR imaging, SIH continues to be frequently misdiagnosed. Suboccipital craniotomies for Chiari 1 malformation, catheter angiography for unexplained headache, and craniotomies for

meningeal biopsy or subdural hematoma evacuation have been performed in cases of undiagnosed SIH (Fig. 7). A 2003 study reported that 17 of 18 consecutive patients referred to a surgical practice for treatment of SIH with a documented CSF leak were initially misdiagnosed by a physician despite typical symptoms.[41] A 2007 study showed that, in a 3-year period, 11 patients who presented to an urban emergency room with SIH were all initially incorrectly diagnosed.[48]

Conservative Treatment

Some cases of SIH resolve spontaneously; thus conservative treatment consisting of bedrest, oral caffeine, and hydration to treat symptoms while waiting for possible spontaneous closure of the leakage site may make sense initially. Intravenous caffeine has also been documented to be effective in post–lumbar puncture headache,[49,50] one study showing relief of headache in 75% of patients compared with a control group treated with intravenous saline.[51] However, unlike the post–lumbar puncture headache, the diagnosis

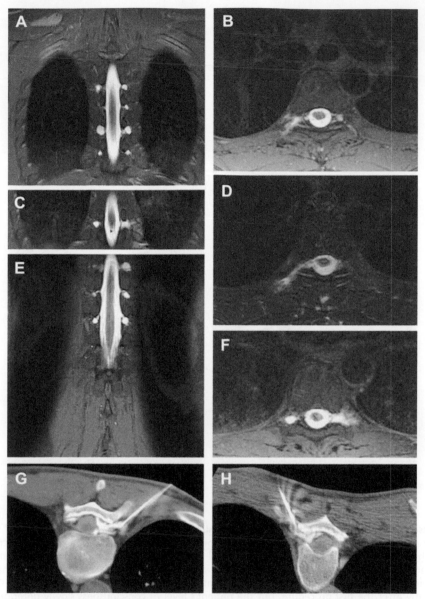

Fig. 6. MR myelography in SIH. 50-year-old man with a 6-year history of progressive neurologic decline, beginning with severe headache and progressing to gait disorder and cranial neuropathies. Coronal (*A, C, E*) and axial (*B, F*) axial fat-suppressed T1-weighted postintrathecal contrast images and (*D*) axial T2-weighted image show two sites of CSF leakage: right T5-T6 perineural cyst (*B*) and left T9-T10 perineural cyst (*F*). Meningeal diverticula are noted at essentially all spinal levels, a frequent finding in SIH believed to be attributable to the higher incidence of connective disorders that predispose patients to this condition. CT myelogram performed earlier the same day failed to show the CSF leak. (*G, H*) Following MR myelographic evidence of sites of CSF leakage, epidural blood patches were applied at the right T5-T6 and left T9-T10 perineural cysts.

of SIH is often made in the setting of longstanding unexplained headaches. Once the diagnosis of SIH is made, epidural blood patch is recommended if conservative treatments fail to reduce headache symptoms.

Epidural Blood Patch

The epidural blood patch is performed by administering autologous blood into the epidural space, usually at a lumbar level (Fig. 8). Typically, 5 to 30 mL of blood are administered slowly to avoid

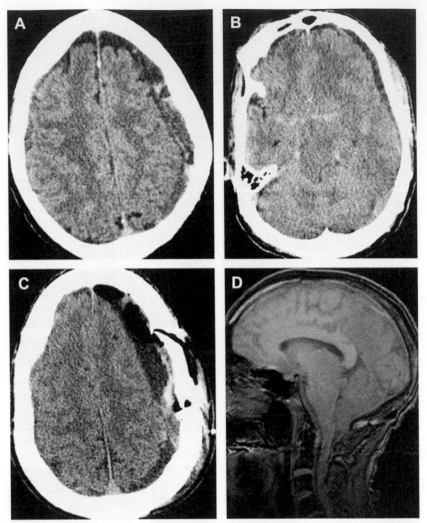

Fig. 7. SIH misdiagnosed as isolated mass effect from a subdural hematoma. Noncontrast head CT (*A, B*) in a 74-year-old man presenting with decreased level of consciousness, progressing to coma. Following craniotomy (*C*) for subdural hematoma evacuation, the patient's clinical status was only minimally improved. Correct diagnosis of SIH was made on review of outside brain MR imaging, which showed characteristic sagging of the brain on T1-weighted sagittal imaging (*D*). The patient underwent 2 epidural blood patch procedures. Clinical status improved briefly after the first procedure, but the patient's level of consciousness slowly deteriorated in the 2 days following the procedure. A second, larger-volume epidural blood patch was performed, resulting in complete return to baseline status, with no known residual neurologic deficits upon hospital discharge.

abrupt local mass effect on the thecal sac that can result in sudden severe back pain or radiculopathy. We use CT guidance to place the needle, and mix a small quantity of iodinated contrast with the blood to visualize the blood as it is injected. The patient is placed in the Trendelenburg position to promote the dispersal of epidural blood cranially along the epidural space. The epidural blood has been shown to spread over many spinal levels, with larger-volume patches traversing a greater number of levels.[52] How this mainstay

treatment of SIH works is not entirely clear. Two mechanisms have been proposed for the efficacy of epidural blood patch. The first is that the blood may increase ICP, by increasing the volume of the epidural space, and the second is that the clot tamponades the site of CSF leakage, sealing off the leakage. These two mechanisms are likely complementary: headache relief is often immediate following blood patch, and, because the formation of CSF is only 0.35 mL/min, this would not be possible if the leak were simply sealed by

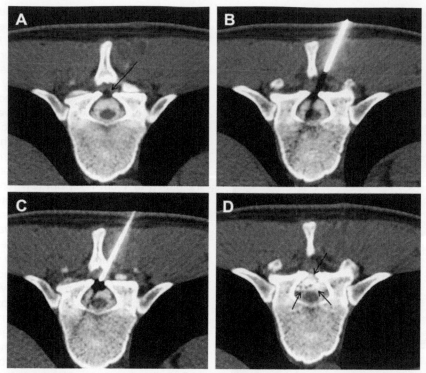

Fig. 8. Epidural blood patch (procedure). Axial CT images showing application of an epidural blood patch. The blood patch is usually performed at a lumbar level, followed by Trendelenburg position, when the site of CSF leak is unknown. However, in cases in which a site of CSF leak is identified at a higher level, blood patches can be performed at a thoracic (as shown here) or cervical level. (*A*) The posterior epidural fat is identified. (*B, C*) Percutaneous needle access to the posterior epidural space. Needle tip location within the posterior epidural space is confirmed by administration of a small quantity (0.2–0.4 mL) of air, with expected indentation of the posterior aspect of the thecal sac. (*D*) Blood patch, consisting of autologous blood mixed with a small quantity of iodinated contrast, has been administered to the posterior epidural space.

a patch. Rapid closure of the leakage site can occur (Fig. 9), with rapid resolution of symptoms, sometimes seen before the patient leaves the examination table. Direct targeting of the blood patch administration to a specific site of known CSF leakage identified through CT or MR myelography is associated with a higher success rate.[53] If an epidural blood patch fails, a repeat large-volume patch can be attempted.

Resolution or significant relief of symptoms is achieved in the majority of patients with SIH. A 2005 study reported that resolution or near-complete resolution of symptoms was achieved in 79% of a series of 33 consecutive patients with SIH symptoms and a confirmed spinal CSF leak on CT myelography through conservative treatment, epidural blood patch, percutaneous fibrin sealant placement, or surgical repair.[36] Targeted epidural blood patch fails to relieve symptoms in approximately one-quarter to one-third of cases with a documented site of CSF leakage. In these cases, percutaneous

application of fibrin glue to the leakage site has proven effective.[4,54]

Surgery is performed rarely for CSF leak, and is reserved for cases in which there has been failure of the percutaneous procedures and when the site of the CSF leakage is known. Most types of meningeal diverticula can be ligated.[4,37,55–57] Pledgets consisting of muscle applied with fibrin sealant to the site of leak, gelfoam, or fibrin sealant alone is also used to pack the epidural space overlying the leak; larger dural tears may be sutured.

Rarely, rebound intracranial hypertension can develop after treatment of intracranial hypertension. In the few reported cases of this phenomenon, orthostatic headache was supplanted by a constant nonorthostatic headache, and nausea, vomiting, blurred vision,[6,8] papilledema, and/or retinal hemorrhages developed.[6,56] An association between SIH and dural venous sinus or cerebral vein thrombosis has been reported, although a definite causal relationship or pathophysiologic mechanism remains to be confirmed.[58–61]

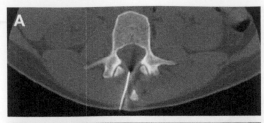

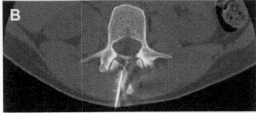

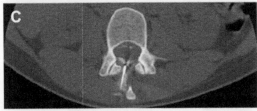

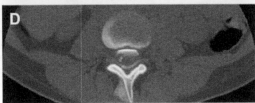

Fig. 9. Epidural blood patch with contrast seen flowing into the thecal sac via a dural tear. Rapid localization of the administered epidural blood to the site of leakage can occur, as shown here. Several minutes after blood patch administration to the posterior epidural space (*A, B*), intrathecal contrast appears within the thecal sac because of imbibation of the administered blood (*C, D*). The clinical correlate of this is rapid resolution of symptoms following the patch of the site of leakage, sometimes observed before the patient leaves the examination table.

Emergent Treatment of Severe Intracranial Hypotension

Whether spontaneous or resulting from surgical or percutaneous intervention, intracranial hypotension is usually not life threatening; however, downward herniation with progressive mental status decline, coma,[10–16] and, rarely, death[17] have been reported in untreated severe cases. In such cases, increase of intracranial and intraspinal pressure by intrathecal infusion of mock CSF (Elliot B solution) or preservative-free saline can be lifesaving if instituted rapidly.[11,16]

Continuous measurement of lumbar CSF pressure to monitor the course of the lumbar saline or Elliot B infusion is performed. In addition, simultaneous monitoring of intracranial as well as lumbar CSF pressure may be helpful. Binder and colleagues[11] reported a case of postural headache that progressed over the course of several weeks to constant headache, and ultimately to declining mental status leading to hospital admission for coma and hyperreflexia. Preservative-free saline was instilled via lumbar catheter, consisting of a 50-mL bolus followed by 30 mL/h continuous infusion. Initial lumbar and ICP were 0. After 2 hours of infusion, lumbar spinal pressure had increased to 1 cm H_2O, but ICP remained at 0. After 5 hours of infusion, ICP abruptly increased to 18 cm H_2O with return of a normal ICP waveform. The sudden increase in ICP was attributed to the time at which continuity between the supra- and infratentorial spaces (or possibly the intracranial and intraspinal subarachnoid spaces and CSF flow through the foramen magnum) was reestablished. The patient's recovery was complete, with no residual neurologic deficits. CT myelography ultimately showed a large upper thoracic extrathecal collection, which was subsequently successfully treated with a 30 mL epidural blood patch.

Complete recovery without residual neurologic deficits is common, even in cases of SIH that have progressed to severe neurologic deficits such as decerebrate posturing, nonreactive pupils, encephalopathic pattern on electroencephalogram, and coma with Glasgow Coma Scale score as low as 4.[11–13,15,16] Rare cases of permanent neurologic deficits, or even death,[17] caused by Duret hemorrhage,[14] have been reported.

INTRACRANIAL HYPERTENSION

Intracranial hypertension can occur in chronic or acute forms in a large variety of neurologic and systemic disorders, including intracranial mass lesions such as tumor or abscess, traumatic brain injury, ischemic or hemorrhagic stroke, dural venous sinus thrombosis, dural arteriovenous fistula, hydrocephalus, or diffuse cerebral edema such as in liver failure. A diagnosis of IIH is made in the setting of chronic elevated ICP when a specific cause cannot be defined. Normal values of ICP in adults are in the range of 5 to 15 mm Hg (6–20 mm H_2O).[1] ICP in the range of 20 to 30 mm Hg is mildly increased and warrants treatment, whereas ICP persistently exceeding 40 mm Hg is severe and life threatening.

CLINICAL PRESENTATION

Acute, abnormal increase of ICP results in headache, nausea and vomiting, blurred vision, and, in severe cases, reflex bradycardia and altered level of consciousness or death caused by cerebral hypoperfusion and/or brain herniation.

In IIH, characterized by mild to intermediate chronic increase of ICP, the most common presenting symptom is chronic daily headache.[62,63] Other common presenting symptoms in IIH are pulsatile tinnitus (60%) and transient visual obscurations (75%),[64] the latter consisting of episodes of transient monocular or binocular vision loss that may occur with changes in head position. Diplopia caused by sixth nerve palsy has also been reported.[62,63] Patients may also present with more sustained, sometimes irreversible, vision impairment caused by longstanding untreated papilledema.[65]

PATHOPHYSIOLOGY
Idiopathic Intracranial Hypertension

IIH, also known as pseudotumor cerebri, is chronically increased ICP in the absence of a specific known cause. Modified Dandy criteria for IIH[66] include increased opening pressure on lumbar puncture, with normal CSF composition and no known specific cause of increased ICP. The overall

Table 1
Causes of intracranial hypertension

Idiopathic Intracranial Hypertension		
Intracranial mass lesion		
Traumatic brain injury	Epidural or subdural hematoma	Hydrocephalus
	Brain parenchymal contusion	Anoxia (cytotoxic edema)
	Cerebral edema caused by vasomotor paralysis/loss of cerebrovascular autoregulation	Cerebral edema caused by brain parenchymal injury (vasogenic, cytotoxic)
	Postoperative (vasogenic and cytotoxic edema, impaired autoregulation)	Hypoxia/hypercarbia (results in cerebral vasodilatation)
Ischemic stroke	Cytotoxic edema, hemorrhagic transformation of infarct	
Nontraumatic intracranial hemorrhage	Hypertensive vasculopathy	Dural venous sinus thrombosis
	Metastatic or primary brain tumor	Dural arteriovenous fistula
	Aneurysmal subarachnoid hemorrhage	Arteriovenous malformation
	Coagulopathy	Cerebral amyloid angiopathy
Intracranial infection	Intracranial abscess	Meningoencephalitis
Hydrocephalus	Obstructive or communicating	
Impaired venous outflow from brain	Increased central venous pressure (heart failure, central venous obstruction, increased intrathoracic pressure from mechanical ventilation or agitation, neck flexion/extension with compression of large cervical veins) Dural venous sinus thrombosis Dural or other intracranial arteriovenous fistula	
Hypoxemia/hypercarbia (causes cerebral vasodilation)	Cardiogenic causes, coma, respiratory depression Airway obstruction, sleep apnea	High-altitude sickness
Drugs and metabolic	Hyponatremia, other electrolyte imbalances	Tetracycline, rofecoxib, divalproex sodium, lead intoxication
Other causes of diffuse cerebral edema	Acute liver failure, end-stage liver disease Severe systemic hypertension, eclampsia	Renal failure including dialysis dysequilibrium syndrome
Secondary factors that may exacerbate intracranial hypertension	Fever	Seizure

Adapted from Rangel-Castilla L, Gopinath S, Robertson CS. Management of intracranial hypertension. Neurol Clin 2008;26(2):521–41.

annual incidence of IIH is 1 to 2 per 100,000,[65,67] although the incidence in women in the 20- to 44-year age range who are more than 20% heavier than ideal body weight is as much as 20 times higher.[65] IIH is likely heterogeneous in cause, given its association with numerous clinical features. In addition to obesity, these also include dural venous sinus thrombosis, sleep apnea, vitamin A toxicity, and withdrawal from steroid medications.[65] African American patients with IIH have been shown to develop severe visual loss more frequently, possibly because of a more aggressive clinical course.[68]

Acute Intracranial Hypertension

In addition to the idiopathic chronic form, acute intracranial hypertension can result from a large number of neurologic and systemic disorders (Table 1).[2] Intracranial mass lesion, traumatic

brain injury, ischemic stroke, hemorrhagic stroke, and other nontraumatic intracranial hemorrhage, hydrocephalus, and liver failure are common causes. In some cases, notably acute traumatic brain injury, increased ICP can be multifactorial (see Table 1).

Acute or severe increase of ICP causes brain damage through several mechanisms. Brain herniation syndromes (Figs. 10 and 11), including downward or upward transtentorial herniation, cerebellar tonsillar herniation, and subfalcine or temporal lobe herniation, result in further compression of critical structures and may lead to death. Cerebral ischemia and stroke (Fig. 12) may occur when cerebral perfusion pressure, defined as the difference between mean arterial pressure and ICP, is reduced to less than the autoregulatory capacity of the brain vasculature. Normal cerebral blood flow is maintained for cerebral perfusion pressures of 50 to 150 mm Hg

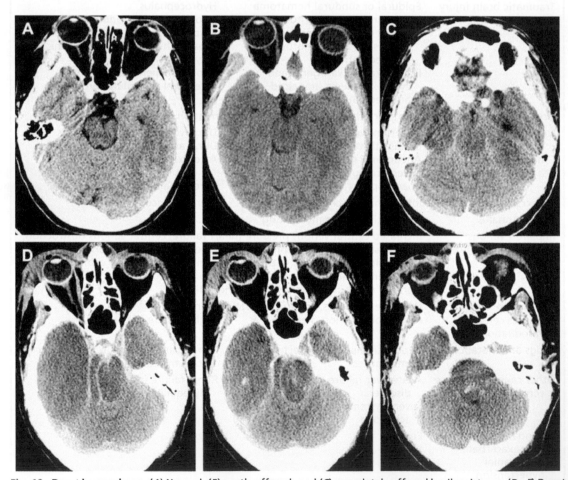

Fig. 10. Duret hemorrhage. (A) Normal, (B) partly effaced, and (C) completely effaced basilar cisterns. (D–F) Duret hemorrhages in the midbrain and pons caused by severe downward herniation in a 50-year-old woman with intracranial hypertension caused by massive subarachnoid hemorrhage from right ophthalmic artery aneurysm rupture.

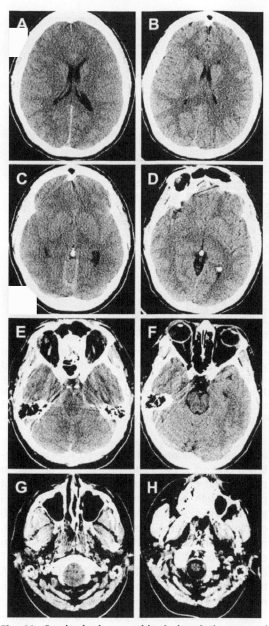

Fig. 11. Cerebral edema and brain herniation caused by increased ICP. (*A, C, E, G*) Cerebral edema in a 24-year-old woman with acute liver failure following acetaminophen overdose. CT demonstrates complete effacement of basal cisterns, as well as mild obstructive hydrocephalus, caused by severe downward transtentorial herniation. Cerebellar tonsillar herniation is seen in (*G*). (*B, E, F, H*) Corresponding head CT 24 hours earlier on admission (*B, D, F, H*) was interpreted as normal.

through autoregulation. When cerebral perfusion pressure is reduced to less than 50 mm Hg, as in sustained increased ICP without a corresponding increase in mean arterial pressure, cerebral blood flow is reduced. This reduced flow can result in

large-territory ischemia or infarction. Increased systemic blood pressure in response to reduced cerebral perfusion pressure may result in or exacerbate existing intracranial hematomas. Reflex bradycardia may further reduce brain perfusion via a reduction in systemic blood pressure and a corresponding reduction in perfusion pressure.

DIAGNOSIS
Idiopathic Intracranial Hypertension: Lumbar Puncture

An increased CSF opening pressure is the essential diagnostic criterion for IIH; imaging studies may be normal despite markedly increased ICP. In contrast, in SIH, CSF pressures can be within the normal range and imaging tests frequently play a key and decisive role in both diagnosis and treatment. IIH is suspected when opening pressure is in excess of 20 cm H_2O (10 cm H_2O in young children, and 25 cm H_2O in obese patients). Asymptomatic presentations of IIH are common, for example when papilledema is noted during routine ophthalmologic examination.[65]

Acute Intracranial Hypertension and Idiopathic Intracranial Hypertension: Imaging

Severe increase in ICP of any cause can result in diffuse effacement of sulci, small or slitlike ventricles, and/or brain herniation. Downward cerebral herniation is manifested as compressed or completely effaced basal cisterns, and subfalcine herniation is manifested as displacement of midline structures. Critically serious abnormalities include brainstem compression; Duret hemorrhages (midbrain and pontine hemorrhage believed to be caused by stretching and laceration of pontine perforating branches of the basilar artery, or less likely to venous thrombosis and infarction[69]); compression of the posterior cerebral artery near the incisura, with resulting infarction; obstructive hydrocephalus secondary to compression of the foramen of Monro; anterior cerebral artery infarction secondary to subfalcine herniation; and cerebellar tonsillar and upward transtentorial cerebellar herniation. If cerebral perfusion pressure falls below 50 mm Hg, as in severely increased ICP without a corresponding increase in mean arterial pressure, a reduction in cerebral blood flow may result in large-territory or global ischemia or infarction (see **Fig. 12**).

Imaging studies in patients with more modest increases of ICP, both acute and chronic, are often normal. In moderate elevation of ICP, as can occur in IIH, small sulci and/or small ventricles, dural venous sinus stenosis or occlusion (**Fig. 13A–C**)

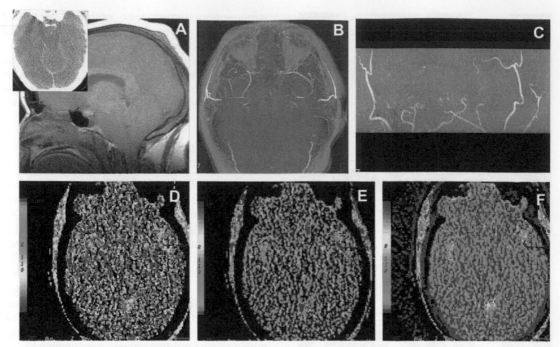

Fig. 12. Inadequate cerebral perfusion pressure caused by severe intracranial hypertension. Patient with renal failure with severe hypermagnesemia and metabolic alkalosis became acutely obtunded. (*A*) Both CT (*inset*) and sagittal T1 image showed downward brain herniation. (*B, C*) Three-dimensional time-of-flight MR angiography maximum-intensity projection (MIP) showed no flow-related enhancement within the circle of Willis. Only external carotid artery branches were seen. (*D–F*) CT perfusion color maps: (*D*) mean transit time; (*E*) cerebral blood flow; (*F*) cerebral blood volume showed markedly reduced blood flow, evidence of inadequate cerebral perfusion pressure.

or an enlarged and/or apparently empty sella[70] (Fig. 13D) are occasionally seen. Narrowing or occlusion of the dural venous sinus increases ICP, and is believed to be a cause for chronically increased ICP. However, dural venous sinus stenosis and occlusion may be a consequence rather than a cause of IIH.

Eye findings may also be present on brain imaging studies in a minority of cases of both chronic and acute intracranial hypertension.[71–73] Flattening of the posterior sclera at the lamina cribrosa (Fig. 14A, B), dilated, fluid-filled optic nerve sheaths (Fig. 14C, D), and enlargement and tortuosity of the superior ophthalmic veins (Fig. 14E, F) are infrequent but specific imaging findings of increased ICP of any cause.

Acute Intracranial Hypertension: Intracranial Pressure Monitoring

ICP monitoring is indicated whenever there is a significant risk of acute intracranial hypertension.[2] Invasive ICP monitoring using implanted measurement devices carries modest associated risk, including intracranial infection (5%–14%), hemorrhage (1.4%), and malposition.[2] Although ICP is not reliably determined by current imaging

techniques, evidence of increased ICP is sometimes present on imaging studies (see above). In the context of acute closed head injury, 60% of patients with admission head CT that demonstrates evidence of acute intracranial injury (intracranial hemorrhage, basal cistern effacement, midline shift) develop intracranial hypertension. In contrast, only 13% of those with normal head CT develop increased ICP. Thus, abnormal admission head CT in patients with acute head trauma often results in invasive ICP monitor placement.[2,74]

ICP monitoring can be performed with a ventriculostomy catheter, subarachnoid screw or bolt, or with one of several transducer-tipped catheters.[2] Ventriculostomy catheters are used most commonly, because they also allow for therapeutic ventricular CSF drainage, are inexpensive, and can be recalibrated to atmospheric pressure without removal. Disadvantages of ventriculostomy catheters include the requirement that the externally located pressure transducer be maintained level with the patients' head, obstruction of the fluid column within the catheter tubing leading to inaccurate pressure measurements, and the difficulty of inserting the catheter into a compressed or displaced ventricular system. Other options include

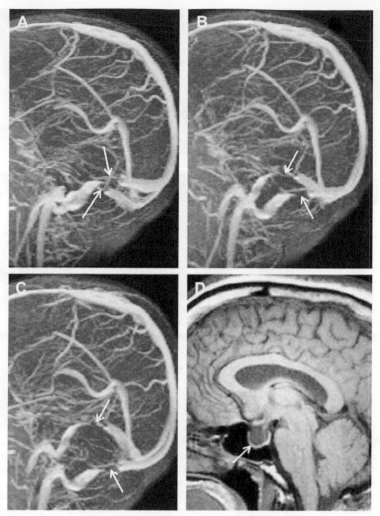

Fig. 13. Imaging findings occasionally seen in idiopathic intracranial hypertension. (*A–C*) Dural venous sinus stenosis in a 7-year-old girl with orthostatic headaches and papilledema. (*D*) Enlarged, partly empty sella in a 40-year-old man with chronic severe headaches. This has been attributed to chronic pituitary gland compression and remodeling of bone by CSF pulsations.

transducer-tipped catheters, in which pressure in the brain parenchyma is measured through either a microsensor transducer or fiberoptic transducer on the catheter tip itself. A key advantage of these devices is that they do not need to be inserted into the ventricular system. Subdural and epidural space pressure monitors exist but are less accurate.[2]

TREATMENT
Acute Intracranial Hypertension

Treatment of acute intracranial hypertension has the following goals:

1. Maintenance of ICP at <20 to 25 mm Hg

2. Maintenance of cerebral perfusion pressure at greater than 60 mm Hg
3. Avoidance of factors that exacerbate intracranial hypertension, including obstruction of venous return through head malpositioning or agitation, hypoxia/hypercarbia, fever, anemia, seizures, and hyponatremia

For patients with persistently increased ICP of more than 20 to 25 mm Hg, aggressive treatment, including hyperosmolar therapy (mannitol, hypertonic saline) or surgical intervention, is indicated. Surgical interventions include ventricular CSF drainage, which immediately and often significantly reduces ICP; however, this technique cannot be used in the setting of diffuse brain swelling resulting in ventricular collapse.

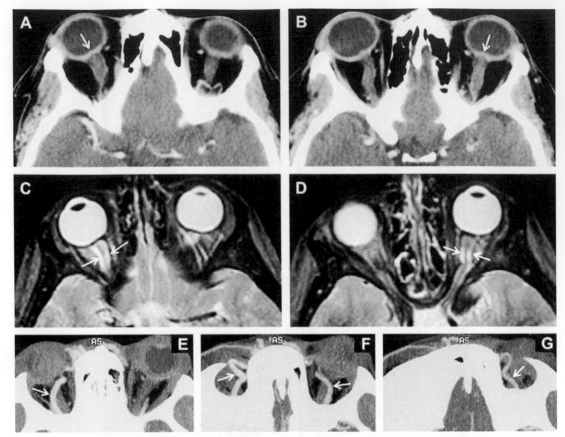

Fig. 14. Imaging findings occasionally seen in both idiopathic and acute intracranial hypertension. (*A, B*) Flattening of the posterior sclera at the lamina cribrosa in a 34-year-old woman with a 2-week history of progressive severe visual loss, headache, nausea, and vomiting. Ophthalmologic examination showed severe bilateral papilledema, and opening CSF pressure on lumbar puncture was 24 cm H_2O. Patient underwent emergent lumbar drain, later converted to lumboperitoneal shunt. (*C, D*) Dilated, fluid-filled optic nerve sheaths. (*E–G*) Dilated, tortuous superior ophthalmic veins in a 41-year-old man with chronic headaches, progressive visual impairment, and suspected chronic hypoventilation syndrome related to severe obesity. Opening CSF pressure was 60 cm H_2O. Patient underwent bilateral optic nerve sheath fenestration to prevent further vision loss.

Decompressive craniectomy relieves increased ICP through evacuation of any intracranial hemorrhagic space-occupying lesions, and by allowing external herniation of the brain, circumventing the Monro-Kellie doctrine. Decompressive craniectomy is still undergoing clinical trials, but has been shown in some studies to increase brain tissue oxygenation and cerebral blood flow and to reduce mortality and increase favorable outcome in acute stroke patients.[75–78] This technique is typically performed in patients with acute traumatic brain injury, intracranial mass lesion, nontraumatic acute intracranial hemorrhage, and, less commonly, malignant edema secondary to middle cerebral artery infarction.

Idiopathic Intracranial Hypertension

Imaging is useful in excluding some treatable causes of intracranial hypertension (see **Table 1**).

Conservative treatment of IIH includes weight reduction, acetazolamide, topiramate, and furosemide.[65,79] The major long-term complication of IIH is irreversible partial or complete vision loss. Therefore, for those failing conservative treatment measures, optic nerve sheath fenestration and CSF shunting are sometimes performed.

REFERENCES

1. Steiner LA, Andrews PJ. Monitoring the injured brain: ICP and CBF. Br J Anaesth 2006;97(1):26–38.
2. Rangel-Castilla L, Gopinath S, Robertson CS. Management of intracranial hypertension. Neurol Clin 2008;26(2):521–41.
3. Mokri B. The Monro-Kellie hypothesis: applications in CSF volume depletion. Neurology 2001;56(12): 1746–8.

4. Schievink WI. Spontaneous spinal cerebrospinal fluid leaks. Cephalalgia 2008;28(12):1345–56.

5. Headache Classification Subcommittee of the International Headache Society. International classification of headache disorders, 2nd edition. Cephalalgia 2004;24:1–160.

6. Schievink WI. Spontaneous spinal cerebrospinal fluid leaks and intracranial hypotension. JAMA 2006;295(19):2286–96.

7. Schievink WI, Wijdicks EF, Meyer FB, et al. Spontaneous intracranial hypotension mimicking aneurysmal subarachnoid hemorrhage. Neurosurgery 2001;48(3):513–6 [discussion: 516–7].

8. Tsui H, Wu S, Kuo H, et al. Rebound intracranial hypertension after treatment of spontaneous intracranial hypotension. Eur J Neurol 2006;13(7):780–2.

9. Mokri B. Intracranial hypertension after treatment of spontaneous cerebrospinal fluid leaks. Mayo Clin Proc 2002;77(11):1241–6.

10. Pleasure SJ, Abosch A, Friedman J, et al. Spontaneous intracranial hypotension resulting in stupor caused by diencephalic compression. Neurology 1998;50(6):1854–7.

11. Binder DK, Dillon WP, Fishman RA, et al. Intrathecal saline infusion in the treatment of obtundation associated with spontaneous intracranial hypotension: technical case report. Neurosurgery 2002;51(3):830–6 [discussion: 836–7].

12. Beck CE, Rizk NW, Kiger LT, et al. Intracranial hypotension presenting with severe encephalopathy. Case report. J Neurosurg 1998;89(3):470–3.

13. Schievink WI, Maya MM. Quadriplegia and cerebellar hemorrhage in spontaneous intracranial hypotension. Neurology 2006;66(11):1777–8.

14. Chi NF, Wang SJ, Lirng JF, et al. Transtentorial herniation with cerebral infarction and duret haemorrhage in a patient with spontaneous intracranial hypotension. Cephalalgia 2007;27(3):279–82.

15. Sayer FT, Bodelsson M, Larsson EM, et al. Spontaneous intracranial hypotension resulting in coma: case report. Neurosurgery 2006;59(1):E204 [discussion: E204].

16. Aghaei Lasboo A, Hurley MC, Walker MT, et al. Emergent image-guided treatment of a large CSF leak to reverse "in-extremis" signs of intracranial hypotension. AJNR Am J Neuroradiol 2008;29(9):1627–9.

17. Han SR, Kim YJ, Kim YI, et al. A case report of unexpected clinical course of spontaneous intracranial hypotension. J Korean Neurol Assoc 1995;13:129–32.

18. Kandel ER. Principles of neural science. New York: McGraw-Hill; 2000.

19. Huang TY, Chung HW, Chen MY, et al. Supratentorial cerebrospinal fluid production rate in healthy adults: quantification with two-dimensional cine phase-contrast MR imaging with high temporal and spatial resolution. Radiology 2004;233(2):603–8.

20. Bier A. Versuche uber Cocainisirung des Ruckenmarkes. Deutsch Ztschr Chir 1899;51:361–9.

21. Oshio K, Watanabe H, Song Y, et al. Reduced cerebrospinal fluid production and intracranial pressure in mice lacking choroid plexus water channel Aquaporin-1. FASEB J 2005;19(1):76–8.

22. Mokri B, Krueger B, Miller GM, et al. Meningeal gadolinium enhancement in low pressure headaches [abstract]. Ann Neurol 1991;30:294–5.

23. Fishman RA, Dillon WP. Dural enhancement and cerebral displacement secondary to intracranial hypotension. Neurology 1993;43(3 Pt 1):609–11.

24. Sable SG, Ramadan NM. Meningeal enhancement and low CSF pressure headache. An MRI study. Cephalalgia 1991;11(6):275–6.

25. Hochman MS, Naidich TP, Kobetz SA, et al. Spontaneous intracranial hypotension with pachymeningeal enhancement on MRI. Neurology 1992;42(8):1628–30.

26. Pannullo SC, Reich JB, Krol G, et al. MRI changes in intracranial hypotension. Neurology 1993;43(5):919–26.

27. Raskin NH. Lumbar puncture headache: a review. Headache 1990;30(4):197–200.

28. Fernandez E. Headaches associated with low spinal fluid pressure. Headache 1990;30(3):122–8.

29. Hadizadeh DR, Kovács A, Tschampa H, et al. Postsurgical intracranial hypotension: diagnostic and prognostic imaging findings. AJNR Am J Neuroradiol 2010;31(1):100–5.

30. Winter SC, Maartens NF, Anslow P, et al. Spontaneous intracranial hypotension due to thoracic disc herniation. Case report. J Neurosurg 2002;96(Suppl 3):343–5.

31. Binder DK, Sarkissian V, Dillon WP, et al. Spontaneous intracranial hypotension associated with transdural thoracic osteophyte reversed by primary. Dural repair. Case report. J Neurosurg Spine 2005;2(5):614–8.

32. Rapport RL, Hillier D, Scearce T, et al. Spontaneous intracranial hypotension from intradural thoracic disc herniation. Case report. J Neurosurg 2003;98(Suppl 3):282–4.

33. Eross EJ, Dodick DW, Nelson KD, et al. Orthostatic headache syndrome with CSF leak secondary to bony pathology of the cervical spine. Cephalalgia 2002;22(6):439–43.

34. Vishteh AG, Schievink WI, Baskin JJ, et al. Cervical bone spur presenting with spontaneous intracranial hypotension. Case report. J Neurosurg 1998;89(3):483–4.

35. Schievink WI, Maya MM, Louy C, et al. Diagnostic criteria for spontaneous spinal CSF leaks and intracranial hypotension. AJNR Am J Neuroradiol 2008;29(5):853–6.

36. Schievink WI, Maya MM, Louy C. Cranial MRI predicts outcome of spontaneous intracranial hypotension. Neurology 2005;64(7):1282–4.

37. Schievink WI, Meyer FB, Atkinson JLD, et al. Spontaneous spinal cerebrospinal fluid leaks and intracranial hypotension. J Neurosurg 1996;84(4): 598–605.

38. Hoxworth JM, Patela AC, Boschb EP, et al. Localization of a rapid CSF leak with digital subtraction myelography. AJNR Am J Neuroradiol 2009;30(3):516–9.

39. Schievink WI, Maya MM, Tourje J. False localizing sign of C1-2 cerebrospinal fluid leak in spontaneous intracranial hypotension. J Neurosurg 2004;100(4): 639–44.

40. Dillon WP. Spinal manifestations of intracranial hypotension. AJNR Am J Neuroradiol 2001;22(7):1233–4.

41. Schievink WI. Misdiagnosis of spontaneous intracranial hypotension. Arch Neurol 2003;60(12):1713–8.

42. Albayram S, Kilica F, Ozera H, et al. Gadolinium-enhanced MR cisternography to evaluate dural leaks in intracranial hypotension syndrome. AJNR Am J Neuroradiol 2008;29(1):116–21.

43. Dillon WP. Intrathecal gadolinium: its time has come? AJNR Am J Neuroradiol 2008;29(1):3–4.

44. Wagner M, du Mesnil de Rochemont R, Ziemann U, et al. Localization of thoracic CSF leaks by gadolinium-enhanced MR-myelography and successful MR-targeted epidural blood patching: a case report. J Neurol 2010;257:1398–9.

45. Li L, Gao FQ, Zhang B, et al. Overdosage of intrathecal gadolinium and neurological response. Clin Radiol 2008;63(9):1063–8.

46. Wang YF, Lirng JF, Fuh JL, et al. Heavily T2-weighted MR myelography vs CT myelography in spontaneous intracranial hypotension. Neurology 2009;73(22): 1892–8.

47. Schievink WI. A novel technique for treatment of intractable spontaneous intracranial hypotension: lumbar dural reduction surgery. Headache 2009; 49(7):1047–51.

48. Schievink WI, Maya MM, Moser F, et al. Frequency of spontaneous intracranial hypotension in the emergency department. J Headache Pain 2007;8(6): 325–8.

49. Choi A, Laurito CE, Cunningham FE. Pharmacologic management of postdural puncture headache. Ann Pharmacother 1996;30(7–8):831–9.

50. Yucel A, Ozyalçin S, Talu GK, et al. Intravenous administration of caffeine sodium benzoate for postdural puncture headache. Reg Anesth Pain Med 1999;24(1):51–4.

51. Sechzer P, Abel L. Post-spinal anesthesia headache treated with caffeine. Evaluation with demand method. Part 1. Curr Ther Res 1978;24:307.

52. Szeinfeld M, Ihmeidan IH, Moser MM, et al. Epidural blood patch: evaluation of the volume and spread of blood injected into the epidural space. Anesthesiology 1986;64(6):820–2.

53. Kroin JS, Nagalla SK, Buvanendran A, et al. The mechanisms of intracranial pressure modulation by epidural blood and other injectates in a postdural puncture rat model. Anesth Analg 2002;95(2): 423–9.

54. Patel MR, Louie W, Rachlin J. Postoperative cerebrospinal fluid leaks of the lumbosacral spine: management with percutaneous fibrin glue. AJNR Am J Neuroradiol 1996;17(3):495–500.

55. Schievink WI, Reimer R, Folger WN. Surgical treatment of spontaneous intracranial hypotension associated with a spinal arachnoid diverticulum. Case report. J Neurosurg 1994;80(4):736–9.

56. Schievink WI, Morreale VM, Atkinson JL, et al. Surgical treatment of spontaneous spinal cerebrospinal fluid leaks. J Neurosurg 1998;88(2):243–6.

57. Mokri B. Expert commentary: role of surgery for the management of CSF leaks. Cephalalgia 2008; 28(12):1357–60.

58. Schievink WI, Maya MM. Cerebral venous thrombosis in spontaneous intracranial hypotension. Headache 2008;48(10):1511–9.

59. Albayram S, Tasmali KM, Gunduz A. Can spontaneous intracranial hypotension cause venous sinus thrombosis? J Headache Pain 2007;8(3):200–1.

60. Lan MY, Chang YY, Liu JS. Delayed cerebral venous thrombosis in a patient with spontaneous intracranial hypotension. Cephalalgia 2007;27(10): 1176–8.

61. Savoiardo M, Armenise S, Spagnolo P, et al. Dural sinus thrombosis in spontaneous intracranial hypotension: hypotheses on possible mechanisms. J Neurol 2006;253(9):1197–202.

62. Radhakrishnan K, Ahlskog JE, Garrity JA, et al. Idiopathic intracranial hypertension. Mayo Clin Proc 1994;69(2):169–80.

63. Wall M. Idiopathic intracranial hypertension. Neurol Clin 1991;9(1):73–95.

64. Giuseffi V, Wall M, Siegel PZ, et al. Symptoms and disease associations in idiopathic intracranial hypertension (pseudotumor cerebri): a case-control study. Neurology 1991;41(2 [Pt 1]):239–44.

65. Randhawa S, Van Stavern GP. Idiopathic intracranial hypertension (pseudotumor cerebri). Curr Opin Ophthalmol 2008;19(6):445–53.

66. Friedman DI, Jacobson DM. Diagnostic criteria for idiopathic intracranial hypertension. Neurology 2002;59(10):1492–5.

67. Jones JS, Nevai J, Freeman MP, et al. Emergency department presentation of idiopathic intracranial hypertension. Am J Emerg Med 1999;17(6): 517–21.

68. Bruce BB, Preechawat P, Newman NJ, et al. Racial differences in idiopathic intracranial hypertension. Neurology 2008;70(11):861–7.

69. Parizel PM, Makkat S, Jorens PG, et al. Brainstem hemorrhage in descending transtentorial herniation (Duret hemorrhage). Intensive Care Med 2002;28(1):85–8.

70. Yuh WT, Zhu M, Taoka T, et al. MR imaging of pituitary morphology in idiopathic intracranial hypertension. J Magn Reson Imaging 2000;12(6):808–13.

71. Agid R, Farb RI. Neuroimaging in the diagnosis of idiopathic intracranial hypertension. Minerva Med 2006;97(4):365–70.

72. Agid R, Farb RI, Willinsky RA, et al. Idiopathic intracranial hypertension: the validity of cross-sectional neuroimaging signs. Neuroradiology 2006;48(8):521–7.

73. Brodsky MC, Vaphiades M. Magnetic resonance imaging in pseudotumor cerebri. Ophthalmology 1998;105(9):1686–93.

74. O'Sullivan MG, Statham PF, Jones PA, et al. Role of intracranial pressure monitoring in severely head-injured patients without signs of intracranial hypertension on initial computerized tomography. J Neurosurg 1994;80(1):46–50.

75. Hutchinson PJ, Corteen E, Czosnyka M, et al. Decompressive craniectomy in traumatic brain injury: the randomized multicenter RESCUEicp study (www.RESCUEicp.com). Acta Neurochir Suppl 2006;96:11–6.

76. Timofeev I, Kirkpatrick PJ, Corteen E, et al. Decompressive craniectomy in traumatic brain injury: outcome following protocol-driven therapy. Acta Neurochir Suppl 2006;96:11–6.

77. Vahedi K, Hofmeijer J, Juettler E, et al. Early decompressive surgery in malignant infarction of the middle cerebral artery: a pooled analysis of three randomised controlled trials. Lancet Neurol 2007;6(3):215–22.

78. Aarabi B, Hesdorffer DC, Ahn ES, et al. Outcome following decompressive craniectomy for malignant swelling due to severe head injury. J Neurosurg 2006;104(4):469–79.

79. Wall M. Idiopathic intracranial hypertension (pseudotumor cerebri). Curr Neurol Neurosci Rep 2008;8(2):87–93.

Seizures: Emergency Neuroimaging

Christopher P. Hess* and A. James Barkovich

KEYWORDS

- Seizures • Epilepsy • Peri-ictal changes
- Posttraumatic epilepsy • Mesial temporal sclerosis

The term seizure refers to an abrupt but transient interruption in normal brain function that comes about as the result of an unregulated discharge of neurons. Seizures are so common that nearly 10% of the population of the United States will have at least one seizure by age 80. New unprovoked seizures or seizures that are not rapidly controlled are viewed as a neurologic emergency, and thus in the emergent setting often undergo computed tomography (CT) scanning or less commonly, magnetic resonance (MR) imaging. Epilepsy, in contrast, is a term reserved for the chronic brain disorder characterized by recurrent and unpredictable seizures without evidence for a reversible systemic cause. The prevalence of this disorder in the United States is estimated at 0.5% to 1%. For the evaluation of patients with epilepsy, MR imaging is almost always the first-line imaging modality. Positron emission tomography (PET) with ^{18}F fluorodeoxyglucose (FDG) and magnetoencephalography (MEG) may also be used in some centers to increase diagnostic sensitivity and specificity in cases where high-quality MR imaging is negative or equivocal.

This article focuses on CT and MR imaging of unusual and potentially reversible causes for acute seizures in the emergency setting. Because many patients who develop seizures after trauma, infection, or metabolic derangements may eventually develop epilepsy, some of the chronic brain conditions that result secondarily from an acute event are also included in this review. In particular, posttraumatic epilepsy and mesial temporal sclerosis (MTS) are discussed in some detail. The interested reader is referred to several excellent articles[1-6] and texts[6-8] for a more comprehensive review of imaging in epilepsy, especially with regard to malformations of cortical development, phakomatoses, and emerging advanced MR imaging, MEG, and nuclear medicine techniques for improving localization of seizure substrates when MR imaging is unrevealing.

SEIZURE TYPES AND INDICATIONS FOR IMAGING

As a single symptom of a broad range of neurologic disorders ranging from Alzheimer to Zellweger disease, seizures have a variety of imaging manifestations. Some of these are common and some are exceedingly rare. Many findings that have been observed represent the secondary hemodynamic, metabolic, or excitotoxic effects of seizures on the brain. Others such as MTS, infarcts, tumors, or cortical dysplasia can represent the primary underlying cause of seizures. When imaging patients presenting with new or recurrent seizures, it is important that the radiologist be able to confidently distinguish between potential causes and the secondary effects of seizure activity, especially with regard to recognizing causes that may be reversible with the institution of appropriate treatment. In the emergency setting, imaging is commonly performed with CT. When CT is contraindicated or unhelpful, MR imaging may also reveal reversible causes for seizures, or may

UCSF Department of Radiology & Biomedical Imaging, 505 Parnassus Avenue, Room L-358, San Francisco, CA 94143-0628, USA
* Corresponding author.
E-mail address: christopher.hess@ucsf.edu

Neuroimag Clin N Am 20 (2010) 619–637
doi:10.1016/j.nic.2010.07.013
1052-5149/10/$ — see front matter © 2010 Elsevier Inc. All rights reserved.

disclose findings that suggest the next step in the workup of seizures.

As detailed in the recently revised terminology for classification of epilepsy developed by the International League Against Epilepsy (ILAE),[9] 2 principal seizure types are recognized: focal seizures (or partial seizures), which show clinical or electroencephalographic (EEG) evidence for origin from a discrete location within the cortical or subcortical gray matter of one hemisphere, and generalized seizures, which may also arise from a single discrete location but in contrast to focal seizures rapidly propagate through both hemispheres and thus clinically do not have consistently localizing features. (Modern imaging, methods for genomic analysis, and molecular biology have significantly altered our understanding of seizures since the initial ILAE classification was published in 1960, and updated for seizures in 1981 and for epilepsy in 1989. The latest proposed revision of the ILAE classification can be found in Ref.[9]) This distinction is important, as the causes, treatment, and outcomes for these 2 types of seizures differ significantly and vary by age. Chronic generalized seizures often present in childhood and usually have normal imaging; acute generalized seizures in the adult are more ominous, as they are more likely to have significant structural lesions evident on routine CT. In contrast, both acute and chronic partial seizures are more likely to have imaging abnormalities that are occult on CT and sometimes exceedingly subtle on MR imaging. In this regard, it is important to recognize the limitations of CT. Adults with acute generalized seizures should be evaluated clinically for evidence of trauma, metabolic abnormalities, or toxic ingestion, with a low threshold for CT imaging when a significant intracranial process such as infection, tumor, or hemorrhage is suspected. In some cases, however, the evaluation should not stop when CT does not disclose any significant abnormality, but rather should include additional imaging with MR.

Multidisciplinary guidelines developed through the process of expert review have led to the development of well-defined criteria for determining whether CT and/or MR imaging are indicated in the emergency setting.[10] As a general rule, *imaging is recommended for any patient in whom a serious structural lesion is suspected based on history and physical examination, or when a clear systemic cause for seizures has not been identified*. Recommendations differ based on age and clinical presentation, with imaging strongly suggested after first-time seizures in patients older than 40, in cases of known malignancy or immune compromise, or when symptoms suggest a partial onset (all conditions that increase the likelihood of a focal brain lesion). Even in patients known to have epilepsy, repeat imaging is recommended when the seizure pattern or type changes, when seizures result in significant head trauma, or when prolonged postictal confusion or declining mental status are present. Appropriateness criteria issued by the American College of Radiology also serve as a useful resource to aid in the selection of patients for imaging.[11]

Patients with acute intracranial hemorrhage, brain tumors, infections, dural venous sinus thrombosis, traumatic brain injury (TBI), developmental abnormalities, and vascular lesions such as cavernous and arteriovenous malformations may all present with seizures. These entities are discussed in other articles in this issue.

In a cohort of 880 individuals from the city of Rochester, Minnesota, no specific cause for seizures was found in 65.5% of patients[12]; however, disorders with abnormalities that could potentially be identified by imaging were also common in this cohort. These abnormalities included cerebrovascular disease in 10.9%, congenital lesions in 8.0%, trauma in 5.5%, tumors in 4.1%, neurodegenerative disease such as Alzheimer disease in 3.5%, and infection in 2.5%. The proportion of cases with underlying brain structural abnormalities varied by age, with tumors and infarcts far more common among patients older than 65 than among those in younger age groups, where infection and trauma were more frequent. Metabolic derangements and alcohol withdrawal collectively represented common causes for seizures among the middle-aged population. In children between the ages of approximately 5 months and 6 years, many series have shown that most seizures represent simple febrile seizures. Imaging in this patient population is usually unwarranted at first presentation, especially in light of growing concerns regarding radiation exposure[13] and the availability of established clinical practice guidelines that do not routinely include CT.[14]

Logistic and cost issues aside the diagnostic yield of MR imaging is far higher than that of CT in both patients with acute seizures and patients with long-standing epilepsy. Not all MR imaging examinations are equivalent, however. The accuracy of MR imaging increases with the field strength used for acquisition, as the higher signal-to-noise and contrast-to-noise afforded by 3-T imaging allow visualization of smaller structures and more small variations in signal intensity than conventional 1.5-T imaging.[15,16] MR imaging studies performed for the evaluation of seizures should also be tailored to optimize detection of seizure foci, as routine brain protocols may miss lesions responsible for seizures. Finally, although there is evidence that general radiologists consistently detect critical structural abnormalities, subtle abnormalities may be detected at higher rates by subspecialty-trained neuroradiologists practicing in dedicated epilepsy centers. According to one study, for example, the diagnosis of hippocampal sclerosis was missed prospectively in 86% of initial imaging reports.[17] Although controversial, this study at the very least reiterates the need for all radiologists to: (1) increase their familiarity with the MR imaging diagnosis of MTS (discussed later in this article), (2) employ dedicated high-resolution seizure protocols, and (3) incorporate clinical and EEG information regarding seizure type and localization into the process of interpretation.

Modern seizure evaluation should routinely include coronal thin-section T2-weighted images of the medial temporal lobes and a volumetric T1-weighted evaluation of the entire brain to allow critical assessment of regional sulcal anatomy, cortical thickness, and definition of gray-white boundaries.[18] In addition, it is important to include sequences sensitive to magnetic susceptibility to identify calcification and chronic blood products from prior trauma, cavernous malformations, and infections such as neurocysticercosis (one of the most important causes for seizures worldwide). New three-dimensional (3D) phase-sensitive susceptibility-weighted techniques likely have higher sensitivity in this regard than conventional

gradient echo T2* sequences. Of note, high spatial resolution, formerly possible only with specialized surface coils,[19] can now be routinely obtained with most sequences on 3-T scanners using phased-array receive coils.[20] Gadolinium-enhanced images are not typically required for evaluation of chronic seizures unless a tumor is suspected. In the acute setting, however, contrast-enhanced sequences may be useful to evaluate for underlying infections, tumors, or vascular lesions (Table 1).

PERI-ICTAL CHANGES ON IMAGING

Independent of cause, seizures are associated with dramatic alterations in cellular metabolism, disruptions in normal cerebral autoregulation, shifts in relative compartmental water distributions, and changes in intracellular ion concentrations. The variety of pathophysiological events that take place as the direct result of seizure activity is reflected in the myriad imaging findings that have been described with ongoing or recent seizure activity. These "peri-ictal" imaging abnormalities may be reversible or irreversible, depending on the nature and duration of seizures and, like the underlying electrochemical events that cause them, may affect the brain in a focal or diffuse fashion.

Often mild or absent on unenhanced CT, peri-ictal changes commonly appear as patchy areas of high signal on T2, fluid-attenuated inversion recovery (FLAIR), or diffusion-weighted MR

Table 1
Adult epilepsy/seizure protocol

	Sequence	TR/TE/TI (ms)	FOV (mm)	Matrix	Slice/Gap (mm)
1	Axial DWI (b = 1000 s/mm²)	10000/MIN	220 × 220	128 × 128	3 skip 0
2	Coronal T2 FSE-IR	5000/120 (ETL 16)	220 × 160	512 × 256	3 skip 0
3	Coronal 3D T1[a]	36/MIN	220 × 160	230 × 230	1.2 skip 0
4	Coronal T2 FLAIR[b]	10000/140/2200	220 × 160	256 × 192	3 skip 0
5	Axial T2 FSE	5850/100 (ETL 17)	220 × 220	384 × 384	3 skip 0
6	Coronal T2* GRE[c]	787/25	220 × 160	256 × 192	5 skip 1
7	Gad axial T1 SE	600/MIN	220 × 220	256 × 192	5 skip 1
8	Gad coronal T1 SE	600/MIN	220 × 160	256 × 192	5 skip 1

Coronal acquisitions should be acquired along the hippocampal axis.

Abbreviations: DWI, diffusion-weighted imaging; ETL, echo train length; FLAIR, fluid-attenuated inversion recovery; FOV, field of view; FSE, fast spin echo; Gad, acquired following administration of gadolinium; GRE, gradient echo; MIN, minimum possible TE; SE, spin echo; TE, echo time; TI, inversion time; TR, repetition time.

[a] Volumetric spoiled gradient echo (SPGR) or magnetization-prepared rapid acquisition gradient echo (MPRAGE) sequences are recommended to optimize gray-white contrast with high spatial resolution. Images should be reformatted and reviewed in 3 planes.

[b] Volumetric FLAIR sequences are also useful when available, as they facilitate review in 3 planes at high spatial resolution.

[c] 3D susceptibility-sensitive sequences may be substituted for conventional T2* gradient echo imaging.

imaging (**Fig. 1**).[21–26] Typically involving gray matter, either within the cerebral cortex or in the deep gray nuclei, these abnormalities are frequently bilateral and may be migratory on serial imaging. Peri-ictal changes may arise within a localized epileptogenic region of the brain or remotely within areas of the brain distant from the actual seizure focus. Changes in the region of seizure onset are thought to be the direct result of localized metabolic and vascular changes associated with abnormal neuronal discharge[27]; the precise cause for remote changes is more difficult to understand. Frequent involvement of limbic structures, especially the hippocampus, suggests that seizures preferentially involve neuronal populations with a lower intrinsic seizure threshold. Alternatively, as suggested by signal changes in the thalamus or cerebellum, seizures may propagate secondarily through distributed networks in the brain.

The signal abnormalities related to seizures on MR imaging are commonly associated with mild mass effect, causing subtle sulcal effacement within involved areas. Occasionally, seizures may be associated with more pronounced mass effect. In these cases, imaging may erroneously lead to the diagnosis of a mass lesion[28] or, in patients with known tumors, be mistaken for tumor progression.[29] The transient and migratory nature of these changes on serial imaging and associated clinical picture may provide the only clues that the abnormalities are related to seizures. Other reported, but less common, findings include transient sulcal hyperintensity on FLAIR sequences, leptomeningeal

enhancement, cross-cerebellar diaschisis, and asymmetric enlargement of arterial branches on MR angiography. These less common findings may confound the diagnosis of postictal changes; follow-up imaging can be useful in assessing the degree to which abnormalities are reversible and in differentiating postictal changes from other disorders that may have similar imaging features, such as encephalitis and infarction. Short-term follow-up imaging and/or lumbar puncture may be warranted to differentiate among these different possibilities.

The observation of peri-ictal changes on MR imaging depends on the duration of seizures and the time between the cessation of seizure activity and imaging. Transient partial seizures are infrequently associated with peri-ictal changes whereas prolonged, refractory seizures or status epilepticus are more likely to exhibit these abnormalities. The exact timing and duration of seizure activity is often difficult to establish with certainty because whereas generalized tonic-clonic seizures are dramatic and more readily documented, partial or nonconvulsive seizures may be clinically occult. In the authors' experience, patients with underlying comorbid diseases such as lupus, immunocompromised patients, solid organ transplant patients, and patients on chemotherapy agents are also more likely to show peri-ictal changes on MR imaging.

Peri-ictal changes may be transient and reversible, or they may progress to permanent cell death and gliosis. The extent of brain injury may be evident clinically. However, longitudinal follow-up

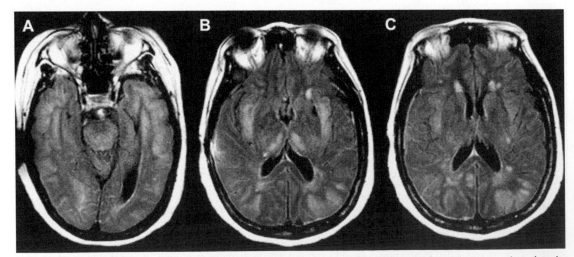

Fig. 1. Peri-ictal changes. Axial T2-weighted FLAIR images show multifocal bilateral frontal, temporal, and occipital abnormal hyperintensity in a patient presenting with medically refractory status epilepticus 2 days before MR imaging. Note widespread involvement of both cortex and white matter. Involvement of the brainstem (*A*), thalami (*B*), and insulae (*B, C*) is characteristic of severe seizure-related changes.

in some cases after prolonged seizures can provide supplementary evidence for permanent brain injury, usually manifest as focal or global cerebral atrophy or cortical injury, including laminar necrosis on T1-weighted images (Fig. 2). Cytotoxic edema, as implied by the presence of reduced diffusion, is a more ominous finding, but does not necessarily imply irreversible injury.[30–32] One interesting location for high T2 signal and reduced diffusion that is typically reversible is the splenium of the corpus callosum (Fig. 3), in which a rare circumscribed lesion has been variably ascribed to certain antiepileptic medications such as vigabatrin or to seizures themselves.[33–35] The reversibility of this finding suggests that reduced diffusion in this lesion does not reflect cytotoxic edema; a transient disturbance in energy metabolism and ionic transport that results in reversible myelin vacuolization or intramyelinic edema has been proposed.[35]

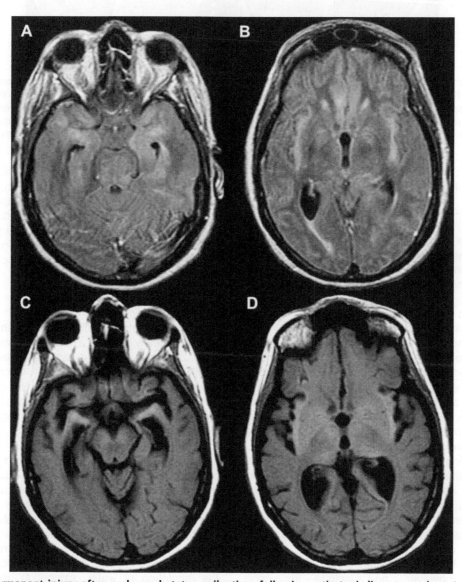

Fig. 2. Permanent injury after prolonged status epilepticus following orthotopic liver transplant. Initial axial FLAIR images obtained shortly following transplant during nonconvulsive status epilepticus (*A, B*) show abnormal hyperintensity of the medial temporal lobes, medial frontal cortex, thalami, and insulae bilaterally. Noncontrast T1-weighted images obtained several months later (*C, D*) illustrate interval development of bilateral cerebral atrophy, especially within the medial temporal lobes, as well as intrinsic T1 shortening in the anterior temporal lobes, insulae, and thalami.

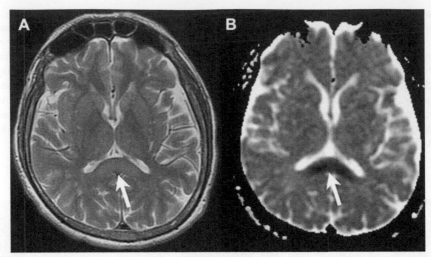

Fig. 3. Signal abnormalities in the splenium of the corpus callosum. Axial T2-weighted (*A*) and apparent diffusivity coefficient (*B*) images show subtle high T2 signal and reduced diffusion within the splenium of the corpus callosum (*arrows*). This reversible signal abnormality has been described both in the setting of recent seizure activity and in patients on certain antiepileptic medications with well-controlled seizures. The finding is not specific to seizures, however, and has also been described in infectious and inflammatory encephalitis.

POSTERIOR REVERSIBLE ENCEPHALOPATHY SYNDROME

Peri-ictal changes may overlap with the so-called posterior reversible encephalopathy syndrome (PRES), a controversial entity that may also be associated with seizures. Several conditions have been associated with this disorder, including hypertension, eclampsia, certain medications, infection, autoimmune diseases, hypercalcemia, hemolytic uremic syndrome, and renal failure.[36–38] Seizures in PRES clinically may initially show focal onset, though frequently generalize and often recur. The pathogenesis of PRES is poorly understood and controversial. One popular hypothesis is that the disorder results from loss of normal cerebral autoregulation with consequent hyperperfusion. Another suggests vasoconstriction with hypoperfusion, and yet another implicating endothelial cell dysfunction.

Following the brain watershed zones,[39] signal abnormalities in cases in PRES are most often bilateral and symmetric. As implied by the acronym, typical findings are reversible focal or patchy areas of T2/FLAIR hyperintensity in the subcortical white matter, especially within the parietal and occipital lobes. The imaging manifestations are broader than the moniker implies, however, and include irreversible cytotoxic injury, abnormalities in both gray and white matter, and involvement of not only the parietal and occipital lobes but also the frontal lobes, the inferior temporo-occipital junction, thalami and basal ganglia, brainstem, and cerebellum.

Cross-sectional and catheter angiographic studies may show vasospasm, vasodilation, and/or beading. Hemorrhage occurs in 15% to 20% of cases. These less common imaging findings may be mistaken for other disorders such as infarct or tumor, especially when reduced diffusion, marked asymmetry, mass effect, and/or enhancement is present (**Fig. 4**).[39–41]

METABOLIC ABNORMALITIES

Because laboratory analysis in the emergency setting routinely includes a metabolic panel, metabolic derangements that lead to seizures are usually diagnosed clinically. Occasionally, however, imaging may provide the first clue as to the initial severity of a corrected metabolic abnormality, or alternatively may show findings related to a known metabolic abnormality that are mistaken for another process.

Metabolic derangements may occur spontaneously or may be precipitated by organ failure, diet, medications, hormonally active tumors, or systemic stress. Most of these abnormalities result in generalized seizures. The underlying physiologic mechanisms for seizure induction depend on the specific metabolite in question and its role in the brain. For example, because of its critical role in the regulation of water distribution and serum osmolarity, rapid changes in serum sodium can be associated with changes in brain volume that result in acute seizures. With hyponatremia, movement of water from the interstitial space into cells results in cellular swelling. When hyponatremia

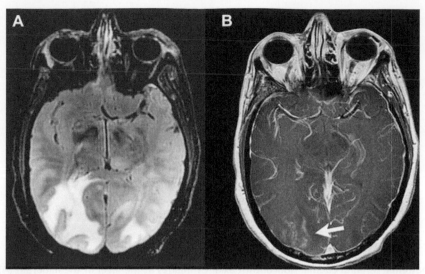

Fig. 4. Atypical PRES in a patient presenting with altered mental status and acute-onset seizures. Axial FLAIR image (*A*) shows hyperintensity within both occipital lobes. Note the asymmetric involvement and additional high signal intensity within the left thalamus. T1-weighted image obtained following administration of gadolinium contrast (*B*) shows patchy areas of enhancement (*arrow*), which can be observed in between 30% and 40% of cases.

develops slowly, this is typically compensated and does not result in cerebral edema, and as a result has no imaging correlate. However, in severe cases with rapid development of low serum sodium, this phenomenon results in an overall increase in brain volume and elevated intracranial pressure. However, as the changes in parenchymal volume observed with hyponatremic brain edema are usually mild, comparison with prior studies may provide the only clue that a change in brain volume has occurred. Subtlety notwithstanding, an assessment of overall brain parenchymal volume, ventricular size, and cisternal spaces should be included in all cases of acute seizures with low serum sodium (**Fig. 5**). Rapid correction of hyponatremia resulting in pontine or extrapontine myelinolysis may also cause seizures.

The most common cause of hypoglycemic seizures is overzealous use of parenteral or oral hypoglycemic treatments for diabetes mellitus, but low serum glucose can also be caused by other medications, hepatic failure, or insulin-secreting tumors. Imaging abnormalities related to hypoglycemia are uncommon, but have a relatively unique appearance on MR imaging. Within the first several days after a severe hypoglycemia episode, symmetric high T2 signal and reduced diffusion may appear within the corona radiata, corpus callosum, and internal capsules (**Fig. 6**).[42,43] Other cases may show high T2 signal within the hippocampi and cortical gray matter.

Reduced diffusion can be reversible in many cases.[44,45] Involvement of the basal ganglia tends to appear in the days to weeks following the initial insult, and may portend a less favorable outcome.[43,46] The thalami and cerebellum are typically spared. The appearance and time course of hypoglycemic injury differ between adults and neonates; neonatal hypoglycemia results in extensive edema and infarcts that affect the parietal and occipital lobes most severely, reflecting regional hypoperfusion and cell-specific excitotoxic injury. As in adults, the most severe cases of hypoglycemia in neonates also show abnormalities within the basal ganglia.

Although rare as a presenting symptom of hyperglycemia, seizures may also occur with high serum glucose. It is speculated that elevated blood sugar lowers γ-aminobutyric acid levels, thus diminishing the seizure threshold.[47] Because ketosis and intracellular acidosis actually increase the seizure threshold,[48] seizures are more frequently seen in nonketotic hyperglycemia than in diabetic ketoacidosis. An interesting constellation of MR imaging findings that have been ascribed to hyperglycemia includes T1 hyperintensity, T2 hypointensity, and reduced diffusion within the putamen but sparing other structures. Involvement of the putamen in this case is hypothesized to reflect selective metabolic vulnerability of neurons within this structure, and subsequent deposition of tissue manganese and reactive astrocytosis and/or ischemic injury.[49,50] The clinical

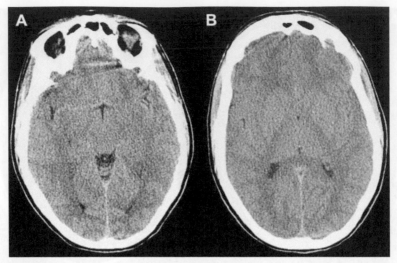

Fig. 5. Hyponatremic cerebral edema. Noncontrast axial CT images at the level of the midbrain (*A*) and thalami (*B*) in a marathon runner presenting with seizures and altered mental status. The patient consumed large quantities of water and was found to be hyponatremic (serum sodium 119). The images show poor visualization of sulci and effaced Sylvian fissures.

presentation in reported cases with these imaging findings is usually hemiballism rather than seizures, however.

STROKE

It is not uncommon that patients with acute seizures present with symptoms that can be confused clinically for acute infarcts. For example, in epileptic hemiplegia or so-called Todd paralysis, transient hemiparesis follows an episode of seizure activity. Especially in patients who also

have postictal aphasia and sensory deficits, the disorder may masquerade as a dominant hemisphere middle cerebral artery infarct. Conventional CT and MR imaging are typically unrevealing in this clinical scenario, but may occasionally show subtle asymmetries in sulcal morphology (Fig. 7). Regional abnormal sulcal FLAIR hyperintensity has also been described. Postictal hypoperfusion and hyperfusion have been described on CT perfusion imaging, both distinguished from ischemia by their atypical vascular distribution and the absence of associated arterial occlusion

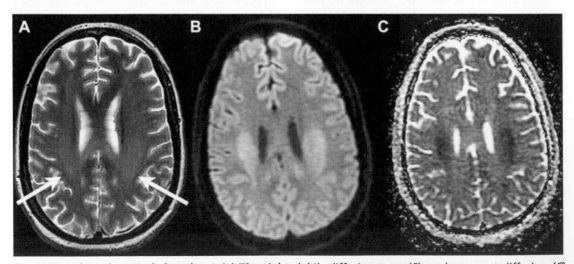

Fig. 6. Hypoglycemic encephalopathy. Axial T2-weighted (*A*), diffusion trace (*B*), and apparent diffusion (*C*) images obtained in a patient with hepatic abscess and severe hypoglycemic event. Note the subtle symmetric hyperintensity (*arrows*) on T2-weighted imaging (*A*) involving the posterior body of the corpus callosum and corona radiata with high signal on diffusion trace and reduced diffusion on apparent diffusion images.

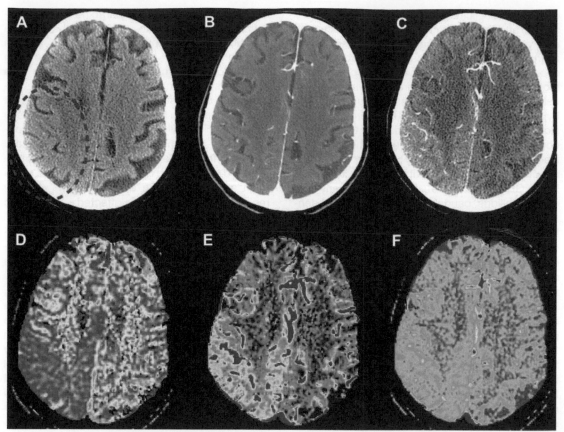

Fig. 7. Postictal Todd's paralysis. Noncontrast (*A*) and postcontrast (*B*) axial CT images at the level of the centrum semiovale show relative effacement of right parietal and posterior frontal sulci (*circle*) and subtle prominence of vessels in this region in a patient presenting with left hemiparesis. CT perfusion image (*C*) from at a single time point during bolus injection of contrast reveals hyperemia in the same region. Processed perfusion maps show reduced mean transit time (*D*), increased cerebral blood flow (*E*), and increased cerebral blood volume (*F*) relative to the remainder of the brain.

or narrowing on accompanying bolus CT angiography.[51–53] As is the case for other reversible postical abnormalities on imaging, perfusion is less likely to be abnormal as the time between the cessation of seizures and imaging increases, during the usual period of clinical recovery from symptoms.

Although neonates with infarcts commonly present with seizures, seizures are rare as the initial presenting symptom of acute infarct in adults. However, the likelihood of seizures increases shortly after the onset of stroke symptoms, and in the days to years that follow. The multicenter Seizures After Stroke Study Group found an overall incidence of seizures of 8.9% following stroke, although only 2.5% of patients went on to develop epilepsy.[54] Because of the focal nature of most infarcts, postinfarct seizures commonly have a focal onset, although secondary generalization is common. In clinical terms, seizures after stroke are arbitrarily divided at

a time point of 2 weeks into those of early or late onset.[55] Almost half of the patients with the early-onset subset of seizures have their first seizure within the first 24 hours after presenting with stroke, although few of these patients will ultimately develop chronic seizures. Late-onset seizures, by contrast, are less common overall, but are associated with a considerably higher incidence of epilepsy. Seizures in both cases are more likely to be associated with larger infarcts, with cortical as opposed to subcortical injury, and in cases where significant hemorrhage has occurred. Infarcts involving the hippocampus and posterior insula, and venous infarcts are also reported to be associated with a higher incidence of developing seizures.

Global anoxic injury is one of the most common causes for status epilepticus and recurrent seizures, especially following respiratory or cardiac arrest. Roughly one-third of patients will have seizures or myoclonus (uncontrolled muscle contractions elicited by movement or sensory stimuli) after resuscitation. Imaging in this scenario may prove useful in documenting that significant injury has taken place. The spectrum of brain injury seen depends on both the partial pressure of blood oxygen and the degree to which normal cerebral autoregulation was disrupted. Pure hypoxic injury, in which adequate cerebral perfusion pressure is maintained but the oxygen concentration in the blood is either insufficient or inadequately extracted by tissue, selectively affects areas of the brain with the highest metabolism. Gray matter structures, particularly the globus pallidus, caudate nuclei, thalami, and dentate nuclei of the cerebellum, are more vulnerable to this type of injury than white matter. Typical causes for hypoxic injury include carbon monoxide poisoning, anemia, and primary lung disease such as severe pneumonia and acute respiratory distress syndrome. By contrast, ischemic injury, in which blood flow to the brain is reduced but blood oxygen concentration is preserved disproportionately, involves areas of the brain for which the blood supply is most tenuous. These "watershed" areas of the brain include both gray and white matter located at the boundary zones between primary arterial territories. The deep white matter, supplied by small-caliber, perfusion-pressure sensitive penetrating arteries, is a boundary zone that is particularly vulnerable to this type of injury. On imaging, hypoperfusion injury may show changes at the boundaries between major vascular territories or in the deep white matter, the latter frequently seen as an anteroposteriorly oriented "string of pearls" (Fig. 8). In the majority of cases, both hypoperfusion and hypoxic injury are present together. The extent of injury depends on the duration and magnitude of hypoxia and circulatory collapse. The most severe cases show diffuse cerebral swelling, poor gray-white differentiation, "pseudo-subarachnoid hemorrhage," and in the worst cases, reversal of normal gray and white matter signal.

AUTOIMMUNE AND PARANEOPLASTIC ENCEPHALITIS

In a patient with known systemic malignancy, the most common underlying cause for a first-time seizure includes metastasis and associated hemorrhage or mass effect. However, even in the absence of intracranial metastatic disease, patients with cancer remain at higher risk for developing seizures. During the course of chemotherapy, many antineoplastic agents and adjuvant medications, including alkylating agents,

high-dose methotrexate, cytarabine, and ondansetron, are known to decrease the seizure threshold and may precipitate seizures. Certain malignancies have also been associated with immunologically mediated seizures.[56–58] The immune system in these cases mounts a cell-mediated response to remove tumor cells that express certain cell surface proteins. When these cells coincidentally also target normal, non-neoplastic neurons that express antigenically similar surface proteins, the brain may be the unanticipated target of the response. The regions of the brain affected in these disorders vary, and any region of the brain may be affected.[59] The limbic system, however, is most frequently affected.

Paraneoplastic limbic encephalitis (PLE) is characterized by the clinical triad of seizures, antegrade memory loss, and psychiatric symptoms (usually depression, psychosis, or personality changes). As with other autoimmune disorders, females are disproportionately affected. The most common tumors associated with PLE are small-cell lung carcinoma, testicular and ovarian cancer, thymoma, and breast cancer. Many patients exhibit symptoms in the face of a normal MRI. In others, unilateral or bilateral T2 signal abnormalities may be found within the mesial temporal lobes (Fig. 9). Atrophy of the same structures may be present in patients with long-standing disease. Because clinical symptoms of PLE usually precede the diagnosis of underlying cancer, whole-body FDG PET or CT may be indicated for the evaluation of patients with unexplained limbic signal abnormalities. Several autoantibody markers have been developed to assist in the diagnosis, though many of these are not widely available in the community and up to a third of patients with pathologically confirmed paraneoplastic encephalitis have negative antibody studies.

Clinical history and lumbar puncture may be necessary to differentiate PLE from infectious encephalitis, particularly herpes encephalitis, which also has a predilection for the limbic system and frequently present with seizures. Although the hippocampus, amygdala, insula, and sometimes the cingulate gyrus may be involved in both disorders, PLE tends to be more symmetric than herpes encephalitis in cases with bilateral temporal lobe involvement. Signal abnormalities also tend to be less dramatic in PLE than herpes encephalitis on MR imaging. Finally, although enhancement is present in up to 30% of cases,[60] hemorrhage and reduced diffusion, typical findings in herpes, have not been described in PLE. Other types of non-paraneoplastic autoimmune encephalitis, in particular that caused by antibodies to neuronal

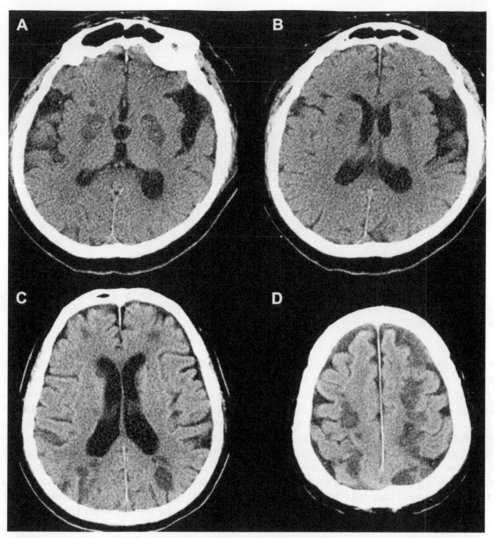

Fig. 8. Hypoxic and hypoperfusion injury. Noncontrast axial CT images (*A, B*) in a patient with respiratory arrest whose circulation was maintained by cardiopulmonary resuscitation show low density primarily confined to the globi pallidi and caudate nuclei, typical sites of hypoxic injury. In a different patient with cardiac arrest and ventricular fibrillation, low blood flow to the brain resulted in bilateral anterior cerebral artery/middle cerebral artery and middle cerebral artery/posterior cerebral artery watershed infarction on noncontrast CT (*C, D*).

voltage-gated potassium channels (VGKC antibodies), can also overlap clinically and radiologically with PLE. VGKC autoantibodies, however, are more likely to occur in males and are frequently associated with hyponatremia. Furthermore, the disorder is more frequently responsive to high-dose corticosteroids than PLE.

MALFORMATIONS OF CORTICAL DEVELOPMENT

Most malformations of cortical development (MCD) are identified in childhood when patients present with recurrent seizures together with developmental delay or congenital hemiparesis. However, the clinical phenotype of MCD is broad, and other patients have occult MCD that is found only incidentally or manifests later in life, when the seizure threshold is lowered for other reasons. Although a full discussion of the imaging appearance of MCD is beyond the scope of this article, it is important to recognize that CT may be the initial modality obtained when these patients present with a first-time seizure or when patients with otherwise quiescent MCD experience seizures. As a result, review of CT scans in patients with seizures should routinely include a careful inspection of the appearance of gray and white

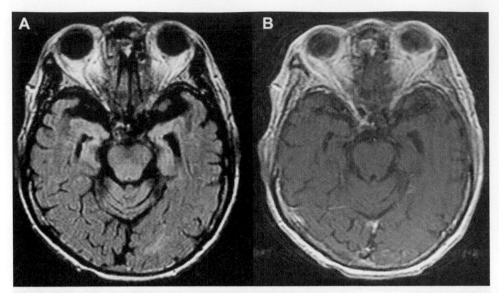

Fig. 9. Paraneoplastic limbic encephalitis. 67-year-old woman with a thymoma. Axial T2 FLAIR (*A*) and gadolinium-enhanced T1-weighted (*B*) images show symmetric high T2 signal and atrophy of the medial temporal lobes without enhancement.

matter, particularly along the cortical surface and the margins of the ventricular system. Subtle abnormalities in sulcation or gyral contour may provide the only clue on noncontrast CT that MCD may be present (**Fig. 10**). When seizures are attributed to systemic causes such as hypertension, alcohol withdrawal, or metabolic abnormality, these abnormalities may be easily overlooked. It is incumbent on the radiologist to remind referring physicians that MR imaging is more sensitive in detecting an underlying substrate for seizures, especially when recurrent, as CT misses significant abnormalities in more than 30% of affected patients.[61]

POSTTRAUMATIC EPILEPSY

Posttraumatic epilepsy (PTE) accounts for 4% of focal epilepsy, and is the leading cause of epilepsy with onset in young adulthood. Seizure onset may be shortly after injury or after a latent period of months or years. The disorder is classified clinically into early and late types, depending on the timing of initial seizure onset. Early posttraumatic seizures, which are further divided into immediate (within the first 24 hours) and delayed (within the first week) subtypes, are usually attributable to the direct effects of brain injury. Chronic PTE, by contrast, first occurs 1 week or later after TBI and often is associated with a developing meningocerebral cicatrix as the underlying epileptogenic substrate. Most early-onset seizures are of the generalized tonic-clonic type, whereas late PTE

has a more variable clinical presentation. Although an initial early seizure does not correlate with the development of late recurrent seizures, patients with a single late seizure have between a 65% and 90% chance of progressing to recurrent seizures. Unfortunately, both early and late PTE are less likely to be controlled with medical therapy than other causes of chronic seizures.

First described by Jennet and Lewin[62] in a landmark study on military head injuries, several of the risk factors for the development of PTE have been enumerated.[63-65] Penetrating injury is associated with a higher risk of developing seizures (50% cumulative incidence) than nonpenetrating injury (30%). Other risk factors for PTE include depressed skull fracture, intracranial hematoma, prolonged unconsciousness, prolonged antegrade amnesia, and low Glasgow Coma Scale score. Other factors include genetic influences and age at the time of trauma; patients with ApoE4 and haptoglobin 2-2 alleles appear to be more vulnerable to developing epilepsy after trauma, and injuries later in life appear less likely to be associated with the development of PTE than childhood trauma.

Although direct injury to the hippocampus is rare after TBI, several surgical series implicate trauma, especially trauma during early childhood, as a significant risk factor for the development of MTS. In a series of 259 patients undergoing temporal lobectomy for treatment of medically refractory seizures, Mathern and colleagues[66] found that 10% had prior traumatic injury as the

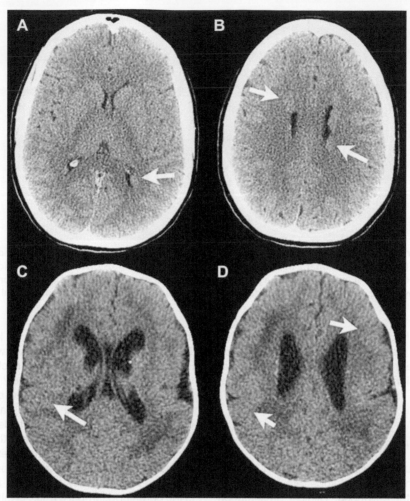

Fig. 10. **Malformations of cortical development on unenhanced CT.** Images from a postpartum woman (*A, B*) and an infant (*C, D*) presenting with first-time seizures. CT was performed in the first patient to evaluate for PRES, but showed multiple lesions (*arrows*) along the surface of both ventricles with the same density as cortical gray matter, consistent with periventricular nodular heterotopia. The second patient was initially thought to have venous sinus thrombosis clinically, but was later found to have thickened areas of cortex bilaterally (*arrows*) consistent with bilateral perisylvian polymicrogyria.

major risk factor, at a mean age of 6.3 years. Among this subgroup, 50% had hippocampal sclerosis on pathologic analysis of surgical specimens. A smaller series by Marks and colleagues[67] found that among 21 patients undergoing surgery for treatment of PTE, 6 patients with pathologically confirmed MTS had excellent outcomes, in contrast to 8 patients without MTS on pathology in whom seizures continued after surgery. There is a controversial relationship between the age at the time of TBI and MTS, with some investigators suggesting that MTS is more likely to develop in younger patients after TBI.

From an imaging standpoint, MTS is also one of the most common abnormalities observed in patients with PTE. Other imaging findings that have a reported association with seizures in this setting include hemorrhagic contusions and reactive astrogliosis (**Fig. 11**). Angeleri and colleagues[63] studied MR imaging scans from 104 patients with TBI 1 year following initial trauma to identify risk factors for PTE. In this cohort, a significant association was identified between cortical or subcortical T2 hyperintense lesions and development of PTE. It is interesting that hemosiderin deposition, by contrast, was not by itself associated with an increased risk of late seizures in this study. Other modalities may also be useful in assessing the risk of PTE following TBI. In a study of 143 patients with TBI, 27 of whom ultimately developed PTE after a mean follow-up of

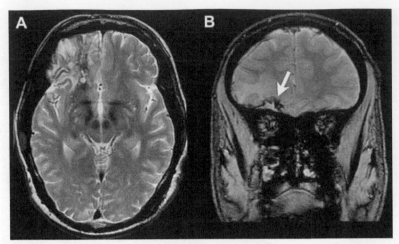

Fig. 11. Late-onset posttraumatic epilepsy. Axial T2 (*A*) and coronal T2*-weighted gradient echo (*B*) images in a patient who initially had traumatic injury resulting in hemorrhagic contusions and then developed medically refractory seizures several months later. Images show right frontal encephalomalacia with subcortical T2 hyperintensity and overlying hemosiderin staining (*arrow*). The patient was free of seizures after local resection.

11.9 months, Mazzini and colleagues[68] found that patients with temporal lobe hypoperfusion on ^{99m}Tc-hexamethylpropylene amine oxime single-photon emission CT (SPECT) developed PTE at a higher rate than patients with normal SPECT scans.

MESIAL TEMPORAL SCLEROSIS

A frequent cause of seizures after TBI, MTS is also the most common overall substrate for epilepsy with onset after childhood. Clinical presentation is heterogeneous, but most affected patients present during or after the adolescent period. Specific symptoms range from abnormal sensations to automatisms and autonomic nervous system dysfunction. All patients have partial seizures, though many ultimately develop secondary generalized tonic-clonic seizures. Partial seizures related to MTS are controlled by antiepileptic medications in most cases. However, approximately 25% of patients with MTS suffer from medically refractory seizures. Up to 80% of patients in this subgroup become seizure free following temporal lobectomy. MR imaging plays a critical role in the selection of patients for temporal lobectomy, with the highest postresection seizure-free rates occurring in patients with positive MR imaging and concordant EEG and clinical localization of seizure onset.

An understanding of normal hippocampal and surrounding temporal lobe anatomy is critical to the MR imaging diagnosis of MTS.[69,70] The 2 primary structures of interest in this regard are the hippocampus and amygdala, both found along the medial surface of the temporal lobe (**Fig. 12**). The amygdala, the smaller of the two structures, is an almond-shaped group of nuclei anterior to the hippocampus and immediately lateral to the uncus of the temporal lobe. The amygdala lies along the anterior and superior aspect of the temporal horn of the lateral ventricle and, as part of the limbic system, plays a role in the processing of memory and emotion. Other useful landmarks for localization are best seen on coronal images. The gyrus immediately below the hippocampus is the parahippocampal gyrus. As this gyrus wraps around the posterior aspect of the lateral ventricles, it is continuous with the cingulate gyrus, the gyrus immediately above the corpus callosum. Within the medial temporal lobe, the parahippocampal gyrus is separated from the more inferior fusiform gyrus by the collateral sulcus. This gyrus is lateral to the lateral temporal gyri (superior, middle, and inferior temporal gyri).

The hippocampal formation, responsible for the formation of new memories and spatial navigation, is a complex, 3-dimensional structure that is anatomically divided into 3 segments. From anterior to posterior, these are the head (or pes), body, and tail. (For reference, the red nuclei within the midbrain are located at the approximate level of the mid-hippocampal body.) The most anterior portion, the hippocampal head, lies posterior to the amygdala and exhibits undulating "digitations" along its superior surface that form a series of ridges along the floor of the anterior temporal horn. Posterior to the hippocampal pes, the body and tail of the hippocampus have a smooth superior contour along the inferomedial ventricular

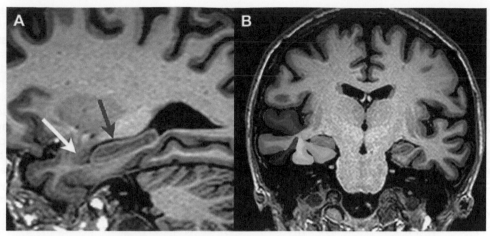

Fig. 12. Normal medial temporal lobe anatomy (Images from a volumetric gradient echo T1 sequence). Sagittal image (*A*) shows the normal hippocampus located along the floor of the temporal horn of the lateral ventricle (*red arrow*), as well as the amygdala along the anterosuperior surface of the temporal horn (*white arrow*). Coronal imaging (*B*) best shows the gyral anatomy of the temporal lobe. The superior temporal (*red*), middle temporal (*blue*), inferior temporal (*purple*), fusiform (*yellow*), and parahippocampal (*green*) gyri of the right temporal lobe are labeled. The body of the right hippocampus (*orange*) is located directly above the parahippocampal gyrus.

surface. On coronal images at the level of the hippocampal body and tail, the inner portion of the hippocampus, the dentate gyrus, is continuous with and encircled by the gray matter of the cornu Ammonis (Ammon's horn) (Fig. 13). Ammon's horn is comprised histologically of 4 sectors (CA1 through CA4), and continues medially and inferiorly along the medial surface of the temporal lobe as the subiculum, presubiculum, parasubiculum, and entorhinal cortex (the cortex of the parahippocampal gyrus). A vestigial sulcus, the

hippocampal sulcus, separates the dentate gyrus superiorly from the CA1 sector of Ammon's horn and subiculum inferiorly. Tiny cystic foci of T2 hyperintensity are occasionally seen incidentally within this sulcus and have no association with seizures.

On high-resolution T2-weighted MR imaging, the normal hippocampus consistently exhibits a well-defined laminar architecture comprising concentric layers of gray and white matter. At a minimum, 3 layers should be seen. The

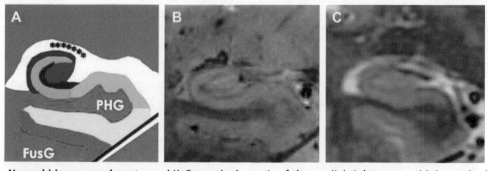

Fig. 13. Normal hippocampal anatomy. (*A*) Coronal schematic of the medial right temporal lobe at the level of the hippocampal body. The hippocampus at this level is appreciated as a curvilinear structure bordered by cerebrospinal fluid within the temporal horn laterally and the choroidal fissure superiorly (*asterisks*). Although the internal architecture of the hippocampus is better visualized at 7 T (*B*) than at 3 T (*C*), several layers can be discerned on both images. These layers include the dentate gyrus (*red*) and Ammon's horn (*green*), which are separated by several internal layers (*dark blue*). The superficial aspect of Ammon's horn is invested with a thin white matter layer called the alveus (*dark purple*). The gray matter of Ammon's horn is continuous with the subiculum (*light blue*), which continues around the medial surface of the temporal lobe as the entorhinal cortex (*yellow*); these comprise the cortex of the parahippocampal gyrus (PHG). The fusiform gyrus (FusG) lies below the PHG, separated by the collateral sulcus.

outermost white matter layer, the alveus, is darker on T2 than the adjacent dentate gyrus and cornu Ammonis, and appears isointense to white matter elsewhere in the brain. This outer layer extends along the subependymal surface of the inferomedial temporal horn, and continues posteriorly as the ipsilateral fornix. Deep to the alveus, the gray matter of the cornu Ammonis appears brighter on T2, with a similar signal to gray matter elsewhere in the brain. The innermost white matter layer between the dentate gyrus and Ammon's horn and subiculum consists of several internal hippocampal white matter layers with darker T2 signal. These layers, which consist primarily of the stratum radiatum, stratum lacunosum, and stratum moleculare, are not visualized separately on in vivo clinical 3-T MR imaging but together can be seen as a single layer of white matter on high-quality images.

Corresponding to the neuropathological abnormalities described on surgical specimens with confirmed mesial sclerosis,[71-73] several imaging features of MTS have been described on high-resolution T1-, T2-, and FLAIR images of the medial temporal lobes. The triad of (1) hippocampal atrophy, (2) loss of normal internal laminar architecture, and (3) high T2 signal intensity on MR imaging can be used to make this diagnosis. Thin-section T2-weighted images best demonstrate the derangement of the normal internal hippocampal architecture and may show asymmetric T2 hyperintensity (Fig. 14). FLAIR sequences are often more sensitive to subtle asymmetries in T2 signal and high resolution, however, and volumetric T1-weighted images may best show the degree of associated hippocampal atrophy. Atrophy of the hippocampus may also been seen as loss of the digitations of the hippocampal head and enlargement of the ipsilateral temporal horn and

choroidal fissure. In addition to the characteristic T2 signal abnormality within the hippocampus, high T2 signal and atrophy may also be evident within the amygdala. Correlative pathology studies have shown that T2 signal in MTS is directly related to the presence of astrogliosis, whereas volume loss is a feature of hippocampal cell loss.

Secondary findings that have been described with hippocampal sclerosis mirror the propagation of seizures along ipsilateral networks that project from the medial temporal lobe. Like the hippocampus, the ipsilateral fornix may also appear atrophic, as may the ipsilateral mammillary body to which the fornix ultimately projects. Similarly, as a major hub for connections between the limbic system and the remainder of the cortex, the ipsilateral thalamus may appear atrophic. Ipsilateral atrophy of the entire temporal lobe has also been described as a feature of MTS, typically seen in more advanced cases. Unfortunately, there is considerable variability in volume of the fornices, mammillary bodies, and temporal lobes across the hemispheres, and these imaging findings are not useful for diagnosis in the absence of other features of MTS.

Although the finding of MTS increases the overall likelihood of surgical success, is important to critically assess MR imaging sequences for additional seizure substrates. Between 5% and 30% of cases of MTS are accompanied by "dual pathology," defined by the presence of a second extrahippocampal area of epileptogenic cortex.[74] Prospective identification of dual pathology is important for surgical planning and patient counseling, as it significantly lowers the success rate of temporal lobectomy, and in some cases may obviate surgery entirely. MCD, contusion, cavernous malformation, glial or glioneuronal tumor, or contralateral hippocampal sclerosis all

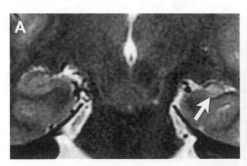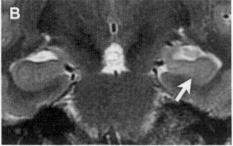

Fig. 14. **Hippocampal sclerosis.** High-resolution coronal T2-weighted images illustrate severe (*A*) and mild (*B*) findings of left MTS (*arrows*). In *A*, the sclerotic left hippocampus is tiny and shows abnormal T2 hyperintensity and poor visualization of internal layers. In *B*, mild volume loss is appreciated by asymmetric increase in size of the choroidal fissure and temporal horn, along with effacement of the normal internal architecture and mild increase in T2 signal.

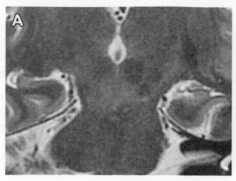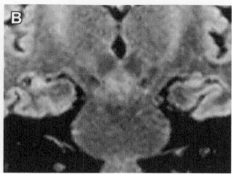

Fig. 15. Bilateral MTS. Coronal T2 (*A*) and FLAIR (*B*) images obtained in a woman presenting with chronic seizures after a prolonged episode of status epilepticus. Decreased volume and abnormal T2 hyperintensity of the hippocampus are more pronounced on the left, and only subtle derangement of the normal hippocampal laminar architecture is evident on the right.

represent important causes for dual pathology. Bilateral hippocampal sclerosis, also implicated as a cause for recurrent seizures after temporal lobectomy, may be overlooked because of the apparent visual symmetry between the sclerotic hippocampi (**Fig. 15**).

CT AND MR IMAGING FOR SEIZURES

As the clinical end point of a variety of acute and chronic neurologic insults, seizures are a common symptom that may or may not require imaging. When imaging is obtained in the acute setting, CT is useful to exclude that require emergent surgical intervention, and may in some cases suggest a cause for seizures. However, because CT may miss important sources of seizures and epilepsy, MR imaging remains the diagnostic modality of choice. For both CT and MR imaging, images should be interpreted together with the knowledge of the seizure type and onset, and in cases with partial onset, particular attention should be given to available clinical and EEG-localizing information. Even in patients presenting acutely with first-time seizures, it is important to exclude epileptogenic structural lesions such as mesial sclerosis, the most common cause for seizures after childhood and a frequent cause for seizures following TBI.

REFERENCES

1. Bronen RA, Fulbright RK, Kim JH, et al. A systematic approach for interpreting MR images of the seizure patient. AJR Am J Roentgenol 1997;169:241–7.
2. Duncan JS. Imaging and epilepsy. Brain 1997; 120(pt 2):339–77.
3. Bronen RA, Knowlton R, Garwood M, et al. High-resolution imaging in epilepsy. Epilepsia 2002;43(S1): 11–8.
4. Vattipally VR, Bronen RA. MR imaging of epilepsy: strategies for successful interpretation. Neuroimaging Clin N Am 2004;14(3):349–72.
5. Wieshmann UC. Clinical application of neuroimaging in epilepsy. J Neurol Neurosurg Psychiatry 2003;74(4):466–70.
6. Gupta V, Bronen RA. Epilepsy. In: Atlas SW, editor. Magnetic resonance imaging of the brain and spine. 4th edition. Philadelphia: Lippincott Williams & Wilkins; 2009. p. 307–42.
7. Kuzniecky RI, Jackson GD, editors. Magnetic resonance in epilepsy: neuroimaging techniques. 2nd edition. Burlington (MA): Elsevier Academic Press; 2004.
8. Duncan JS, editor. Epilepsy. Neuroimag Clin N Am 2004;14(3).
9. Berg AT, Berkovic SF, Brodie MJ, et al. Revised terminology and concepts for organization of seizures and epilepsies: report of the ILAE Commission on Classification and Terminology, 2005–2009. Epilepsia 2010;51(4):676–85.
10. American College of Emergency Physicians, American Academy of Neurology, American Association of Neurological Surgeons, et al. Practice parameter: neuroimaging in the emergency patient presenting with seizure (summary statement). Ann Emerg Med 1996;28(1):114–8.
11. Karis JP, Seidenwurm DJ, Davis PC, et al. Expert panel on neurologic imaging Epilepsy. [online publication]. Reston (VA): American College of Radiology (ACR); 2006.
12. Hauser WA, Annegers JF, Kurland LT. Incidence of epilepsy and unprovoked seizures in Rochester, Minnesota: 1935-1984. Epilepsia 1993;34(3): 453–68.
13. Brenner DJ, Hall EJ. Computed tomography—an increasing source of radiation exposure. N Engl J Med 2007;357(22):2277–84.
14. Practice parameter: the neurodiagnostic evaluation of the child with a first simple febrile seizure.

American Academy of Pediatrics. Provisional Committee on Quality Improvement, Subcommittee on Febrile Seizures. Pediatrics 1996;97(5):769–72.

15. Briellmann RS, Pell GS, Wellard RM, et al. MR imaging of epilepsy: state of the art at 1.5 T and potential of 3 T. Epileptic Disord 2003;5(1):3–20.

16. Phal PM, Usmanov A, Nesbit GM, et al. Qualitative comparison of 3-T and 1.5-T MRI in the evaluation of epilepsy. AJR Am J Roentgenol 2008;191(3): 890–5.

17. Von Oertzen J, Urbach H, Jungbluth S, et al. Standard magnetic resonance imaging is inadequate for patients with refractory focal epilepsy. J Neurol Neurosurg Psychiatry 2002;73(6):643–7.

18. Barkovich AJ, Rowley HA, Andermann F. MR in partial epilepsy: value of high-resolution volumetric techniques. AJNR Am J Neuroradiol 1995;16(2): 339–43.

19. Grant PE, Barkovich AJ, Wald LL, et al. High-resolution surface-coil MR of cortical lesions in medically refractory epilepsy: a prospective study. AJNR Am J Neuroradiol 1997;18(2):291–301.

20. Knake S, Triantafyllou C, Wald LL, et al. 3T phased array MRI improves the presurgical evaluation in focal epilepsies: a prospective study. Neurology 2005;65(7):1026–31.

21. Yaffe K, Ferriero D, Barkovich AJ, et al. Reversible MRI abnormalities following seizures. Neurology 1995;45:104–8.

22. Chan S, Chin SS, Kartha K, et al. Reversible signal abnormalities in the hippocampus and neocortex after prolonged seizures. AJNR Am J Neuroradiol 1996;17:1725–31.

23. Silverstein AM, Alexander JA. Acute postictal cerebral imaging. AJNR Am J Neuroradiol 1998;19: 1485–8.

24. Briellmann RS, Wellard RM, Jackson GD. Seizure-associated abnormalities in epilepsy: evidence from MR imaging. Epilepsia 2005;46:760–6.

25. Huang YC, Weng HH, Tsai YT, et al. Periictal magnetic resonance imaging in status epilepticus. Epilepsy Res 2009;86(1):72–81.

26. Goyal MK, Sinha S, Ravishankar S, et al. Peri-ictal signal changes in seven patients with status epilepticus: interesting MRI observations. Neuroradiology 2009;51:151–61.

27. Cole AJ. Status epilepticus and periictal imaging. Epilepsia 2004;45(Suppl 4):72–7.

28. Hicdonmez T, Utku U, Turgut N, et al. Reversible postictal MRI change mimicking structural lesion. Clin Neurol Neurosurg 2003;105(4):288–90.

29. Finn MA, Blumenthal DT, Salzman KL, et al. Transient postictal MRI changes in patients with brain tumors may mimic disease progression. Surg Neurol 2007; 67(3):246–50.

30. Kim JA, Chung JI, Yoon PH, et al. Transient MR signal changes in patients with generalized tonic-clonic seizure or status epilepticus: peri-ictal diffusion-weighted imaging. AJNR Am J Neuroradiol 2001;22:1149–60.

31. Moritani T, Smoker WRK, Sato Y, et al. Diffusion-weighted imaging of acute excitotoxic brain injury. AJNR Am J Neuroradiol 2005;26:216–28.

32. Katramados AM, Burdette D, Patel SC, et al. Peri-ictal diffusion abnormalities of the thalamus in partial status epilepticus. Epilepsia 2009;50(2): 265–75.

33. Kim SS, Chang KH, Kim ST, et al. Focal lesion in the splenium of the corpus callosum in epileptic patients: antiepileptic drug toxicity? AJNR Am J Neuroradiol 1999;20:125–9.

34. Polster T, Hoppe M, Ebner A. Transient lesion in the splenium of the corpus callosum: three further cases in epileptic patients and a pathophysiological hypothesis. J Neurol Neurosurg Psychiatry 2001; 70:459–63.

35. Oster J, Doherty C, Grant PE, et al. Diffusion-weighted imaging abnormalities in the splenium after seizures. Epilepsia 2003;44(6):1–3.

36. Hinchey J, Chaves C, Appignani B, et al. A reversible posterior leukoencephalopathy syndrome. N Engl J Med 1996;334:494–500.

37. Casey SO, Sampaio RC, Michel E, et al. Posterior reversible encephalopathy syndrome: Utility of fluid-attenuated inversion recovery MR imaging in the detection of cortical and subcortical lesions. AJNR Am J Neuroradiol 2000;21:1199–206.

38. Lee VH, Wijdicks EF, Manno EM, et al. Clinical spectrum of reversible posterior leukoencephalopathy syndrome. Arch Neurol 2008;65(2):205–10.

39. Covarrubias DJ, Luetmer PH, Campeau NG. Posterior reversible encephalopathy syndrome: prognostic utility of quantitative diffusion-weighted MR images. AJNR Am J Neuroradiol 2002;23(6): 1038–48.

40. Bartynski WS, Boardman JF. Distinct imaging patterns and lesion distribution in posterior reversible encephalopathy syndrome. AJNR Am J Neuroradiol 2007;28(7):1320–7.

41. McKinney AM, Short J, Truwit CL, et al. Posterior reversible encephalopathy syndrome: incidence of atypical regions of involvement and imaging findings. AJR Am J Roentgenol 2007;189:904.

42. Hasegawa Y, Formato JE, Latour LL, et al. Severe transient hypoglycemia causes reversible change in the apparent diffusion coefficient of water. Stroke 1996;27:1648–55.

43. Fujioka M, Okuchi K, Hiramatsu KI, et al. Specific changes in human brain after hypoglycemic injury. Stroke 1997;28:584–7.

44. Finelli PF. Diffusion-weighted MR in hypoglycemic coma. Neurology 2001;57:933–5.

45. Bottcher J, Kunze A, Kurrat C, et al. Localized reversible reduction of apparent diffusion coefficient

in transient hypoglycemia-induced hemiparesis. Stroke 2005;36:20–2.

46. Maekawa S, Aibiki M, Kikuchi K, et al. Time-related changes in reversible MRI findings after prolonged hypoglycemia. Clin Neurol Neurosurg 2006;108: 511–3.

47. Hennis A, Corbin D, Fraser H. Focal seizures and non-ketotic hyperglycaemia. J Neurol Neurosurg Psychiatry 1992;55:195–7.

48. Singh BM, Strobos RJ. Epilepsia partialis continua associated with nonketotic hyperglycemia: clinical and biochemical profile of 21 patients. Ann Neurol 1980;8:155–60.

49. Shan DE, Ho DM, Chang C, et al. Hemichorea-hemi-ballism: an explanation for MR signal changes. AJNR Am J Neuroradiol 1998;19:863–70.

50. Wintermark M, Fischbein NJ, Mukherjee P, et al. Unilateral putaminal CT, MR, and diffusion abnor-malities secondary to nonketotic hyperglycemia in the setting of acute neurologic symptoms mimicking stroke. AJNR Am J Neuroradiol 2004; 25(6):975–6.

51. Mathews MS, Smith WS, Wintermark M, et al. Local cortical hypoperfusion imaged with CT perfusion during postictal Todd's paresis. Neuroradiology 2008;50(5):397–401.

52. Royter V, Paletz L, Waters MF. Stroke vs. status epi-lepticus: a case report utilizing CT perfusion. J Neu-rol Sci 2008;266:174–7.

53. Gelfand JM, Wintermark M, Josephson SA. Cerebral perfusion-CT patterns following seizure. Eur J Neurol 2010;17(4):594–601.

54. Bladin C, Alexandrov A, Bellavance A, et al. Seizures after stroke: a prospective multicenter study. Arch Neurol 2000;57:1617–22.

55. Silverman IE, Restrepo L, Mathews GC. Poststroke seizures. Arch Neurol 2002 Feb;59(2):195–201.

56. Gultekin SH, Rosenfeld MR, Voltz R, et al. Paraneo-plastic limbic encephalitis: neurological symptoms, immunological findings and tumour association in 50 patients. Brain 2000;123(Pt 7):1481–94.

57. Ances BM, Vitaliani R, Taylor RA, et al. Treatment-responsive limbic encephalitis identified by neuro-pil antibodies: MRI and PET correlates. Brain 2005; 128(8):1764–77.

58. Vernino S, Geschwind M, Boeve B. Autoimmune encephalopathies. Neurologist 2007;13(3):140–7.

59. McKeon A, Ahlskog JE, Britton JA, et al. Reversible extralimbic paraneoplastic encephalopathies with large abnormalities on magnetic resonance images. Arch Neurol 2009;66(2):268–71.

60. Bien CG, Urbach H, Schramm J, et al. Limbic enceph-alitis as a precipitating event in adult-onset temporal lobe epilepsy. Neurology 2007;69:1236–44.

61. Raymond AA, Fish DR, Sisodaya SM, et al. Abnor-malities of gyration, heterotopias, tuberous

sclerosis, focal cortical dysplasia, microdysgenesis, dysembryoplastic neuroepithelial tumour and dysgenesis of the archicortex in epilepsy. Clinical, EEG and neuroimaging features in 100 adult patients. Brain 1995;118:629–60.

62. Jennett WB, Lewin W. Traumatic epilepsy after closed head injuries. J Neurol Neurosurg Psychiatry 1960;23:295–301.

63. Angeleri F, Majkowski J, Cacchib G, et al. Posttrau-matic epilepsy risk factors: one-year prospective study after head injury. Epilepsia 1999;40(9): 1222–30.

64. Diaz-Arrastia R, Agostini MA, Frol AB, et al. Neuro-physiologic and neuroradiologic features of intrac-table epilepsy after traumatic brain injury in adults. Arch Neurol 2000;57(11):1611–6.

65. Messori A, Polonara G, Carle F, et al. Predicting posttraumatic epilepsy with MRI: prospective longi-tudinal morphologic study in adults. Epilepsia 2005;46(9):1472–81.

66. Mathern GW, Babb TL, Vickrey BG, et al. Traumatic compared to non-traumatic clinical-pathologic asso-ciations in temporal lobe epilepsy. Epilepsy Res 1994;19:129–13927.

67. Marks DA, Kim J, Spencer DD, et al. Seizure locali-zation and pathology following head injury in patients with uncontrolled epilepsy. Neurology 1995;45:2051–7.

68. Mazzini L, Cossa FM, Angelino E, et al. Posttrau-matic epilepsy: neuroradiologic and neuropsycho-logical assessment of long-term outcome. Epilepsia 2003;44(4):569–74.

69. Naidich TP, Daniels DL, Haughton VM, et al. Hippo-campal formation and related structures of the limbic lobe: anatomic-MR correlation. Part I. Surface fea-tures and coronal sections. Radiology 1987;162(3): 747–54.

70. Naidich TP, Daniels DL, Haughton VM, et al. Hippo-campal formation and related structures of the limbic lobe: anatomic-MR correlation. Part II. Sagittal sections. Radiology 1987;162(3):755–61.

71. Jackson GD, Berkovic SF, Tree BM, et al. Hippo-campal sclerosis can be reliably detected by magnetic resonance imaging. Neurology 1990;40: 1869–75.

72. Meiners LC, van Gils A, Jansen GH, et al. Temporal lobe epilepsy: the various MR appearances of histo-logically proven mesial temporal sclerosis. AJNR Am J Neuroradiol 1994;15(8):1547–55.

73. Lee DH, Gao FQ, Rogers JM, et al. MR in temporal lobe epilepsy: analysis with pathologic confirmation. AJNR Am J Neuroradiol 1998;19(1): 19–27.

74. Li LM, Cendes F, Andermann F, et al. Surgical outcome in patients with epilepsy and dual pathology. Brain 1999;122:799–805.

Spine and Spinal Cord Emergencies: Vascular and Infectious Causes

Vincent Y. Wang[a], Dean Chou[a] and Cynthia Chin[b],*

KEYWORDS

- Spinal cord emergencies • Spine infections
- Spine vascular emergencies

EPIDURAL ABSCESS

Spinal epidural abscess can develop primarily or after spinal surgery. *Primary* spinal epidural abscess is a rare entity, with an estimated prevalence of 0.2 to 2.0 cases per 10,000 hospital admissions.[1] However, its incidence has increased over the last 20 years as a result of better diagnostic methods, an aging population, an increase in the number of patients with medical comorbidities, and an increase in intravenous drug use.[1,2] Most cases occur in middle-aged to elderly adults, with a predilection for men.[1–3] Risk factors include diabetes, intravenous drug use, previous invasive procedures to the spine, superficial infections of the back, immunocompromised state, and infections at distant sites.[1–4] *Staphylococcus aureus* is the most common pathogen and is found in approximately 70% of cases.[1–3,5] Gram-negative rods were previously reported to be associated with a significant number of spinal epidural abscesses and vertebral osteomyelitis; however, its prevalence has been decreasing over the years.[1,6] In rare cases, other pathogens, such as tuberculosis, fungal, and parasitic agents, can also be associated with a spinal epidural abscess.[1,7]

The classic clinical triad of fever, back pain, and neurologic deficits is found in only a small fraction of patients.[2] Almost all patients have back pain, but fever occurs in only about two-thirds of patients, and neurologic deficits occur in 25% to 60% of patients.[1,3,8] Therefore, many patients do not seek medical treatment with the onset of symptoms and a delay in diagnosis is not uncommon.[4,9]

In terms of location, epidural abscess can occur in all 3 regions of the spine (cervical, thoracic, and lumbosacral). Of the 3 regions of the spine, the thoracic and the lumbosacral regions are affected more commonly than the cervical spine.[1,5,8] There are also cases of a spinal epidural abscess involving the entire spine.[8,10]

The spinal epidural abscess can cause neurologic deficits by either direct compression or by vascular compromise through thrombophlebitis or thrombosis.[11] Thus, sudden neurologic deterioration can occur and prompt diagnosis is important. MR imaging is the initial study of choice for identifying a spinal epidural process of any etiology. In the case of an abscess, the diagnosis is often straightforward: isointense or hypointense on T1-weighted images and hyperintense on T2-weighted images.[3,8] The collection usually partially enhances with gadolinium-based intravenous contrast media (Gad).[3,8] The fluid portion of the abscess is typically hyperintense on T2-weighted images.[12] The enhancement pattern sometimes helps to define the consistency of the collection. Specifically, liquid purulent material is associated with a central area of low T1 signal intensity; whereas, a rim of tissue that enhances after Gad represents granulation tissue.[12] Recently, diffusion-weighted imaging (DWI) has been used

[a] Department of Neurological Surgery, University of California, 505 Parnassus Avenue, MS112, San Francisco, CA 94143, USA
[b] Section of Neuroradiology, Department of Radiology, University of California, San Francisco, San Francisco, CA 94143, USA
* Corresponding author.
E-mail address: cynthia.chin@radiology.ucsf.edu

Neuroimag Clin N Am 20 (2010) 639–650
doi:10.1016/j.nic.2010.07.006

in the spine; on DWI, the abscess is markedly hyperintense to the surrounding tissue and hypointense on the apparent diffusion coefficient map (Fig. 1).[13] More than 80% of patients with spinal epidural abscess have concomitant osteomyelitis.[2,3] Therefore, in patients with a suspected spinal epidural abscess, it is important to look for additional findings of osteomyelitis or diskitis.

Patients who are unable to undergo MR imaging can be studied with CT myelography (CTM), which has been shown to have similar sensitivity to MR imaging for detecting an epidural abscess.[14] MR imaging has the advantage of being more specific in its ability to differentiate the epidural mass from other pathologies. In addition, it is superior for evaluating the adjacent paraspinal soft tissues. Moreover, CTM requires intrathecal injection of contrast material and therefore has the theoretical risk of introducing the infectious agents into the intrathecal space in cases of lumbosacral abscess. Nevertheless, CTM may be an alternative diagnostic method for patients who are unable to undergo an MR imaging examination and for patients in whom MR imaging may be difficult to interpret because of previous spinal instrumentation. Although MR imaging, and to a lesser extent CTM, is a key diagnostic study to establish the diagnosis of a spinal epidural abscess, plain radiographs or CT of the spine are often the first diagnostic tests that are obtained, especially in patients who are afebrile without neurologic deficits. Surgical decompression with antibiotic treatment have historically been the mainstay of treatment for spinal epidural abscess.[1-5,8] Recently, nonsurgical treatment has been used to treat patients with no neurologic deficits, significant comorbidities, or complete spinal cord injury at the affected level below the level of epidural abscess.[2,3]

EPIDURAL HEMATOMA

Spinal epidural hematoma (EDH) can compress the spinal cord or nerve roots and result in neurologic deficits. Spinal EDHs occur most commonly after spinal surgery.[15] After discectomy or decompression, EDH can be identified in 33% to 100% of the patients when evaluated by postoperative CT or MR imaging.[15] However, despite the radiographic appearance of compression by many of these lesions, neurologic symptoms associated with postoperative EDH are extremely rare.[15] It is estimated that the incidence of symptomatic EDH after spinal surgery is only 0.1% to 0.2%.[15] Risk factors associated with EDH formation include advanced patient age, multilevel surgery,

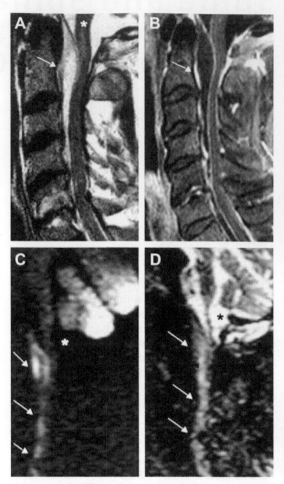

Fig. 1. **Methicillin-resistant Staphylococcus aureus spinal epidural abscess.** 58-year-old man with diabetes with progressive weakness. Sagittal fast spin echo T2 (A) and postgadolinium T1 with fat saturation (B) sequences through the cervical spine demonstrate extensive circumferential peripherally enhancing epidural abscess (arrow) with cord compression and associated cord edema (asterisk). Sagittal diffusion-weighted imaging (C) demonstrates increased signal, and apparent diffusion coefficient map (D) demonstrates decreased signal (arrows) relative to cerebrospinal fluid (asterisk) compatible with reduced diffusion within the epidural abscess.

and coagulopathy (increased international normalized ratio).

In contrast, spontaneous EDHs of the spine are rare. The incidence of spontaneous spinal epidural hematomas is estimated to be 0.1/100,000 population per year.[16] They usually occur in older patients (aged 50–80 years) with a slight predominance of male patients.[16] Limited evidence suggests that the spontaneous spinal EDH is caused by bleeding from the valveless venous plexus, although some investigators postulate that arterial rupture may be the cause.[16] In most cases, there is no clear source of hemorrhage or a causative event. There have been several case reports of spinal epidural hematomas occurring after chiropractic manipulation, epidural anesthesia, and steroid injection.[17,18] The incidence of spinal EDH after chiropractic manipulation is extremely low, with fewer than 10 cases reported in the literature.[17] The risk of spinal EDH after epidural anesthesia is also low, estimated to be about 1:220,000.[19] It is thought that coagulopathy increases the risk of spinal EDH in these latter cases.[17,18]

The classic clinical presentation of a spinal EDH consists of the sudden onset of back or neck pain. Neurologic symptoms related to the compression of nerve roots or spinal cord may also occur.[20] Many pathologic conditions, including intervertebral disc herniation, infection, pathologic fractures associated with tumor, transverse myelitis, and other vascular malformations, may mimic the clinical presentation of a spinal EDH. Therefore, prompt evaluation with MR imaging is important to establish the diagnosis.

The typical imaging appearance of an acute spinal EDH is that of a homogenously isointense to hyperintense mass on T1-weighted images, and hyperintensity on T2-weighted images.[20] The hematoma can have homogenous or heterogeneous hyperintensity on T2-weighted images.[20] Atypical appearance of the hematoma usually involves a shift from isointense to hyperintense on T1-weighted images.[20] Importantly, the acute spinal EDH *should not* enhance with gadolinium-based intravenous contrast media.[20] In one series of 19 subjects with a diagnosis of spinal EDH, 2 cases showed Gad enhancement on MR imaging and the intraoperative findings revealed that neither case was an EDH.[20] Most hematomas occur in the cervical or the thoracic region (Fig. 2).[18]

In the majority of cases, emergent surgical evacuation of the hematoma is the treatment of choice. Patients with small hematomas and without neurologic deficit may be managed conservatively.[17,20] For patients with neurologic deficits, it is important to remove the hematoma. Further, because neurologic improvement has been observed even in patients presenting with complete injury, prompt recognition, diagnosis, and treatment are essential for the optimal management of the spinal EDH.[20]

ARTERIOVENOUS SHUNTS

Arteriovenous shunts and vascular malformations in the spinal cord region are classified based on

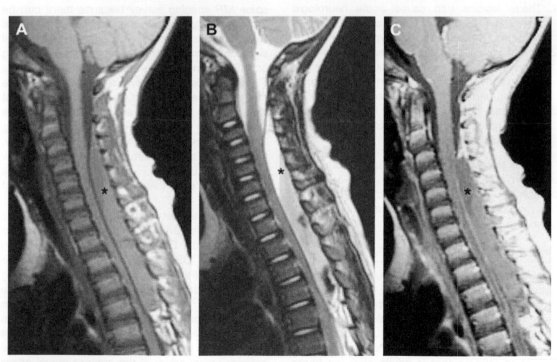

Fig. 2. Spontaneous epidural hematoma. 3-year-old healthy girl with 4-day history of back pain progressing to lower extremity weakness and inability to ambulate. Sagittal T1 (A) fast spin echo T2 (B) and postgadolinium T1 with fat saturation (C) images of the cervical spine demonstrate extensive nonenhancing dorsal epidural hematoma compressing the spinal cord. A hematocrit level is present within the epidural hematoma (asterisks).

their nidus location, vascular supply, and drainage pattern. In one of the most commonly used classifications, developed by Oldfield and Doppman, the lesions are divided into 4 types:[21]

> Type I lesions are the typical dural arteriovenous fistula (DAVF), and usually arise near nerve roots.
> Type II lesions are glomus arteriovenous malformations (AVM), with a mass of dysmorphic arteries and veins without an intervening capillary bed. These lesions can be partial or entirely intramedullary.
> Type III lesions are juvenile AVMs that are composed of a network of arteries and veins, without an obvious nidus. These lesions can be extensive and involve the spinal cord, spine, and paravertebral tissue.
> Type IV lesions are perimedullary DAVF.

Combined, these 4 types of arteriovenous shunts or vascular malformations account for 3% to 16% of all space-occupying lesions of the spinal cord, with the Type 1 DAVF being the most common.[22] Each of these types are subsequently discussed.

Spinal vascular malformations/arteriovenous shunts can cause neurologic symptoms by 3 mechanisms:

1. These lesions can cause acute neurologic symptoms by hemorrhage, and the risk of hemorrhage varies for the 4 types of lesions.
2. Spinal vascular malformations and arteriovenous shunts can result in venous hypertension. Venous hypertension, in turn, can lead to reduced perfusion, and thus ischemia.
3. They can cause symptoms by direct mass effect, resulting in a progressive myelopathy or radiculopathy.

In one study of 78 subjects with myelopathy of unknown cause, 22 subjects had an AVM on angiography.[23] Importantly, 5 subjects in this series had previous MR imaging that was interpreted as normal.[23]

Type I: Dural Arterial Venous Fistula

The spinal dural arterial venous fistula is an acquired arteriovenous shunt in the dura.[22] It is most commonly located near the exiting nerve root.[22] In some cases, the fistulous vessel may penetrate the dura at a more distant site and have a significant extradural component.[24] Spinal DAVFs usually present in adults after the fourth or the fifth decade, have a significant male predominance, and most commonly affect the thoracic spine.[22] Patients often present with vague complaints of back pain or radicular pain, followed by progressive lower-extremity paresis, and bowel and bladder sphincter dysfunction.[22,25,26] Hemorrhage is extremely rare.[22,26] Histologically, spinal DAVFs are supplied by a normal dural branch artery and drain into a single, dilated vein.[27] This drainage results in retrograde flow into the venous plexus surrounding the spinal cord. Physiologic studies have shown that venous pressure is approximately 75% of systemic arterial pressure.[25] The resultant venous hypertension and venous congestion cause a reduction in the arterial-venous pressure gradient, and thus a reduction in tissue perfusion pressure. A reduction in tissue perfusion pressure then leads to hypoxia, and further vasodilation may occur as a result of autoregulation.[22] Eventually, compensatory mechanisms from autoregulation are exhausted, the spinal cord tissue becomes ischemic. Cord edema and progressive loss of function then develops.

Although most patients present with *progressive myelopathy*, acute worsening of motor or sphincter function can also occur.[24] It is important to evaluate patients with an unclear cause of myelopathy, because 50% of untreated patients with a spinal DAVF can become disabled in 3 years.[28] MR imaging is the initial screening test of choice, and it is important to obtain a *whole-spine MR imaging survey* because there can be a discrepancy between the location of the spinal DAVF and the spinal level as suggested by clinical signs and symptoms.[28] The most common finding on MR imaging in patients with DAVF is abnormal T2 signal hyperintensity within the cord.[22,28] There can also be enlargement of the cord, consistent with swelling from cord edema.[29] The T2 signal changes can be extensive, extending over 6 to 7 vertebral levels in some cases.[30] Occasionally, prominent, lacelike tortuous and ectatic flow voids may be seen.[22,31] There can also be nonspecific enhancement with Gad contrast (Fig. 3).[22]

None of the aforementioned imaging findings are specific for DAVF. The current gold standard for imaging the DAVF is with digital subtraction angiography (DSA). Angiography allows a clear definition of the anatomy of the DAVF, including its location, arterial supply, and venous drainage pattern.[22,24–26] In some cases, the DAVF can obtain arterial supply from 2 arteries located in adjacent nerve roots.[22] One of the most important angiographic details to assess is the *origin of the anterior spinal artery*. If the anterior spinal artery shares a common origin with the supply to the DAVF, then the DAVF is not amendable to endovascular treatment.[25]

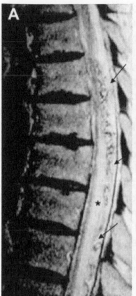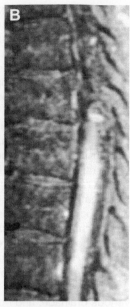

Fig. 3. **Spinal dural arterial venous fistula.** 65-year-old man with progressive lower extremity weakness. Sagittal fast spin echo T2 (*A*) images of the thoracic cord demonstrate extensive cord edema (*asterisk*) with flow voids along the dorsal spinal cord (*black arrows*). There is associated cord enhancement demonstrated on sagittal postgadolinium T1 fat saturated sequences (*B*).

Although DSA provides high temporal and spatial resolution imaging information of the DAVF, it is not without its drawbacks. DSA is often time consuming, as many as 40 injections can be needed to catheterize the bilateral intercostal, lumbar, and sacral arteries.[30] This procedure requires a high dose of iodinated contrast and increased radiation exposure. In addition, each catheterization also poses a small risk of vascular injury and can cause transient neurologic symptoms.[31] Thus, there is interest in developing noninvasive imaging technology to optimally evaluate the spinal DAVF. Two main technologies, CT angiography and MR angiography, have shown some promising developments. Lai and colleagues[32] reported their experience of 8 subjects with 16-row multidetector CT (MDCT) angiography for DAVF. In all 8 subjects, MDCT angiography correctly identified the enlarged radiculomedullary draining vein, the fistula, and the feeding artery.[32] Only 1 subject had an additional feeding artery identified on the subsequent DSA that was not identified on the MDCT angiography.[32] Similarly, Yamaguchi and colleagues[33] reported the successful identification of 2 out of 3 subjects with a DAVF. In the one case where MDCT angiography failed to identify the fistula, DSA also failed to identify the DAVF,

and the fistula was only identified at surgery.[33] In a more recent report, Si-jia and colleagues[31] noted that the spinal DAVF could be readily identified by MDCT angiography using a 64-row detector. In their series of 9 subjects, all of the draining veins were identified, and in 7 of 9 subjects, the feeding artery was also found.[31] Another recent study by Yamaguchi and colleagues[34] evaluated 10 subjects with 16-row detector MDCT angiography and DSA. Dilated perimedullary veins were found in all 10 subjects, focal enhancement of nerve root and intradural draining veins were noted in 8 subjects, and localization of the feeding artery was correctly depicted in 6 subjects. In 2 subjects, there were additional feeding arteries from the contralateral side that were not depicted on the MDCT angiography but were visualized on conventional angiography.[34] Although these findings are promising in that MDCT angiography can reveal a spinal DAVF, the temporal and spatial resolution of MDCT is still inferior to that of DSA. Therefore, the anterior or posterior spinal artery cannot be distinguished easily from that of the feeding artery.[29,31] In addition, the field of view is often more limited and it is difficult separating the arterial from venous phase.[29] MDCT angiography also exposes patients to radiation.

MR angiography (MRA) has been gaining attention in the diagnosis of spinal DAVFs. Rapid multiphase dynamic MRA with gadolinium and parallel imaging can achieve better temporal and spatial resolution than MDCT angiography.[29] However, increase in temporal resolution may come at an expense of the spatial resolution and signal-to-noise ratio is reduced.[30] Using time-resolved MRA, Ali and colleagues[30] studied 12 subjects with suspected DAVF based on clinical symptoms and MR imaging findings. In 6 subjects with a DAVF confirmed by DSA, all of them also demonstrated arteriovenous shunting on the time-resolved MRA.[30] Furthermore, the location of the arteriovenous shunting identified on MRA was within one vertebral level as identified on DSA.[30] Others have used contrast-enhanced MRA to study DAVFs. Using elliptic centric contrast-enhanced MRA, Luetmer and colleagues[35] depicted DAVFs in 20 out of 22 subjects who had DAVFs identified on conventional angiography. In 14 subjects, the level of the fistula was within the volume of imaging, and MRA correctly located the fistula to within one level of the spine in 13 subjects.[35] However, MRA does not always correctly identify the type of lesion. In one case, Sharma and Westesson reported that although the MRA showed a convincing type I DAVF, subsequent conventional angiography revealed a type IV perimedullary AVF.[36]

Although both MDCT angiography and MRA show promising results, they are still considered to be inferior to conventional angiography; however, both techniques help demonstrate the location of the fistula, which may minimize the number of catheterizations during DSA. Furthermore, newer techniques will continue to improve the temporal and spatial resolution of MDCT and MRA. These developments may one day enable these noninvasive techniques to become the primary diagnostic modality for studying spinal DAVFs.

Because of the potential for neurologic deterioration over time, prompt treatment of the spinal DAVF is advocated. Microsurgery has been the traditional method of treatment. In one meta-analysis, Steinmetz and colleagues[37] showed a 98% success rate of fistula obliteration with microsurgery. During recent years, endovascular treatment has also been used to treat spinal DAVFs. Although early experience demonstrated only limited success, with an overall success rate of only 46%, recent advances in embolization material and the possibility of being able to perform the treatment during the same setting of the diagnostic angiogram make endovascular therapy an option employed as a first line of treatment.[25,37,38] Surgical treatment can then be performed if endovascular therapy is unsuccessful or contraindicated. In addition, endovascular treatment is not advised for patients with a feeding artery that shares a common origin with the anterior or posterior spinal artery.[25]

Type II: Glomus Arteriovenous Malformation

Type II lesions, or glomus AVMs, have a nidus that is located completely or partially *within the spinal cord*.[25] These AVMs can be supplied by either the ventral radiculomedullary or anterior spinal arteries, or the dorsal radiculopial or posterior spinal arteries.[22] In 20% to 40% of cases, there is an associated arterial or venous aneurysm.[25] In 20% of cases, the AVMs are supplied by multiple shunts.[22]

Compared with the Type I spinal DAVF, the Type II glomus AVM tends to present in *younger* age, usually in young adults aged 20 to 30 years.[22,25] In 20% of cases, it affects pediatric patients.[22] In one series of pediatric subjects with spinal vascular malformations/arteriovenous shunts, AVMs were found in 44% of the subjects, representing the most common vascular malformation in children.[39] Also, unlike the DAVF, AVM most commonly presents with hemorrhage and *sudden onset* of neurologic symptoms.[22] There is a high

rebleeding rate if the AVM is not treated; therefore, prompt recognition and treatment is warranted.[22]

MR imaging is currently the imaging modality of choice for the initial evaluation of spinal AVMs. MR imaging may show areas of low signal intensity in the center of the cord (representing either vascular flow voids or blood products) and hyperintensity on T2-weighted images.[22] Moreover, MR imaging can show the relationship between the lesion and the spinal cord and dura, identify recent or remote hemorrhage and thrombosis, and reveal any paravertebral involvement (**Fig. 4**).[22]

DSA remains the definitive test for the diagnosis and treatment planning of spinal AVMs. The goal of angiography is to define the normal vasculature around the lesion as well as the diseased vasculature of the lesion. Features to look for include perimedullary and intramedullary anastomoses, direct and indirect AVM supply, collateral recruitment, associated aneurysms and pseudoaneurysms, venous drainage, and normal spinal cord vascular supply.

The goals of treatment include preservation of neurologic function and minimization of rebleeding. Treatment options include surgical excision, endovascular obliteration, or conservative management. Spetzler and colleagues[40] reported that 92% of subjects who underwent surgery had complete resection, with 68% of subjects experiencing neurologic improvement and 29% of subjects remaining neurologically unchanged. Others have reported favorable experience with endovascular treatment. For example, Da Costa and colleagues[22] reported that in a series of 47 subjects with spinal AVMs treated with endovascular obliteration, 77% of subjects had a favorable result, with about half of the subjects achieving complete obliteration. However, 22% of subjects experienced procedure-related complications, with 50% being permanent.[22] Conservative therapy includes physical therapy, pain control, and possible anticoagulation in patients with thrombosis.[22]

Type III: Juvenile Metameric Vascular Malformation

Type III lesions, also known as juvenile vascular malformations or metameric vascular malformations, are large, high-flow lesions with involvement of the *paraspinal tissues*.[25,40] These are uncommon lesions; among the 48 AVMs treated surgically by Spetzler and colleagues,[40] only 5 were metameric vascular malformations. Similarly, in a series of 72 pediatric subjects with spinal vascular malformations/arteriovenous shunts, only 3 had paravertebral tissue involvement.[00] As

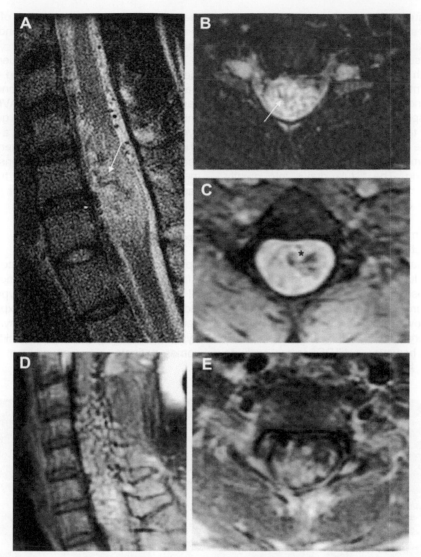

Fig. 4. Glomus arteriovenous malformation. 21-year-old man with right leg weakness. Sagittal (*A*) and axial (*B*) fast spin echo T2 sequences of the cervical spine demonstrate cord expansion, intramedullary edema, and flow voids (*arrows*) with associated enhancement on postgadolinium sagittal (*D*) and axial (*E*) T1 fat saturated images. Axial gradient echo sequence (*C*) shows evidence of cord hemorrhage (*asterisk*).

the name implies, these lesions commonly present in the pediatric population. Neurologic deficits occur from compression, hemorrhage, or vascular steal phenomenon.[40] MR imaging remains the initial diagnostic modality of choice, because it nicely reveals the extent of the lesion in the paravertebral tissue. DSA reveals the flow dynamics and feeder pattern, which are essential for treatment planning. A multidisciplinary approach is often required to address these lesions, with a combination of embolization and surgical resection; however, complete resection and obliteration is often difficult without incurring significant neurologic morbidity.[40]

Type IV: Perimedullary Arteriovenous Fistula

The perimedullary AVF is usually located in the *midline* and *ventrally* in the subarachnoid space.[40] The lesion consists of an abnormal connection between the anterior spinal artery and an enlarged venous network.[25,40] Blood flow through the lesion can be rapid, and therefore flow-related acquired lesions, such as aneurysms or ectatic venous malformations, can develop.[25,40] They most commonly present in young adulthood, but they can also present in the pediatric population.[39,41] The most common presentation is a progressive myelopathy, but rupture of an associated aneurysm resulting in hemorrhage can also be the first sign and symptom.[41]

Perimedullary AVFs have been further subclassified into 3 subtypes. Type I perimedullary AVF are small, with a single feeder and low flow fistula, and mild to moderate venous hypertension.[25,41] Type II perimedullary AVFs are larger, supplied by 1 or 2 spinal medullary arteries, and have a more rapid transit time.[41] Type III perimedullary AVFs are the most common. These are giant lesions with multiple dilated feeding arteries and rapid transiting. The fistula drains into greatly dilated and dysplastic veins.[25,41]

As with all other vascular malformations, MR imaging and conventional angiography remain the primary mode of diagnostics. MR imaging may demonstrate T2-hyperintensity within the spinal cord caused by venous hypertension and edema. Intradural signal voids can often be seen, which represent dilated vascular structures (Fig. 5).[41] More recently, MDCT angiography has also been shown to be effective in correctly diagnosing the perimedullary AVF.[31] The gold standard of evaluation, however, is still DSA to best evaluate the anatomy and flow dynamics of the arterial feeders, fistulas, draining veins, and associated aneurysms.

Treatment is often advised for patients with perimedullary AVFs because untreated lesions may lead to progressive myelopathy and eventually paralysis.[41] Type I perimedullary AVFs are small and are bested treated with surgery.[25,41] For Type II lesions with multiple feeders, a combination of endovascular therapy and surgery should be used.[25,41] For the giant Type III lesions, it is recommended that these lesions be first treated endovascularly , and reserve surgery for patients who fail endovascular treatment.[25,41]

SPINAL CORD INFARCT

Spinal cord infarction is rare in comparison to infarction of brain tissue, comprising only 1% of all strokes.[42] It is a disease that typically affects older adults.[42–44] Most patients experience *pain* before the onset of neurologic symptoms.[42,43] Symptoms usually develop quickly, although some patients may experience a transient

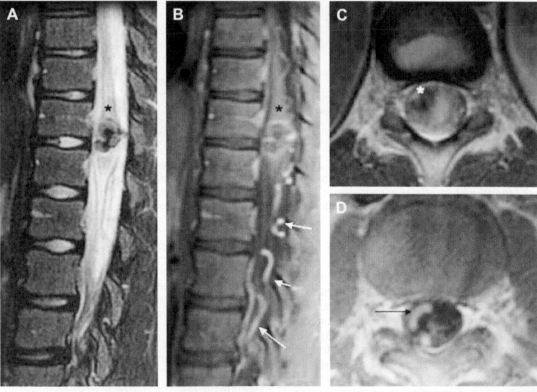

Fig. 5. **Perimedullary arteriovenous malformation.** 13-year-old boy with abrupt onset of back pain and lower extremity weakness. Sagittal and axial fast spin echo T2 (*A, C*) and postgadolinium T1 fat saturated (*B, D*) sequences of the lumbar spine demonstrate focal hemorrhage within the conus (*asterisk*) with numerous prominent, dilated enhancing vessels (*arrows*).

ischemic attack before the actual spinal cord infarct.[42,43] There are 2 potential pathophysiological mechanisms for spinal cord infarction: (1) hypoperfusion from arterial insufficiency and hypotension, and (2) occlusion of a specific arterial branch (anterior spinal artery or, sometimes, posterior spinal artery).[42]

The most common risk factors include aortic disease and atherosclerosis.[45,46] Aortic dissections are associated with an overall 4.2% chance of having paraparesis or paraplegia as a result of spinal cord infarction.[47] Furthermore, aortic surgery also carries a significant risk of spinal cord ischemia, ranging from 1% in the upper and lower levels of the aorta to 10% in the midsection of the aorta, corresponding to the watershed area of the spinal cord.[48] Others have proposed a mechanical cause, as disk protrusions, foraminal fibrosis, and other degenerative spinal disease may put mechanical stress on a radicular artery.[42] It is unclear whether degenerative spinal conditions, such as disk protrusions, can directly cause radicular artery thrombosis/occlusion, because the prevalence of degenerative spine disease is high; whereas, spinal cord infarction is so rare. Degenerative spinal changes may potentially predispose patients to a spinal infarct, but other factors likely also contribute, such as a traumatic event.

Spinal cord infarcts occur at about equal frequency in the cervical and thoracolumbar spine, but they are extremely rare in the upper thoracic spine.[42,43] The most common pattern involves the anterior spinal artery (unilateral or bilateral). Other infarct patterns include the posterior spinal artery territory, a central cord infarct that affects bilateral spinothalamic tracts without any effect on the motor tracts, and a transverse infarct that results in a complete infarct of the level, resulting in bilateral motor function deficits and complete sensory deficits.[42,43] MR imaging is the imaging tool of choice for evaluation of patients with suspected spinal cord infarct. On sagittal T2-weighted images, a pencil-like hyperintensity can be seen in most patients.[44] Cord enlargement caused by swelling may also be seen.[44] In patients with an anterior spinal artery infarct, the owl's sign (T2 signal hyperintensity within anterior horns bilaterally) may be identified (Fig. 6).[49] Another imaging finding pointing to a cord infarct as the cause for an intramedullary signal abnormality is the presence of an adjacent *vertebral body* infarct.[42,43] Recently, diffusion weighted imaging has been used to evaluate spinal cord infarction.[44] Similar to ischemic infarction of the brain, acute spinal cord infarction also shows restricted diffusion with marked hyperintensity on the DWI sequence and a reduction in the apparent diffusion coefficient.[44] Because DWI changes develop before T2 signal changes, the addition of a diffusion sequence may expedite the diagnosis of spinal cord infarction (Fig. 7).[44] In some cases, DSA is

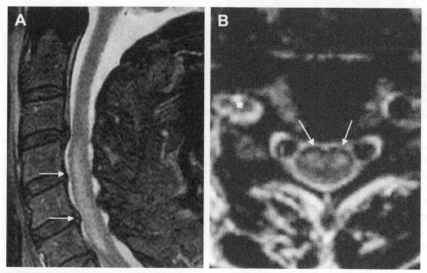

Fig. 6. Cervical spinal cord infarct and right vertebral artery dissection. 61-year-old woman with right shoulder weakness progressing to bilateral shoulder and upper extremity weakness. Sagittal (*A*) and axial (*B*) fast spin echo T2 sequences demonstrate mild cord expansion with increased signal within the bilateral anterior horns involving the anterior spinal artery territory (*arrows*). There is absence of the normal right vertebral artery flow void (*asterisk*).

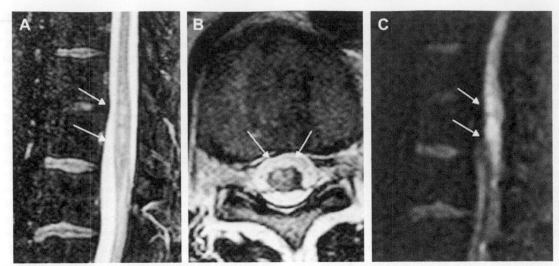

Fig. 7. **Spinal cord infarct.** 49-year-old man with acute back pain, nausea, and lower extremity weakness. Sagittal (A) and axial (B) fast spin echo T2 images through the thoracic cord demonstrate increased signal within the bilateral anterior horns involving the anterior spinal artery territory. (C) Sagittal diffusion-weighted imaging demonstrates reduced diffusion compatible with ischemia (arrows).

used to evaluate for specific arterial occlusions. In addition, DSA can be useful for ruling out treatable conditions, such as the DAVF, which also frequently shows abnormal intramedullary T2 hyperintensity on MR imaging.

The treatment of patients with spinal cord infarction remains supportive. Thrombolytics have not been used. Some patients may receive antiplatelet therapy, such as aspirin.[42] Most patients will have some recovery with supportive care and physical therapy. However, sphincter functions do not recover as well as motor functions.[42,43]

SUMMARY

Like the brain, the spinal cord is composed of neuronal and glial tissue that is vulnerable to trauma, infection, inflammation, ischemia, hemorrhage, and compression. This wide variety of conditions can damage spinal cord tissue and result in permanent paralysis or paraplegia. Certain conditions, such as the epidural abscess, can be treated, and therefore, prompt diagnosis is important. Advances in neuroimaging, especially with MR imaging, allow for improved evaluation of the spine and spinal cord. Noninvasive imaging, including MDCT angiography and MRA, are also likely to become more important in the evaluation of spinal vascular lesions. The development of new neuroradiological techniques and technology will continue to improve the diagnosis and treatment options for patients with spinal cord pathology.

REFERENCES

1. Reihsaus E, Waldbaur H, Seeling W. Spinal epidural abscess: a meta-analysis of 915 patients. Neurosurg Rev 2000;23:175–204 [discussion: 205].
2. Darouiche RO. Spinal epidural abscess. N Engl J Med 2006;355:2012–20.
3. Chen WC, Wang JL, Wang JT, et al. Spinal epidural abscess due to staphylococcus aureus: clinical manifestations and outcomes. J Microbiol Immunol Infect 2008;41:215–21.
4. Chuo CY, Fu YC, Lu YM, et al. Spinal infection in intravenous drug abusers. J Spinal Disord Tech 2007;20:324–8.
5. Pereira CE, Lynch JC. Spinal epidural abscess: an analysis of 24 cases. Surg Neurol 2005;1(Suppl 63):S26–9.
6. Chen WH, Jiang LS, Dai LY. Surgical treatment of pyogenic vertebral osteomyelitis with spinal instrumentation. Eur Spine J 2007;16:1307–16.
7. Alg VS, Demetriades AK, Naik S, et al. Isolated subacute tuberculous spinal epidural abscess of the cervical spine: a brief report of a special case. Acta Neurochir (Wien) 2009;151:695–6.
8. Curry WT Jr, Hoh BL, Amin-Hanjani S, et al. Spinal epidural abscess: clinical presentation, management, and outcome. Surg Neurol 2005;63:364–71 [discussion: 371].
9. Gonzalez-Lopez JJ, Gorgolas M, Muniz J, et al. Spontaneous epidural abscess: analysis of 15 cases with emphasis on diagnostic and prognostic factors. Eur J Intern Med 2009;20:514–7.
10. Gorchynski J, Hwang J, McLaughlin T. A methicillin-resistant Staphylococcus aureus-positive holospinal

epidural abscess. Am J Emerg Med 2009;27(514): e517—9.

11. Lohr M, Reithmeier T, Ernestus RI, et al. Spinal epidural abscess: prognostic factors and comparison of different surgical treatment strategies. Acta Neurochir (Wien) 2005;147:159—66 [discussion: 166].

12. Parkinson JF, Sekhon LH. Spinal epidural abscess: appearance on magnetic resonance imaging as a guide to surgical management. Report of five cases. Neurosurg Focus 2004;17:E12.

13. Eastwood JD, Vollmer RT, Provenzale JM. Diffusion-weighted imaging in a patient with vertebral and epidural abscesses. AJNR Am J Neuroradiol 2002; 23:496—8.

14. Hlavin ML, Kaminski HJ, Ross JS, et al. Spinal epidural abscess: a ten-year perspective. Neurosurgery 1990;27:177—84.

15. Sokolowski MJ, Garvey TA, Perl J 2nd, et al. Prospective study of postoperative lumbar epidural hematoma: incidence and risk factors. Spine (Phila Pa) 1976;2008(33):108—13.

16. Kunizawa A, Fujioka M, Suzuki S, et al. Spontaneous spinal epidural hematoma inducing acute anterior spinal cord syndrome. J Neurosurg Spine 2009;10: 574—7.

17. Heiner JD. Cervical epidural hematoma after chiropractic spinal manipulation. Am J Emerg Med 2009;27(1023):e1021—2.

18. Xu R, Bydon M, Gokaslan ZL, et al. Epidural steroid injection resulting in epidural hematoma in a patient despite strict adherence to anticoagulation guidelines. J Neurosurg Spine 2009;11:358—64.

19. Horlocker TT, Wedel DJ, Benzon H, et al. Regional anesthesia in the anticoagulated patient: defining the risks (the second ASRA Consensus Conference on Neuraxial Anesthesia and Anticoagulation). Reg Anesth Pain Med 2003;28:172—97.

20. Liao CC, Hsieh PC, Lin TK, et al. Surgical treatment of spontaneous spinal epidural hematoma: a 5-year experience. J Neurosurg Spine 2009;11:480—6.

21. Oldfield EH, Doppman JL. Spinal arteriovenous malformations. Clin Neurosurg 1988;34:161—83.

22. da Costa L, Dehdashti AR, terBrugge KG. Spinal cord vascular shunts: spinal cord vascular malformations and dural arteriovenous fistulas. Neurosurg Focus 2009;26:E6.

23. Strom RG, Derdeyn CP, Moran CJ, et al. Frequency of spinal arteriovenous malformations in patients with unexplained myelopathy. Neurology 2006;66:928—31.

24. Clarke MJ, Patrick TA, White JB, et al. Spinal extradural arteriovenous malformations with parenchymal drainage: venous drainage variability and implications in clinical manifestations. Neurosurg Focus 2009;26:E5.

25. Medel R, Crowley RW, Dumont AS. Endovascular management of spinal vascular malformations:

history and literature review. Neurosurg Focus 2009;26:E7.

26. Rosenblum B, Oldfield EH, Doppman JL, et al. Spinal arteriovenous malformations: a comparison of dural arteriovenous fistulas and intradural AVM's in 81 patients. J Neurosurg 1987;67:795—802.

27. Benhaiem N, Poirier J, Hurth M. Arteriovenous fistulae of the meninges draining into the spinal veins. A histological study of 28 cases. Acta Neuropathol 1983;62:103—11.

28. Andres RH, Barth A, Guzman R, et al. Endovascular and surgical treatment of spinal dural arteriovenous fistulas. Neuroradiology 2008;50:869—76.

29. Eddleman CS, Jeong H, Cashen TA, et al. Advanced noninvasive imaging of spinal vascular malformations. Neurosurg Focus 2009;26:E9.

30. Ali S, Cashen TA, Carroll TJ, et al. Time-resolved spinal MR angiography: initial clinical experience in the evaluation of spinal arteriovenous shunts. AJNR Am J Neuroradiol 2007;28:1806—10.

31. Si-jia G, Meng-wei Z, Xi-ping L, et al. The clinical application studies of CT spinal angiography with 64-detector row spiral CT in diagnosing spinal vascular malformations. Eur J Radiol 2009;71: 22—8.

32. Lai PH, Pan HB, Yang CF, et al. Multi-detector row computed tomography angiography in diagnosing spinal dural arteriovenous fistula: initial experience. Stroke 2005;36:1562—4.

33. Yamaguchi S, Eguchi K, Kiura Y, et al. Multidetector-row CT angiography as a preoperative evaluation for spinal arteriovenous fistulae. Neurosurg Rev 2007;30:321—6 [discussion: 327].

34. Yamaguchi S, Nagayama T, Eguchi K, et al. Accuracy and pitfalls of multidetector-row computed tomography in detecting spinal dural arteriovenous fistulas. J Neurosurg Spine 2010;12:243—8.

35. Luetmer PH, Lane JI, Gilbertson JR, et al. Preangiographic evaluation of spinal dural arteriovenous fistulas with elliptic centric contrast-enhanced MR angiography and effect on radiation dose and volume of iodinated contrast material. AJNR Am J Neuroradiol 2005;26:711—8.

36. Sharma AK, Westesson PL. Preoperative evaluation of spinal vascular malformation by MR angiography: how reliable is the technique: case report and review of literature. Clin Neurol Neurosurg 2008;110:521—4.

37. Steinmetz MP, Chow MM, Krishnaney AA, et al. Outcome after the treatment of spinal dural arteriovenous fistulae: a contemporary single-institution series and meta-analysis. Neurosurgery 2004;55: 77—87 [discussion: 87—8].

38. Eskandar EN, Borges LF, Budzik RF Jr, et al. Spinal dural arteriovenous fistulas: experience with endovascular and surgical therapy. J Neurosurg 2002; 96:162—7.

39. Du J, Ling F, Chen M, et al. Clinical characteristic of spinal vascular malformation in pediatric patients. Childs Nerv Syst 2009;25:473–8.

40. Spetzler RF, Detwiler PW, Riina HA, et al. Modified classification of spinal cord vascular lesions. J Neurosurg 2002;96:145–56.

41. Halbach VV, Higashida RT, Dowd CF, et al. Treatment of giant intradural (perimedullary) arterio-venous fistulas. Neurosurgery 1993;33:972–9 [discussion: 979–80].

42. Novy J, Carruzzo A, Maeder P, et al. Spinal cord ischemia: clinical and imaging patterns, pathogenesis, and outcomes in 27 patients. Arch Neurol 2006;63:1113–20.

43. Cheng MY, Lyu RK, Chang YJ, et al. Spinal cord infarction in Chinese patients. Clinical features, risk factors, imaging and prognosis. Cerebrovasc Dis 2008;26:502–8.

44. Thurnher MM, Bammer R. Diffusion-weighted MR imaging (DWI) in spinal cord ischemia. Neuroradiology 2006;48:795–801.

45. Cheshire WP, Santos CC, Massey EW, et al. Spinal cord infarction: etiology and outcome. Neurology 1996;47:321–30.

46. Nedeltchev K, Loher TJ, Stepper F, et al. Long-term outcome of acute spinal cord ischemia syndrome. Stroke 2004;35:560–5.

47. Zull DN, Cydulka R. Acute paraplegia: a presenting manifestation of aortic dissection. Am J Med 1988;84:765–70.

48. Connolly JE. Hume memorial lecture. Prevention of spinal cord complications in aortic surgery. Am J Surg 1998;176:92–101.

49. Mawad ME, Rivera V, Crawford S, et al. Spinal cord ischemia after resection of thoracoabdominal aortic aneurysms: MR findings in 24 patients. AJR Am J Roentgenol 1990;155:1303–7.

Emergency Head & Neck Imaging: Infections and Inflammatory Processes

Jason A. McKellop[a,b,*], Wessam Bou-Assaly[a,c,d] and Suresh K. Mukherji[e]

KEYWORDS

• Deep neck infection • Neck mass • Computed tomography
• Magnetic resonance imaging • Emergency

Emergency neck infections are diverse in both their presentation and their affected patient population; with pathology ranging from a transient enlargement of a child's cervical lymph node to a rapidly spreading necrotizing fasciitis in an adult diabetic. Despite the widespread availability of antibiotics and early surgical intervention, deep neck infections still present significant morbidity and mortality in clinical centers. Complex neck anatomy can frequently obscure or delay diagnoses, so timely and appropriate radiological interpretation are critical to patient care. This article reviews common neck infections that may be encountered in the emergency room and details some of their most salient findings on imaging.

INFECTIONS OF THE LYMPH NODE

The development of the lymphatic system begins in early fetal life and continues through early neonatal growth. The lymphatic system comprises a combination of lymphocytes and surrounding cellular structures that include epithelial and stromal elements. Lymph nodes are a secondary lymphoid structure where primary immune responses are initiated. Like other secondary lymphoid organs of the body, lymph nodes have specialized architecture that promotes controlled interactions of immune cells to facilitate an appropriate immune response to infectious agents.[1] The ultimate anatomy of the head and neck lymphatic system consists of an elegant meshwork of lymphatic drainage. This network can be simplified broadly into 3 groups: the ring of Waldeyer—a circle of adenoidal, tonsillar, and lymphoid tissue; a more superficial ring consisting of the facial groups, parotids, preauricular, postauricular, and occipital nodes; and finally the nodes of the neck, which include the submaxillary, submental, and superficial and deep cervical chains.[2]

Pathologically, an infective agent within the head and neck will spread into the surrounding tissues and be partially inactivated by the host's immune response. A portion of the infective antigenic focus will be passively drained into the afferent lymphatic channels of the lymph node causing a cascade of events including the activation of T and B lymphocytes, the formation of multiple germinal centers with active cell proliferation, and ultimately enlargement of the lymph node. A variety of infectious and noninfectious processes may cause enlargement of the cervical

[a] Department of Radiology at the University of Michigan Health System, 1500 East Medical Center Drive, Ann Arbor, MI 48105, USA
[b] Radiology Department, NYU Langone Medical Center/Bellevue Hospital Center, 462 First Avenue, NBV 3W38, New York, NY 10016, USA
[c] Neuroradiology Division, Department of Radiology, University of Michigan Health System, 1500 East Medical Center Drive, Ann Arbor, MI 48105, USA
[d] Neuroradiology and Nuclear Medicine Division, Department of Radiology, Ann Arbor VA Health System, 2215 Fuller Road, Ann Arbor, MI 48105, USA
[e] Department of Radiology, University of Michigan Health System, B2 A209-0030, 1500 East Medical Center Drive, Ann Arbor, MI 48109-0030, USA
* Corresponding author.
E-mail address: jason.mckellop@nyumc.org

Neuroimag Clin N Am 20 (2010) 651–661
doi:10.1016/j.nic.2010.07.007

lymph nodes. The stimulated node is often referred to as "reactive." Ongoing and untreated infection may eventually result in necrosis of the node leading to suppurative adenitis.

Cervical Adenitis

The term cervical adenitis denotes an inflammation of the lymph nodes of the neck due to an infectious process (Fig. 1A). Suppurative adenitis indicates an infected node that has undergone liquefaction necrosis (Fig. 1B). The likelihood of developing cervical adenitis, especially suppurative forms, decreases with age, although the incidence of suppurative adenitis is increasing in older patients.[3] The pediatric population, not surprisingly, comprises a large proportion of infectious head and neck emergency room presentations.

The most common cause of cervical lymph node enlargement in children is viral infections of the upper respiratory tract.[4] The true incidence of viral infections is unknown because the majority of such infections are benign, and do not require any form of biopsy or incision and drainage. Noteworthy virions include adenovirus, rhinovirus, enterovirus, and herpes simplex virus. Epstein-Barr virus, the causative agent in infectious mononucleosis, is characterized by generalized lymphadenopathy, weakness, fever, and malaise. Infection with cytomegalovirus and Varicella zoster is also a well-documented cause of generalized lymph node enlargement. Another noteworthy viral infection is the acquired immunodeficiency syndrome (AIDS), caused by human T-cell lymphotrophic virus type III (HTLV-III), a potentially devastating disease of childhood. Nearly 90% of human immunodeficiency virus–infected children acquire their infection vertically, during gestation or, more commonly, during labor and delivery.[5] Patients affected by congenital transmission usually develop symptoms during the first year of life. Symptoms include localized or generalized lymphadenopathy, thrush, parotid swelling, interstitial pneumonitis, hepatosplenomegaly, and diarrhea. Affected patients also have an increased risk of bacterial superinfection including meningitis and sepsis.

Bacterial infections are the most common cause of suppurative cervical adenitis, with *Staphylococcus aureus* and Group A streptococcus being the most common etiologic agents.[6–8] Infected patients typically present with fever and upper respiratory tract infections. Early in the course of infection, discrete nodes are palpated. With uncontrolled infection, the firm nodes are replaced by a palpable fluctuant mass (suppurative adenitis), which may require drainage. Other noteworthy bacteria that may cause suppurative cervical lymph nodes include *Streptococcus pyogenes*, Group B streptococcus, and *Pseudomonas aeruginosa*.[4]

Computed tomography (CT) is the preferred modality to evaluate patients suspected of having cervical lymphadenitis. CT has the advantage of a shorter acquisition time relative to magnetic resonance (MR) imaging, which in children may necessitate sedation to reduce motion artifact. Early involvement by infection is characterized by homogeneous enlargement, loss of the fatty hilum, and increased enhancement of the involved lymph node on CT (see Fig. 1A). Reticulation of the

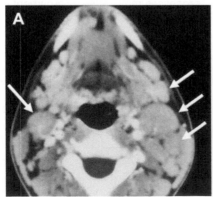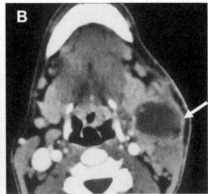

Fig. 1. **Cervical and suppurative adenitis.** (*A*) Axial contrast-enhanced computed tomography (CT) shows homogeneous enlargement of multiple various-sized lymph nodes (*arrows*) in a patient with neck pain due to cervical adenitis. (*B*) Axial contrast-enhanced CT shows a suppurative cervical lymph node (*large arrow*) with surrounding phlegmon.

adjacent fat surrounding a suppurative lymph node or the presence of a circumferential rim of soft tissue may be helpful in differentiating an inflammatory origin as the cause of the abnormal node as opposed to metastases.[3]

Cat-Scratch Disease

Cat-scratch disease (CSD) is a very common cause of enlarged cervical lymph nodes in the pediatric age group, and has been reported to be the most common cause of chronic unilateral regional lymphadenitis in children in the United States.[2,9] The disorder is caused by the bacteria *Bartonella henselae* and usually presents within 3 to 10 days following contact. A prior history of a cat scratch, lick, bite, or other exposure is present in more than 90% of cases.[10] These patients present clinically with tender, enlarged cervical lymph nodes, fever, and malaise. Approximately 10% of patients develop overlying erythema and fluctuant lymph nodes that require drainage. Diagnosis is confirmed by a positive cat-scratch antigen or demonstration of the bacillus on a Warthin-Starry stain of infected material.

The typical findings on CT are a unilateral clumped group of enlarged lymph nodes clustered in the primary echelon drainage of the site of contact. Central areas of decreased attenuation within the lymph nodes are rare (Fig. 2). There may be some subtle reticulation of the fat surrounding the lymph nodes; however, gross findings of extracapsular extension is rare. On MR imaging, the signal characteristics are nonspecific and can be seen in a variety of disorders. The nodes typically enhance with contrast and contain high T2 signal.[3]

Tuberculous Lymphadenitis

There has been a dramatic increase in the prevalence of tuberculosis in industrialized countries due to the AIDS epidemic, drug abuse, and increased migration.[11] The most common form of head and neck tuberculosis is lymphadenitis.[12] This form of tuberculosis represents 15% of cases of extrapulmonary disease and 1% to 2% of all new cases of tuberculosis.[3] Cervical lymphadenopathy is usually painless. Involvement is commonly bilateral and most frequently involves the internal jugular, posterior triangle, and supraclavicular nodes. In advanced stages, the overlying skin may be inflamed and sinus tracts may appear.

Pathologically, tuberculosis typically shows tubercles with marked fibroblastic response. These tubercles show characteristic amorphous caseating necrosis, which may rupture into

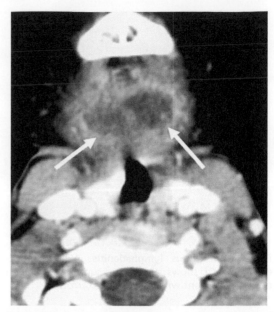

Fig. 2. **Cat-scratch disease.** Axial contrast-enhanced CT shows enlarged level II and V lymph nodes in a patient with pathologically proven cat-scratch disease (*arrows*).

surrounding structures such as the airway and blood stream, causing endobronchial or hematogenous dissemination.

CT imaging of the early stages of tuberculous lymphadenitis reveals nodes with homogeneous contrast enhancement. As the disease evolves, central necrosis can be detected as foci of low density associated with rim enhancement (Fig. 3). One may also note a relative lack of fat stranding and effacement.[13] Healed lesions and nodes undergoing chemotherapy may show calcifications.

MR imaging shows nonspecific homogeneous enhancement on T1-weighted images and high signals on T2-weighted images. In nodes undergoing necrosis, contrast-enhanced MR imaging shows rim enhancement with a central area of no enhancement representing caseating necrosis. These nodes typically show high signal intensity on T2-weighted images. MR imaging, though helpful in demonstrating lymphadenitis, cannot detect nodal calcifications.[3]

SUBLINGUAL SPACE INFECTIONS

The sublingual space (SLS) is located inferior to intrinsic muscles of the oral tongue, lateral to the genioglossus-geniohyoid complex and superomedial to the mylohyoid muscle, forming an attachment to a line on the medial surface of the

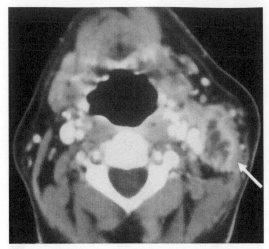

Fig. 3. **Tuberculous lymphadenitis.** Axial contrast-enhanced CT shows a necrotic suppurative lymph node in a patient with tuberculosis (*arrow*).

mandible. Posteriorly, the SLS communicates with the submandibular space (SMS) with no fascia separating these spaces.

Sublingual Space Abscess

\Abscesses originating in this space are usually due to sublingual or submandibular duct stenosis or calculus disease. Dental infection or mandibular osteomyelitis, however, may also extend into the SLS. The most commonly encountered organisms in SLS abscess formation are *Staphylococcus aureus* and *Streptococcus viridans*.

Clinically, patients with SLS abscess usually present with pain, tenderness, and swelling in the anterior floor of the mouth. There may be a history of salivary colic, recent dental disease, or dental manipulation. Treatment of an SLS abscess should commence with antibiotic therapy followed by surgical drainage.

CT remains the imaging modality of choice for such infections.[14] Noncontrast CT may show a rounded low-attenuation lesion on the floor of the mouth (**Fig. 4**) while delayed postcontrast CT may show a peripherally enhancing mass.[15] These lesions are often associated with subcutaneous streaking and thickening of the platysmus muscle. The genioglossus-geniohyoid complex is often displaced medially or across the midline. If an SMS component is present, this abscess may track into the parapharyngeal space where further spread can take place in a craniocaudal axis. Infection may also spread to the medial pterygoid (see **Fig. 4B**) or masseter muscles.[3,14]

MR imaging is rarely used for inflammatory disease of the sublingual space. An SLS abscess shows the typical enhancing mass on T1-weighted images and high signal intensity on T2-weighted images. On contrast-enhanced images, a central area of absent enhancement indicating pus collection can readily be demonstrated. Mandibular marrow edema is more readily demonstrated on MR imaging as intermediate signal tissues replacing high signal intensity fat on T1-weighted images.[3]

Ludwig Angina

The term Ludwig angina refers to cellulitis involving the floor of the mouth. It is an infection

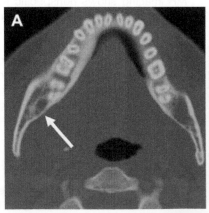
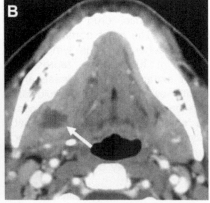

Fig. 4. **Sublingual space abscess after dental extraction.** (*A*) The bone algorithm shows focal cortical erosion in the region of the right second molar, postextraction of a "rotten" tooth (*arrow*). (*B*) Axial contrast-enhanced CT shows abscess extending into the right sublingual space and pterygoid muscles (*arrow*).

of the submental, sublingual, and SMSs causing elevation and posterior displacement of the tongue and tense induration between the hyoid bone and the genu of the mandible. This infection is usually caused by *Streptococcus* or *Staphylococcus* species. Once thought to be only of dental origin, numerous cases arising from the sinuses and pharynx, among other locations, have recently been described.[15,16] Patients usually present with pain, tenderness, and swelling of the mouth floor. The infection is usually precipitated by an odontogenic infection.[17] In neglected cases, Ludwig angina may spread inferiorly through fascial planes into the mediastinum. Hence some patients may present with chest pain.

Because the tongue can rapidly become posteriorly displaced in this condition, securing a patent airway is a priority. Early signs of airway collapse may be subtle and many patients may require awake fiberoptic intubation or tracheostomy.[18] Definitive treatment requires intravenous antibiotics and, if necessary, surgical drainage of secondary abscesses.[19]

Contrast-enhanced CT shows swelling of the floor of the mouth (Fig. 5). This finding is frequently associated with streaky changes in the adjacent subcutaneous fat and thickening of the overlying platysmus muscle. Enlargement of the submental or submandibular lymph nodes may also be seen. In late cases, pus or gas formation may take place and the airway may be compressed.

Contrast-enhanced MR images show a thickened floor of the mouth with strong enhancement. On T2-weighted images, diffuse high signal is evident on the floor of the mouth and adjacent soft tissues.[3]

NECK INFECTIONS
Retropharyngeal Space Infections

The retropharyngeal space is a potential space that lies immediately posterior to the pharynx and extends from the base of the skull superiorly to the upper mediastinum inferiorly. It is bordered anteriorly by the buccopharyngeal fascia, posteriorly by the alar fascia and laterally by the carotid sheaths and parapharyngeal spaces. Pathology within this space can cause rapid airway compromise and requires immediate clinical attention. Infection of this space is usually the consequence of one of two mechanisms: direct inoculation or spreading infection. In adults, infection of the retropharyngeal space is usually caused by a penetrating injury. Iatrogenic causes such as endotracheal intubation and nasogastric tube placement, and incidental causes such as fish bone ingestion, are frequent culprits. Gram-positive cocci are the most common pathogen implicated in such cases.[20] In children, however, retropharyngeal space infections are most commonly the result of a spreading upper respiratory tract infection. Acute pharyngitis, for example, may spread from the pharyngeal space to the retropharyngeal lymph nodes that may ultimately communicate with the retropharyngeal space. Such infections are common in childhood and frequently affect children younger than 3 years.[8] Similarly, microorganisms from the nose, paranasal sinuses, and eustachian tube can drain to the retropharyngeal nodes, resulting in suppurative adenitis. If treatment is delayed, suppurated lymph nodes may rupture and result in formation of retropharyngeal abscess or retropharyngeal cellulitis. Patients with retropharyngeal space infection often present clinically with fever, neck pain, sore throat, and neck mass[21]; they may

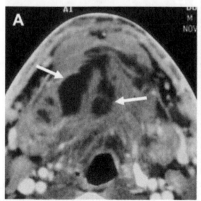
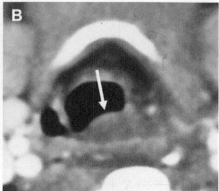

Fig. 5. **Ludwig angina.** (*A*) Contrast-enhanced CT shows multiple abscess (*arrows*) on the mouth floor in a patient with Ludwig angina. (*B*) This patient also had edema of the larynx as demonstrated by thickening of the left aryepiglottic fold (*arrow*).

also complain of a choking feeling and difficulty in swallowing. Inspection of the pharynx reveals edema and redness.

On imaging, plain films typically demonstrate thickening of the soft tissues in the prevertebral space. This finding is nonspecific and may be seen in retropharyngeal cellulitis, retropharyngeal suppurative adenitis, or retropharyngeal abscess.[3,15]

On CT, retropharyngeal cellulitis is identified by symmetric low attenuation in the retropharyngeal space (Fig. 6A). There is anterior displacement of the posterior wall of the pharynx from the prevertebral muscles. However, the symmetric displacement does not typically exceed a few millimeters as compared with retropharyngeal edema of other origin (Fig. 6B). Retropharyngeal suppurative adenitis is identified by enlarged paramedian retropharyngeal lymph nodes that have a low-attenuation center (Fig. 7). A retropharyngeal abscess is identified by a low-attenuation fluid collection that causes anterior displacement of the posterior wall of the pharynx from the prevertebral muscles (Fig. 8). The collection may be asymmetric. Retropharyngeal abscesses usually do not have a thick enhancing wall.[3]

On MR imaging, enlarged retropharyngeal nodes show intermediate signal intensity on T1-weighted images and marked contrast enhancement. Rim enhancement indicates suppurative lymphadenitis. On T2-weighted images, the inflamed nodes show increased signal intensity. Soft tissue thickening, secondary to cellulitis, also shows contrast enhancement and increased signal intensity on T2-weighted imaging.[3]

Tonsillar Abscess

In contrast to acute tonsillitis, which is more common in children, a tonsillar abscess is more common in young adults. The average age is 25 years with more than 65% of patients falling between the ages of 20 and 40 years.[22,23] The most common symptoms are sore throat, dysphagia, fever, and trismus. Nearly all patients have a history of recurrent pharyngitis. Management typically includes incision and drainage with antibiotic coverage.[24]

CT should be used to evaluate a suspected tonsillar abscess because it is quicker and cheaper than MR imaging. CT shows an enhancing mass in the tonsillar fossa that may or may not show pus formation (Fig. 9). MR imaging demonstrates hyperintensity on T2-weighted imaging (and hypointensity on T1) in the region of the abscess (Fig. 10). Extension into the parapharyngeal space may involve the medial pterygoid muscles (leading to trismus). In extensive disease, the inflammatory process may spread posterolaterally to involve the carotid sheath. It is important to evaluate this entity for possible jugular vein thrombosis or carotid artery erosion.[3]

Parapharyngeal Abscess

The parapharyngeal space is the area within the deep neck medial to the masseter muscle and lateral to the superior pharyngeal constrictor. The space is divided into anterior and posterior compartments by the styloid process, the latter of which contains the carotid artery and internal jugular vein. An abscess in this space may arise from direct extension of infection from the pharynx through the pharyngeal wall, as a consequence of odontogenic infection, local trauma, and occasionally tonsillar abscess.[25] Diabetes is the most common systemic condition predisposing one to parapharyngeal abscess.

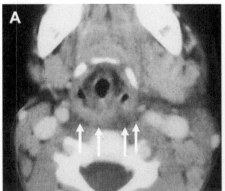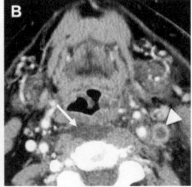

Fig. 6. **Retropharyngeal space cellulitis and edema.** (*A*) Patient with retropharyngeal space cellulitis. There is symmetric low attenuation in the retropharyngeal space (*arrows*) without evidence of a focal fluid collection. (*B*) Retropharyngeal space edema secondary to internal jugular vein thrombosis: there is symmetric low attenuation in the retropharyngeal space (*arrow*) without evidence of a focal fluid collection. Also note ring-enhancing wall of left jugular vein with a nonenhancing lumen, representing thrombus (*arrowhead*).

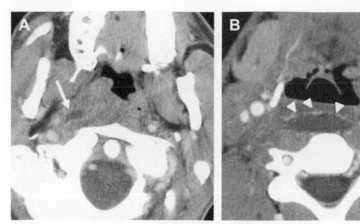

Fig. 7. **Suppurative adenitis of the retropharyngeal lymph node with retropharyngeal space edema.** (*A*) Axial CT shows a suppurative retropharyngeal lymph node (*arrow*). (*B*) Contrast-enhanced axial CT shows low attenuation in the retropharyngeal space (*arrowheads*) representing retropharyngeal space edema.

Parapharyngeal abscess often presents clinically with fever, sore throat, and neck swelling. Erythema, odynophagia, and dysphagia often accompany such infections.[26] Trismus is most commonly associated with anterior compartment abscesses.

On imaging, plain film findings are typically nonspecific, and include thickening of the soft tissues in the prevertebral space and loss of cervical lordosis. Contrast-enhanced CT is the imaging examination of choice to diagnose parapharyngeal abscess. CT shows a single or multiloculated low-density lesion with an air and/ or fluid center (**Fig. 11**). Contrast-enhanced

sequences may occasionally demonstrate enhancement of the abscess wall.

Necrotizing Fasciitis

Cervical necrotizing fasciitis is a rapidly spreading bacterial infection of the soft tissue that can quickly become a life-threatening condition. It is commonly caused by either streptococcal or polymicrobial infections; however, methicillin-resistant *Staphylococcus aureus* species have been seen with increasing prevalence.[27] Patients commonly present with high fevers and appear acutely ill. The overlying skin of the affected tissue

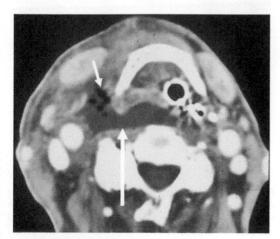

Fig. 8. **Retropharyngeal space abscess.** Contrast-enhanced CT shows fluid (*large arrow*) and gas (*small arrow*) in the retropharyngeal space.

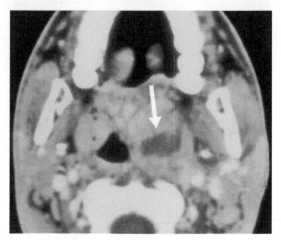

Fig. 9. **Tonsillar abscess.** Contrast-enhanced axial CT demonstrates an abscess involving the left tonsil (*arrow*).

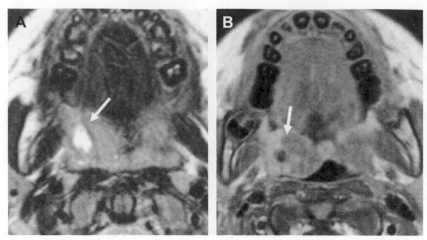

Fig. 10. Tonsillar abscess. (*A*) T2-weighted axial MR imaging image demonstrates an abscess involving the right tonsil (*arrow*). (*B*) Postcontrast T1-weighted image demonstrates hypodense fluid collection within an enhanced abscess wall and swollen right tonsil.

may be erythematous and tender. One might appreciate crepitus with gas-producing bacterium. Patients with necrotizing fasciitis are best managed in the intensive care unit, and are typically treated with parenteral antibiotics and frequent surgical debridement.[28]

CT imaging reveals nonspecific findings of diffuse reticulation of subcutaneous fat along with thickening and enhancement of the platysma. One may also find multiple abscesses extending along the fascial planes. Presence of gas within the soft tissue in the absence of prior surgery or radiation therapy is pathognomonic for necrotizing fasciitis (**Fig. 12**).[3]

Bezold Abscess

A Bezold abscess is a rare complication of otomastoiditis characterized by necrosis of the mastoid tip and spread of infection from bone to the adjacent soft tissue. Inflammatory collections form inferior to the mastoid process and may course along the plane of the sternocleidomastoid muscle to the lower neck. If left untreated, the

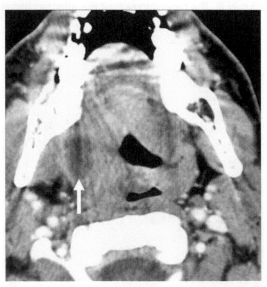

Fig. 11. Parapharyngeal space abscess. Contrast-enhanced CT shows a low-attenuation fluid collection deep to the right tonsil located in the parapharyngeal space (*arrow*).

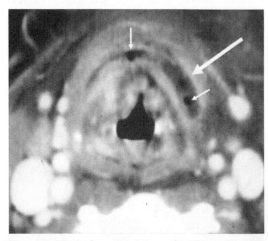

Fig. 12. Cervical necrotizing fasciitis. Contrast-enhanced CT scan showing diffuse thickening of the soft tissues of the neck associated with small fluid collection (*large arrow*). The presence of air (*small arrows*) in a patient with a fever who has never had surgery or radiation therapy is strongly suggestive of necrotizing fasciitis.

abscess may spread as far as the larynx and mediastinum, which results in a poor prognosis. Clinically, patients present with fever, neck pain, restricted neck motion, and otalgia. Because the secondary abscesses lie deep to the superficial fascial planes surrounding the sternocleidomastoid and trapezius muscles, the contours of the fluctuant soft tissue mass may be difficult to palpate.[29]

On CT, one can identify unilateral opacification of the middle ear and mastoid cavities, often associated with bone erosion, especially of the mastoid tip (Fig. 13A). The abscess involves the adjacent musculature surrounding the mastoid and extends inferiorly (Fig. 13B).[25,30] Surrounding the abscess, one may see obliteration of the fat planes, reticulation of the subcutaneous tissues, and thickening of the overlying skin.

OTHER PATHOLOGIES
Foreign Body Ingestion

Among other complications, inadvertent swallowing of foreign objects may also result in retropharyngeal space infections, most notably retropharyngeal abscess formation. Nearly 80% of all swallowed pharyngeal and esophageal foreign bodies take place in the pediatric population.[31] However, adult patients who are stuperous, senile, or have psychiatric illness are also prone to swallowing a variety of foreign objects including animal bones and dentures. These objects are usually lodged in areas of normal anatomic narrowing in the cricopharyngeus area, the aortic arch, or the distal esophagus. Sharp objects may perforate the pharynx or esophagus and migrate along tissue planes and

compartments, which may result in abscess formation in the adjacent spaces such as the retropharyngeal space.

Children present clinically with respiratory distress, drooling, or regurgitation, but adults usually present with pain and dysphagia. Senile, psychiatric, or stuperous patients may present late with evidence of fever or sepsis.

Noncontrast CT of the neck may be performed to confirm the presence or absence of an ingested foreign body. Contrast-enhanced CT demonstrates the site and level of the resultant inflammation or abscess. Frequently, gas translucencies are detected within the retropharyngeal space. MR imaging is seldom used for foreign body ingestion as it cannot define reliably the presence of foreign body or gas collections.[3]

Calcific Tendinitis

Calcific tendinitis is a benign inflammatory condition that may mimic infectious pathology of the neck. Calcific tendinitis is caused by deposition of hydroxyapatite in the tendon fibers of the longus colli muscles.[32] Patients present clinically with either sudden onset or subacute pain in the neck and throat worsened by head movement and swallowing.[33] Due to its rare occurrence, it is often mistaken clinically for traumatic injury, retropharyngeal abscess, or infectious spondylitis, causing patients to frequently undergo unnecessary tests and treatment. The condition, however, is self-limited and resolves after 1 to 2 weeks on calcium resorption.

Lateral neck radiography may show extensive soft tissue swelling between C1 through C4 with amorphous calcific deposits anterior to C1 and C2.[34] Likewise, CT imaging may demonstrate the

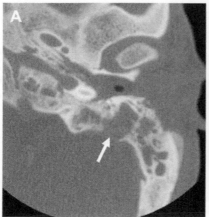 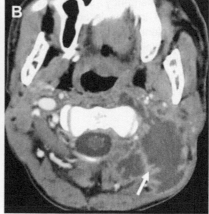

Fig. 13. **Bezold abscess.** (*A*) Axial contrast-enhanced CT shows opacification of the mastoid air cells with associated bone erosion indicating an aggressive inflammatory process. (*B*) The soft tissue algorithm demonstrates a multiloculated abscess involving the paraspinal musculature.

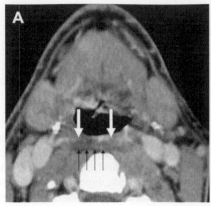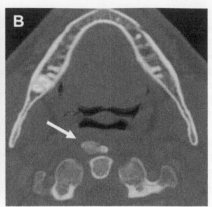

Fig. 14. Calcific tendinitis. (*A*) Axial contrast-enhanced CT of the neck demonstrates retropharyngeal space edema (*large arrows*). Note the preservation of the alar fascia (*small arrows*), which indicates that the low attenuation is edema and not an abscess. (*B*) The bone algorithm shows an ossific mass anterior to the dens, confirming that the edema in the retropharyngeal space is due to calcific tendinitis.

same findings along with prevertebral edema, an image finding that must be distinguished from that found within retropharyngeal space infection (**Fig. 14**).

Though typically unnecessary for diagnosis, MR imaging demonstrates a signal void anterior to C1 and C2 representing an amorphous calcification. In addition, MR may demonstrate marrow edema in adjacent vertebrae.[3]

IMAGING MODALITIES FOR NECK INFECTION

The range of inflammatory and infectious processes of the neck is diverse, requiring a thorough appreciation for neck anatomy as well as the appropriate imaging modalities to investigate such pathology. In the emergency setting, timely interpretation of these images is critical to the care of acutely ill patients, especially those with a threatened airway. While plain film, ultrasonography, and MR imaging play a part in the investigation of inflammatory and infectious pathology of the neck, cross-sectional imaging with CT plays a central role.

REFERENCES

1. Randall TD, Carrhager DM, Rangel-Moreno J. Development of secondary lymphoid organs. Annu Rev Immunol 2008;26:627–50.
2. Long SS, Pickering LK, Prober CG. Principles and practice of pediatric infectious diseases. 3rd edition. Philadelphia: Churchill Livingstone; 2008.
3. Mukherji SK, Chong V. Atlas of head and neck imaging: the extracranial head and neck. New York: Thieme; 2004.
4. Peters T, Edwards K. Cervical lymphadenopathy and adenitis. Pediatr Rev 2000;21:399–404.
5. Murray DL. Infectious diseases. In: Rudolph CD, Rudolph AM, Hostetter MK, et al, editors. Rudolph's pediatrics. 21st edition. New York (NY): The McGraw-Hill Companies Inc; 2003. p. 867–1165.
6. Baker CJ. Group B streptococcal cellulitis-adenitis in infants. Am J Dis Child 1982;136(7):631–3.
7. Dajani AS, Garcia RE, Wolinski E. Etiology of cervical lymphadenitis in children. N Engl J Med 1963;268:1329.
8. Schweinfurth J. Demographics of pediatric head and neck infections in a tertiary care hospital. Laryngoscope 2006;116(6):887–9.
9. Bass JW, Vincent JM, Person DA. The expanding spectrum of Bartonella infections II: Cat-scratch disease. Pediatr Infect Dis J 1997;16:163–79.
10. Heyman DL. Control of communicable diseases manual. 19th edition. Washington, DC: American Public Health Association Press; 2008. p. 98.
11. Frieden TR, Sterling TR, Munsiff SS, et al. Tuberculosis. Lancet 2003;362:887.
12. Menon K, Bem C, Gouldesbrough D, et al. A clinical review of 128 cases of head and neck tuberculosis presenting over a 10-year period in Bradford, UK. J Laryngol Otol 2007;121(4):362–8.
13. Hanck C, Fleisch F, Katz G. Imaging appearance of nontuberculous mycobacterial infection of the neck. AJNR Am J Neuroradiol 2004;25(2):349–50.
14. Branstetter BF, Weissman JL. Infection of the facial area, oral cavity, oropharynx, and retropharynx. Neuroimaging Clin N Am 2003;13:393–410.

15. Hurley MC, Heran MK. Imaging studies for head and neck infections. Infect Dis Clin North Am 2007;21: 305–53.

16. Djupesland P. Necrotizing fasciitis of the head and neck: report of three cases and review of the literature. Acta Otolaryngol 2000;543:186–9.

17. Weed HG, Forest LA. Deep neck infection. In: Cummings CW, Flint PW, Harker LA, et al, editors Otolaryngology: head and neck surgery, vol. 3. 4th edition. Philadelphia: Elsevier Mosby; 2005. p. 2515–24.

18. Marple, BF. Ludwig angina: a review of current airway management. Arch Otolaryngol Head Neck Surg 1999;125(5):600.

19. Bross-Soriano D, Arrieta-Gomez J, Prado-Calleros H, et al. Management of Ludwig's angina with small neck incisions: 18 years experience. Otolaryngol Head Neck Surg 2004;130(6):712–7.

20. Brook I. Microbiology and management of peritonsillar, retropharyngeal, and parapharyngeal abscesses. J Oral Maxillofac Surg 2004;62(12): 1545–50.

21. Craig FW, Schunk JE. Retropharyngeal abscess in children: clinical presentation, utility of imaging, and current management. Pediatrics 2003;111(6): 1394–8.

22. Steyer TE. Peritonsillar abscess: diagnosis and treatment. Am Fam Physician 2002;65(1):937–96.

23. Belleza WG, Kalman S. Otolaryngologic emergencies in the outpatient setting. Med Clin North Am 2006;90(2):329–53.

24. Johnson RF, Stewart MG. The contemporary approach to diagnosis and management of peritonsillar abscess. Curr Opin Otolaryngol Head Neck Surg 2005;13(3):157–60.

25. Glynn F, Skinner LJ, Riley N, et al. Parapharyngeal abscess in an insulin dependent diabetic patient following an elective tonsillectomy. J Laryngol Otol 2007;121(9):e16.

26. Page C, Biet A, Zaatar R, et al. Parapharyngeal abscess: diagnosis and treatment. Eur Arch Otorhinolaryngol 2008;265:681–6.

27. Smouha EE, Levenson MJ, Anand VK, et al. Modern presentations of Bezold's abscess. Arch Otolaryngol Head Neck Surg 1989;115:1126–9.

28. Miller LG, Perdreau-Remington F, Rieg G, et al. Necrotizing fasciitis caused by community-associated methicillin-resistant Staphylococcus aureus in Los Angeles. N Engl J Med 2005;352:1445–53.

29. Castillo M, Albernaz VS, Mukherji SK, et al. Imaging of Bezold's abscess. AJR Am J Roentgenol 1998; 171:1491–5.

30. Gaffney RJ, O'Dwyer TP, Maguire AJ. Bezold's abscess. J Laryngol Otol 1991;105:765–6.

31. Digoy GP. Diagnosis and management of upper aerodigestive tract foreign bodies. Otolaryngol Clin North Am 2008;41(2):485–96.

32. Vieira F, Allen SM, Stocks RM, et al. Deep neck infection. Otolaryngol Clin North Am 2008;41: 459–83, vii.

33. Eastwood JD, Hudgins PA, Malone D. Retropharyngeal effusion in acute calcific prevertebral tendinitis: diagnosis with CT and MR imaging. AJNR Am J Neuroradiol 1998;19:1789–92.

34. Haun CL. Retropharyngeal tendinitis. AJR Am J Roentgenol 1978;130:1137–40.

Pediatric Central Nervous System Emergencies

Sanjay P. Prabhu[a,b] and Tina Young-Poussaint[a,b,*]

KEYWORDS

• Pediatric • Neurologic • Emergencies • MRI • CT • Brain

This article summarizes current state-of-the-art techniques used in the management of pediatric neurologic emergencies. Solutions to challenges faced by the radiologist, including the selection of an appropriate modality for an individual patient, are discussed. Imaging appearances of specific entities are described with an emphasis on conditions unique to the pediatric population.

SPECIAL CHALLENGES IN IMAGING THE PEDIATRIC PATIENT

Neuroimaging of the pediatric patient presenting to the emergency department is most often indicated for evaluating the child who is comatose or obtunded; has a change in neurologic status; presents with prolonged seizures; or suffers the neurologic consequences of a traumatic, infectious/inflammatory, vascular, or metabolic abnormality.

Among the challenges faced by the clinician and radiologist in this situation is the need to decide (1) whether imaging is required emergently, (2) which imaging modality is most appropriate for a particular clinical indication, and (3) whether the available imaging techniques must be modified to ensure a speedy and accurate diagnosis. In addition, there are certain characteristic findings on imaging studies in pediatric patients that deserve special mention.

This review aims to address the neuroimaging issues typically encountered in central nervous system (CNS) emergencies involving the pediatric patient, with illustrative examples and a discussion of the various imaging modalities.

HOW DOES EMERGENCY NEUROIMAGING OF THE ADULT DIFFER FROM THAT OF THE PEDIATRIC PATIENT?

Whereas the adult brain is fully formed from a structural and functional standpoint, the pediatric brain (neonate to young adult) follows a steady and predictable course of development and maturation over the course of approximately 20 years, depending on the individual. Hence, the radiologist's ability to perform and interpret neuroimaging studies in the infant, child, adolescent, and young adult hinges largely on knowledge of normal brain development, an understanding of the biologic and morphologic changes that take place from gestation through adolescence, familiarity with age-specific diagnoses, and a grasp of the specific normative appearances that characterize each stage of development.

It is also well known that the pediatric patient shows greater short- and long-term sensitivity to radiation than the adult patient.[1] In particular, the potential for ionizing radiation (eg, that produced by radiographs and computed tomography [CT]) to harm children, especially those for whom serial imaging may be necessary, forms an especially important consideration when selecting the most appropriate imaging modality in the emergency department. Other factors in selecting the

[a] Department of Radiology, Harvard Medical School, 25 Shattuck Street, Boston, MA 02115, USA
[b] Department of Radiology, Children's Hospital Boston, 300 Longwood Avenue, Boston, MA 02115, USA
* Corresponding author. Department of Radiology, Children's Hospital Boston, 300 Longwood Avenue, Boston, MA 02115.
E-mail address: tina.poussaint@childrens.harvard.edu

Neuroimag Clin N Am 20 (2010) 663–683
doi:10.1016/j.nic.2010.07.008

modality include the availability of equipment, the need for sedation or general anesthesia, and the clinical status of the child. For example, although magnetic resonance imaging (MRI) is ideally suited for evaluating a comatose child, CT or ultrasonography (US) may be considered adequate if the child is clinically unstable and would benefit from the rapid image acquisition and attendant diagnostic information generated by these modalities. When time and circumstances permit, the radiologist may decide to defer the study until the child is stabilized and a more definitive examination can be obtained.

Finally, except in instances of severe illness, cognitive impairment, or dementia, the adult patient is generally able to understand and cooperate with the goals of a neuroimaging study. In contrast, the pediatric patient's ability in this regard depends on his or her developmental stage, on the amount of pain or distress caused by the pathology under investigation, and on the environment in which the study is undertaken.

These factors, separately and in combination, form the decision-making matrix for selecting the most appropriate neuroimaging modality for the pediatric patient in the setting of the emergency department.

NEUROIMAGING TECHNIQUES
Plain Radiographs

Very few indications remain for performing plain radiographs to evaluate the neuraxis in the acutely ill child in the emergency department. Plain radiographs, however, continue to have a role in documenting fractures of the skull and appendicular skeleton in the suspected child abuse victim, but this is usually done after transfer from the emergency department and therefore will not be discussed further in this review. Plain radiographs remain the primary method for visualizing the entire cervical spine in children with traumatic injuries. In most children, anteroposterior and lateral spine radiographs suffice to clear the spine following trauma. The false negative rate for the single cross-table lateral view ranges between 21% and 26%.[2,3] A 3-view series can improve sensitivity to 94% in children.[4] More recent studies suggest that the open-mouth odontoid view is routinely beneficial only in children older than 5 years.[5]

Some investigators have argued that multislice CT with sagittal and coronal reformats may be required in the obtunded patient to clear the cervical spine.[6] At our institution, we reserve focused CT and MRI to clarify areas of abnormality and to define further injuries.[7]

Ultrasound

Ultrasound (US) has numerous imaging advantages, including ready access, portability, real-time and multiplanar capabilities, and reproducible results. Moreover, it is a noninvasive, radiation-free procedure that can be performed at the bedside, in the intensive care unit, or on an intubated, ventilated baby following delivery. Ultrasonography is also useful in evaluating hydrocephalus, extra-axial fluid collections, and large intracranial hemorrhages in the young infant who is too ill to be transported to CT or MRI. Further, transcranial Doppler techniques have been used to correlate resistive indices with elevated intracranial pressure in patients with head trauma.[8]

Computed Tomography

The widespread availability and speed of image acquisition has made CT the neuroimaging modality of choice in the acutely ill child over the past 2 decades.[9] CT can detect acute intracranial hemorrhage, cerebral edema, hypoxic-ischemic injury, infarction, hydrocephalus/shunt dysfunction, neoplasm, or abnormal collections. In addition, modern multidetector CT scanners can acquire submillimeter-thick images, which can be manipulated to produce multiplanar reformats and 3-dimensional (3D) images, thereby facilitating rapid detection of skull and facial fractures. When performed with iodinated contrast media, CT provides information about both inflammatory and infectious lesions and their resultant complications.

CT angiography (CTA) provides accurate information for a variety of arterial and venous abnormalities in the acute setting. CTA also compares favorably with MR angiography (MRA) in evaluating vertebral artery dissection, as shown in a number of adult studies.[10,11] CT venography (CTV) is the initial study of choice in many centers for assessing cerebral venous sinus thrombosis. Further, in evaluating the child presenting after major trauma, multidetector CT (MDCT) has shown great utility in imaging the head, cervical spine, chest, abdomen, pelvis, and, where applicable, the appendicular skeleton.

The primary disadvantage of CT is that it requires the use of ionizing radiation, which can have potentially harmful effects on the tissues of the pediatric patient, particularly if used for multiple studies over the course of weeks, months, or years. It is, therefore, imperative that alternatives to CT be considered in making the diagnosis. When CT is chosen as the imaging modality for a child, the radiologist should follow the ALARA (as low as reasonably acceptable) principle, which entails using appropriate age- and weight-based dose adjustment parameters available on modern scanners. In addition, the scan should be strictly limited to the area of concern.[12]

Magnetic Resonance Imaging

The multiplanar capability of MR to show superior anatomic detail and tissue contrast without the harmful effects of ionizing radiation makes it the imaging modality of choice for evaluating the neuraxis in children of all ages presenting with acute neurologic symptoms in the emergency department. MRI is superior to CT in evaluating the posterior fossa and in detecting early cerebral edema and microhemorrhages. Further, MRI can provide functional and physiologic information about the brain that cannot be generated by other modalities. Use of higher field strengths (most commonly 3-Tesla MRI scanners) has also demonstrated improved diagnostic accuracy for many conditions affecting the CNS.[13]

Advanced MR imaging sequences, including susceptibility-weighted imaging (SWI), diffusion-weighted and diffusion-tensor imaging (DWI and DTI), magnetic resonance spectroscopy (MRS), and perfusion imaging, including arterial spin labeling (ASL), are being increasingly incorporated into acute pediatric neuroimaging protocols.

Susceptibility-weighted imaging
SWI imaging uses the paramagnetic property of blood products and increases visibility of microhemorrhages by accentuating signal dropout by rapid spin dephasing. It has been shown to be more sensitive than conventional MRI in detecting intraparenchymal blood products after traumatic brain injury in children (Fig. 1). The technical aspects of SWI and its role in the detection of venous thrombosis, intracerebral hemorrhage, and vascular malformations have been described in a number of original studies and reviews.[14] SWI has several advantages over conventional gradient-echo sequences, including its potential ability to differentiate between hemorrhage and calcium, as well as its ability to visualize vessel connectivity and microbleed location in relation to the vasculature and other structures in the brain.[15] Methods for evaluating the arterial and venous systems simultaneously at higher field strengths (3 T and higher) using postcontrast SWI sequences have also been described.[16] By optimizing the flip angle and echo times, the arterial and venous circulations can be separately visualized on maximum and minimum intensity projections.[17] The value of this method has not yet been fully evaluated in children.

Diffusion-weighted imaging and diffusion tensor imaging
DWI is being increasingly used in the acutely ill child for early detection of ischemia, differentiating between infectious and inflammatory collections, and predicting of outcome in traumatic brain injury (TBI).[18] The most common cause of decreased diffusion is ischemia, although it is important to remember that decreased diffusion can be seen in cellular tumors, abscesses, encephalitis, TBI,

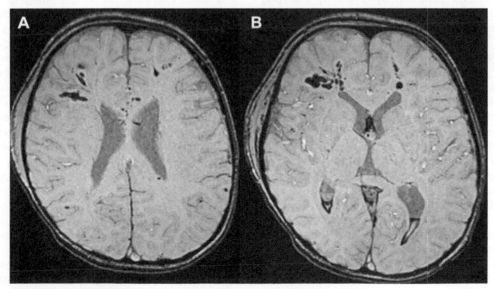

Fig. 1. **Traumatic axonal injury.** 5-year-old child status-post blunt head trauma. Note the multiple foci of hemorrhage within the white matter depicted on SWI images (A, B).

edema caused by astrocyte swelling in metabolic disorders, and in areas of intracerebral hemorrhage. The main advantage of DWI in acute brain injury is that the decrease in apparent diffusion coefficient (ADC) can be appreciated within minutes to hours following the insult. This information is vital to planning therapies for acute stroke and for initiating interventions that are neuroprotective, eg, hypothermia induction in hypoxic-ischemic injury and severe TBI.

DTI provides visualization of fiber bundle direction and integrity with in vivo characterization of the rate and direction of white matter diffusion. In the normal brain, water diffusion is restricted to the axis parallel in the direction of the axons. This property is termed "anisotropy." The proportion of the diffusion tensor that is attributable to anisotropy is termed "fractional anisotropy" (FA). A decrease in FA in the setting of trauma has been shown to indicate white matter damage. By placing regions of interest over specific tracts, valuable information can be gained about the disruption caused to various white matter networks in the setting of acute brain injury.[19–21] The role of DTI in defining the diagnosis, management, and prognosis of children with acute brain injury is being currently investigated.[22,23] Early results indicate a significant decrease of FA in young children with TBI in the genu of the corpus callosum and internal capsules, and that differences in white matter integrity in children after early TBI may persist for several years.[24]

Perfusion imaging

MR perfusion imaging is a technique used to evaluate cerebral perfusion dynamics by analyzing hemodynamic parameters including relative cerebral blood volume, relative cerebral blood flow (CBF), and transit time. It can be performed with a T2*-weighted dynamic susceptibility technique, ASL, or a T1-weighted dynamic contrast-enhanced perfusion technique. We reserve the use of perfusion imaging in the emergency setting at present to the evaluation of new tumors. The feasibility and utility of ASL perfusion MRI for characterizing alterations of CBF in pediatric patients with arterial stroke and other neurologic emergencies are being actively investigated.[25] The short acquisition time, lack of ionizing radiation, widespread availability of MRI scanners, and ability to detect small regional hemodynamic alterations make perfusion techniques a potentially attractive technique to consider in the critically ill neonate.[26,27]

Magnetic resonance spectroscopy

MRS has been used as a noninvasive in vivo technique that measures concentrations of various compounds within a sampled region in the brain to provide metabolic diagnostic indices beyond anatomic information. Its role has been documented in acute ischemic injury, metabolic disorders, and differentiation between abscesses and tumors. An early report indicated that MRS can have a role in differentiating between tumefactive demyelination and neoplastic lesions.[28] More recently, it has been suggested that MRS shows some promise as a quantitative outcome-prediction tool in the subacute phase of TBI.[23] The utility of MRS in making prognoses has not yet been established sufficiently to advocate its use in all routine MRI brain studies performed in the acutely injured pediatric patient.[29]

Magnetic Resonance Angiography and Magnetic Resonance Venography

Magnetic resonance angiography (MRA) has shown considerable utility in the emergency setting for assessing aneurysms and arteriovenous malformations in patients presenting with intracranial hemorrhage, and in identifying dissections of the vertebral and internal carotid arteries following trauma. Recent studies have shown that, in some cases, 2D time-of-flight MRA may not be as sensitive as conventional angiography for detecting vertebral or internal carotid artery dissection in children; however, it is used successfully as an initial screening tool.[30]

MRI with magnetic resonance venography (MRV) is the imaging study of choice in older children being evaluated for dural venous sinus thrombosis owing to their relatively clinically stable condition and their tolerance for longer imaging times compared with infants and toddlers. In addition, MRI/MRV can characterize associated parenchymal lesions without the use of ionizing radiation. One potential pitfall of MRV in neonates, however, is the increased flow gaps in the venous sinuses, particularly affecting the posterior aspect of the superior sagittal sinus, which can be attributed to the age-related smaller caliber of the sinus, smaller venous flow, and skull molding.[31,32] At our institution, postcontrast, 3D, fast spoiled gradient-echo images (3D-FSPGR) have proved especially useful in cases where MRV is equivocal, or is affected by slow flow, in veins proximal to thrombus.

ETIOPATHOLOGY OF NEUROLOGIC EMERGENCIES IN A CHILD

The differential diagnoses in the child considered for emergent neuroimaging can be roughly divided into the following groups, as shown in Table 1. These groups are specific to (1) the

Table 1
Pediatric Central Nervous System Emergencies: Brain
Acute Hydrocephalus
Trauma
Accidental
Nonaccidental
Non-traumatic vascular events
Arterial ischemic stroke
Venous thrombosis
Embolic stroke
Vasculitis
Dissection
Migraine
Hypoxic-ischemic injury
Strangulation
Cardiorespiratory insufficiency
Near-drowning
Electrolyte and hormonal imbalances
Hypoglycemia
Hyponatremia
Hypocalcemia
First-time seizure and status epilepticus
Infection
Congenital
Acquired
Complications and sequelae
Demyelination
Acute disseminated encephalomyelitis (ADEM)
Multiple sclerosis (MS)
Metabolic disease (acute presentation)
Iatrogenic, toxic and drug-related injury
L-asparaginase
Cyclosporine
Methotrexate
Recreational drugs
Carbon monoxide
Neoplastic disease (acute presentation)
Encephalopathy in hematologic and oncologic disease
Posterior reversible encephalopathy (PRES)
Posttransplant lymphoproliferative disorder (PTLD)

pediatric patient, (2) the imaging features of the suspected or known condition, and (3) the diagnostic algorithms that are selected in performing the examination. The pediatric patient differs significantly from the adult patient who may present with a similar pathology, and these differences are presented in the remainder of this article.

HYDROCEPHALUS
Acute Hydrocephalus

Hydrocephalus can be caused by either overproduction of cerebrospinal fluid (CSF) by a tumor such as choroid plexus papilloma, by an obstruction to normal CSF flow, or by decreased CSF absorption. The latter 2 problems result in "obstructive hydrocephalus." Obstructive hydrocephalus can be further divided into *communicating* hydrocephalus, where there is obstruction to CSF flow or diminished CSF absorption, and *noncommunicating* hydrocephalus, where there is intraventricular obstruction to CSF flow. More recent classifications that are based on the effect of pressure-flow derangements in CSF dynamics within the circuit diagram of CSF flow are designed to serve as a template for the study, nomenclature, and treatment of hydrocephalus.[33]

In the emergency setting, there are 2 common scenarios that often warrant imaging: (1) the child with shunted hydrocephalus, and (2) the acute presentation of noncommunicating hydrocephalus.

Child with Shunted Hydrocephalus

The child with known shunted hydrocephalus can present with nausea, vomiting, irritability, fever, altered level of consciousness, or increased seizure frequency. Papilledema, cranial nerve palsies, hyperactive reflexes, and ataxic gait may be found on examination. Infants may present with increased head circumference, a bulging fontanelle, or splayed cranial sutures. Neurosurgical consultation is mandatory if shunt malfunction is clinically suspected.

Ultrasound can be considered in the young infant with large, open fontanelles in this setting. However, in most cases, CT is the modality of choice because of its ready availability, ability to detect changes in ventricular size and configuration, easy identification of intracranial hemorrhage or infarction, shunt catheter discontinuity in the skull and upper neck, and catheter migration.

A low-dose CT technique can be used to minimize radiation risks in these patients, especially those in whom multiple CT scans are required over their life span. Several authors have shown that there is no significant loss in diagnostic accuracy when such techniques are used in this clinical setting.[34,35]

At our institution, a limited axial T2-weighted MRI in an imaging plane similar to that used in prior CT studies is used. This approach offers an attractive imaging alternative for the stable, older child who can lie still for a few minutes in the MR scanner. With the increased availability of MRI, and the advent of faster pulse sequences and motion correction software, hydrocephalus may also be safely and reliably assessed in younger patients without the need for sedation, while being spared the potentially harmful effects of ionizing radiation.

When evaluating a CT in a child with hydrocephalus, comparison with a baseline study obtained after successful shunt placement and serial prior scans can help detect subtle evidence of shunt malfunction. A single shunt may fail in patients with multiple shunts, and comparison with prior studies is essential to determine which shunt is malfunctioning. Ultrasound or MRI examinations performed since the prior CT must be reviewed to avoid errors that result from a failure to recognize changes that may have occurred in the interval between the 2 CTs.

In the patients with suspected shunt malfunction, a plain radiograph shunt series is often performed to differentiate between obstruction and other causes of mechanical shunt malfunction including catheter fracture. It is important not to mistake the radiolucent areas between the intermittent radiopaque markers seen in some shunts for areas of discontinuity. Shunt mechanism disconnection occurs most commonly at the level of the valve where the proximal and distal tubing meet. The actual fracture of the catheter tubing, however, usually occurs in the neck, likely resulting from its increased mobility.[36,37]

Abdominal ultrasound and/or CT may be useful in determining the presence of ascites or an intra-abdominal mass such as a large CSF pseudocyst. In some cases, shunt malfunction may not always cause absolute or relative ventriculomegaly. CT scans performed in children experiencing true shunt malfunction may be normal, have stable ventriculomegaly, or even show decreased ventricular size compared with prior studies.[38] Neurosurgical consultation is mandatory if shunt malfunction is clinically suspected, despite normal imaging.

Acute Presentation of Noncommunicating Hydrocephalus

Noncommunicating hydrocephalus is caused by intraventricular obstruction of CSF flow. Obstruction sites are most commonly located where the CSF pathway is narrowest, namely at the foramen of Monro, cerebral aqueduct, and fourth ventricle and its outflow foramina. In the child, tumors are a common cause of such obstruction.[39]

Tumors obstructing the foramina of Monro can involve the lateral ventricles (eg, choroid plexus tumors, astrocytomas, and ependymomas) or extend anteriorly from the third ventricle (eg, astrocytomas, choroid plexus tumors, and craniopharyngiomas) (Fig. 2). Similarly, third ventricle

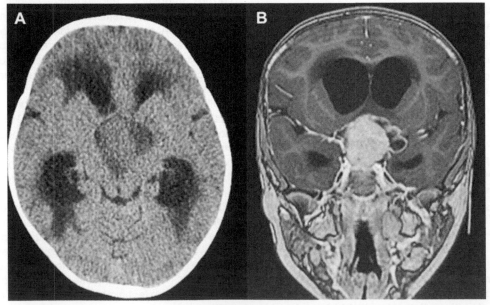

Fig. 2. Optic glioma. 2-year-old girl presenting with sixth nerve palsy. Axial noncontrast CT (A) shows obstructive hydrocephalus, and a large mass filling the third ventricle. On postcontrast T1-weighted MRI (B), the macrolobulated heterogeneously enhancing suprasellar tumor involves the optic pathway and hypothalamus.

tumors can extend posteriorly and inferiorly to obstruct the cerebral aqueduct. Most commonly, aqueductal obstruction is the result of a pineal region tumor including pineal origin tumors; germ cell tumors; astrocytomas arising from the tectal plate, thalamus, or quadrigeminal plate; or tentorial meningiomas and vein of Galen malformations. In patients with tuberous sclerosis, subependymal giant cell tumors originating in the region of the foramen of Monro can grow to obstruct the lateral ventricles.

Posterior fossa tumors in the pediatric population include the medulloblastoma, pilocytic astrocytoma, ependymoma, and, occasionally, cerebellar hemangioblastoma. Lesions of this type can cause fourth ventricle or aqueductal obstruction either by tumor extension into the ventricle, or by extrinsic compression of the ventricular walls.

MRI is the imaging modality of choice in these cases, although CT can identify many of these lesions as an initial screen in the emergency room and can demonstrate hydrocephalus. Though rare, primary and secondary (leptomeningeal metastases) tumors in the spine and spinal cord can cause hydrocephalus. The spine should therefore be imaged in all cases of new-onset unexplained hydrocephalus.

Non-neoplastic causes of noncommunicating hydrocephalus include arachnoid cysts, aqueductal stenosis, aqueductal webs, and congenital anomalies such as Chiari malformations. A discussion of these entities is beyond the scope of this article. In our experience, the 3D FIESTA (fast-imaging employing steady-state acquisition) sequence can play a useful role in evaluating new-onset hydrocephalus. This technique enables detection of arachnoid cysts and septations within the ventricles, and it can help confirm patency of the aqueduct. In some cases of Chiari 1 malformation, a phase contrast, velocity-encoded CSF flow study may also demonstrate CSF flow aberrations at the foramen magnum, eg, decreased flow posterior to the cerebellar tonsils.

Communicating Hydrocephalus (Extraventricular Obstruction to CSF Flow)

Extraventricular obstruction to CSF may result from intracranial hemorrhage, bacterial or granulomatous meningitis, CSF seeding of tumor, venous hypertension, or normal pressure hydrocephalus. Some of these entities are discussed in other parts of this article and in other articles in this issue: "Hemorrhagic Stroke and Nontraumatic Intracranial Hemorrhage," "Central Nervous System Infections," and "Intracranial Hypo- and Hypertension."

NONACCIDENTAL TRAUMA/CHILD ABUSE

Child abuse is a global problem, with head trauma being the leading cause of morbidity and mortality in abused children younger than 2 years. Nonaccidental injury is a leading cause of brain injury in infants, and is associated with high morbidity (up to 45%) and mortality (6%–26%).[40] Nonaccidental injury should be suspected in the infant or young child who presents with the following[41]:

- When there is no history of injury
- When there is a discrepancy between the explanation and nature of lesions
- When there are injuries of various ages
- When there are multiple injuries
- When there are associated retinal hemorrhages
- When there is a change or inconsistency in the history, delay in medical care, repeated injuries, or overall poor care.

The initial presentation varies from an impaired level of consciousness with significant neurologic damage to a child with relatively minor symptoms. The neuroimaging findings in these patients also vary, ranging from skull fractures to extra-axial hemorrhages, with or without concomitant brain parenchymal injury.

The decision to perform acute neuroimaging in the child who presents in the emergency department with suspected abuse is difficult at best. Clinicians agree that neuroimaging must be performed in all children with overt neurologic symptoms, but for those without obvious CNS involvement, the decision is less clear. Some investigators suggest, however, that even children without apparent neurologic signs or symptoms, but who present with other signs of physical abuse, may have intracranial injury and benefit from neuroimaging.[40]

Currently, CT is the recommended initial imaging modality for detection of acute blood and fractures in pediatric patients suspected of abuse. Multiplanar reformatting of MDCT images can help identify small extra-axial and parenchymal contusions. Further, 3D reformats can also increase the ability of CT to detect skull fractures and differentiate fractures from normal variants.

Recent literature suggests that MRI (including DWI, MRS, and T2* and/or SWI imaging) should promptly follow the initial CT.[40] MRI is the modality of choice for determining the sequelae of injury, which can include small extra-axial hemorrhages, brain contusions, shear injury, and infarction that may be difficult to identify on CT. Indeed, additional significant or evolving abnormalities are found on MRI in up to 25% of patients with an abnormal early CT examination.[42] The SWI sequence (described earlier in this article) obtained on higher field strength magnets has also increased the sensitivity of MRI for the detection and differentiation of subarachnoid blood from extra-axial blood.[43]

DWI is invaluable in this scenario, as it identifies hypoxic–ischemic injury in the first few hours after the trauma, and it is more accurate and sensitive in detecting hypoxic injury earlier than CT.[40] MRI with diffusion has demonstrated increased sensitivity in the early detection of injury in children with nonaccidental head trauma.[44] In addition to the well-described findings of extra-axial hemorrhage, global or focal ischemia, and skull fractures in these infants, more recent findings that support inflicted trauma include a small subdural hematoma with a disproportionately larger area of underlying unilateral hemispheric white matter edema (Fig. 3). One group has suggested that this may be a sign of head injury related to abuse, arising specifically from cervical vascular compression, whether from kinking during hyperflexion/hyperextension, or from direct strangulation.[45] Follow-up imaging in these cases demonstrated extensive cortical infarction. The role of MRI/DWI in children with a normal early CT, and the optimal timing of MRI/DWI after early CT in patients with suspected nonaccidental trauma, have not yet been fully determined, however.

In the setting of trauma, including nonaccidental trauma, some authors have reported elevated lactate, reduced N-acetyl aspartate, and elevations in choline-related compounds on MRS, which indicated poor outcome.[15,46]

SEIZURES

Approximately one-third of children in studies from emergency departments evaluated for a "first" seizure will be recognized as having epilepsy.[47] The routine practice of obtaining brain CT scans for all patients with new-onset afebrile seizures has been shown to be of low yield.[47] CT identifies clinically relevant abnormalities in 7% to 24% of children, but alters immediate medical management in only a minority of cases.[47–52]

A detailed clinical history and physical examination can identify patients for whom an emergent CT scan is likely to be appropriate. Prolonged seizures with focal onset and focal neurologic deficits are indicators of focal pathology and warrant emergent imaging. In all other cases, referral to a pediatric neurologist is recommended for a detailed neurologic examination and electroencephalogram (EEG). In this setting, imaging is aimed at detecting acute processes that warrant urgent intervention, and in subacute or chronic processes that warrant further workup. Examples of findings in children presenting with seizures that need urgent intervention include acute hydrocephalus, acute stroke or hemorrhage, encephalitis, and space-occupying neoplastic lesions. Examples of other relevant findings with important diagnostic or prognostic implications include the leukodystrophies, metabolic disorders, mesial temporal sclerosis, and malformations of cortical development.

IMAGING OF CENTRAL NERVOUS SYSTEM INFECTIONS

CNS infections can cause significant mortality and morbidity in children. When a child presents with fever and alteration in mental status, the possibility of CNS infection is high on the list of differential diagnoses. In the emergency setting, neuroimaging can play an important role in clearly diagnosing infectious lesions of the brain and spine and the complications of these infections. Although we continue to rely on CSF analysis, laboratory findings, and, in selected cases, biopsy results to identify the infective agent, characterizing typical lesion patterns can help the clinician come to a rapid and accurate diagnosis and make subsequent therapeutic decisions.

Bacterial Meningitis and Meningoencephalitis

CT findings are usually normal in the early phase of meningitis. Contrast-enhanced CT may show early leptomeningeal enhancement, which becomes more pronounced in the later stages of the disease. Repeat CT may be considered in patients with persistent drowsiness and meningeal signs to rule out obstructive hydrocephalus.

The diagnostic yield of MRI in cases of uncomplicated bacterial meningitis is low.[53] It is important to note, however, that although MRI characterizes leptomeningeal enhancement in many cases, absence of enhancement *does not* preclude the diagnosis of meningitis. Imaging studies can also help in detecting causes of meningitis. For example, CT can identify fractures and infections of the paranasal sinus, petrous temporal bone, middle ear, and mastoid air cells, which can spread by direct extension into the brain. Dermal sinus tracts may be the primary

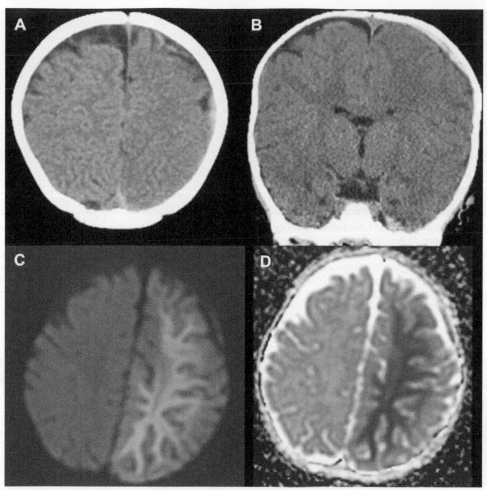

Fig. 3. Nonaccidental trauma. 7-month-old boy with a reported history of mild head trauma presenting with vomiting. There is a very small left subdural hemorrhage with underlying edema in the left cerebral hemisphere seen on axial (*A*) and coronal reformatted (*B*) CT. Restricted diffusion on trace (*C*) and ADC maps (*D*) in the left cerebral hemisphere is out of proportion to the size of subdural hemorrhage.

source of infection affecting the meninges, leading to intracranial complications (Fig. 4).[53] The primary role of imaging in meningitis is to aid in the detection of the various complications that can arise from the brain infection (Fig. 5). These include cerebritis, abscess formation, infarcts, subdural empyema, and epidural abscess. DWI is extremely important in diagnosing these complications.[54] DWI can indicate the presence of infected material within extra-axial collections, differentiate between vascular and cytotoxic edema, and help identify early cerebritis and small abscess cavities. T1 and T2 FLAIR hyperintensity may be seen as a result of protein or pus accumulation in the CSF spaces. The role of imaging in brain abscess and extra-axial collections in patients with meningitis is discussed in the following sections.

Pyogenic Cerebral Abscess

Brain abscess is defined as a focal suppurative process within the brain parenchyma. This diagnosis should be considered in the setting of new-onset acute headaches or first-time seizure, especially when fever and focal neurologic signs are present on examination. In the neonate with brain abscess, a bulging fontanelle and a rapid increase in head circumference may be the presenting features.

Intraparenchymal abscesses have central T2 prolongation and T1 hyperintensity and demonstrate enhancement of the margins of the lesion following gadolinium-based contrast administration. Contrast-enhanced images also aid in identifying additional smaller lesions. DWI and MR spectroscopy can be helpful in cases in which it

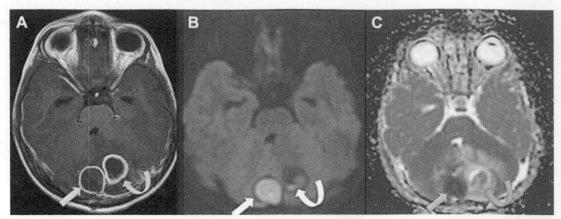

Fig. 4. Cerebellar abscess and infected dermoid cyst. 4-year-old girl presenting with intermittent fever and headaches. Postcontrast T1-weighted image (*A*) demonstrates 2 rounded posterior fossa hypointense lesions with peripheral rim enhancement. On trace diffusion (*B*) and ADC maps (*C*), there is restricted diffusion within both lesions and surrounding white matter edema. The more posterior extra-axial lesion (*straight arrow*) is an infected dermoid cyst. The intraparenchymal lesion within the left cerebellar hemisphere, adjacent to the occipital dermoid, is a cerebellar abscess (*curved arrow*) with surrounding edema and mass effect on the fourth ventricle.

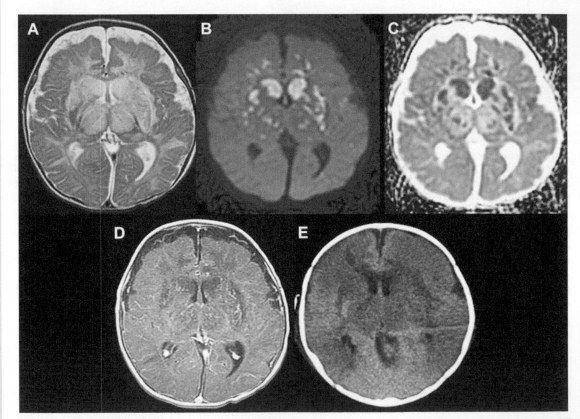

Fig. 5. Pneumococcal meningitis. 4-month-old child presenting with seizures. There is T2 prolongation on axial T2-weighted images (*A*) and extensive areas of restricted diffusion on trace diffusion (*B*) and ADC maps (*C*) involving the periventricular white matter, thalami, and basal ganglia. On postcontrast T1-weighted imaging (*D*), there is enhancement of the leptomeninges and the deep gray matter structures. Axial CT (*E*) obtained 4 days later demonstrates bilateral hypodensities in the basal ganglia, thalami, and frontal and temporal lobes consistent with cerebral infarcts.

is difficult to differentiate a brain abscess from a tumor, and may potentially differentiate between fungal and bacterial sources.[55] DWI is considered the method of choice to accurately differentiate between an abscess and a necrotic tumor, and must be performed in all cases of suspected CNS infection (see **Fig. 4**B). Virtually all pyogenic abscesses demonstrate decreased ADC values, indicating restricted water diffusion compared with nonpyogenic lesions.[55]

In select cases, additional information can be obtained from MRS. The presence of lactate, acetate, and succinate originating from the enhanced glycolysis and fermentation of the infecting microorganisms and amino acids (eg, alanine, glycine, valine, and leucine) that are end products of enzyme proteolysis, are released by neutrophils in pus and can be regarded as an MRS marker for abscess.[56]

Subdural and Epidural Empyema

CT can identify these extra-axial collections as a fluid collection that is slightly hyperdense compared with CSF; however, it is not always possible to define the exact location and nature of the collection. On MRI, empyemas are mildly hyperintense relative to CSF on T1-weighted images, hyperintense relative to CSF and white matter on T2-weighted images, and show peripheral enhancement after gadolinium administration. Presence of displaced dura, seen as a hypointense rim between the lesion and brain, is suggestive of an epidural empyema. Surrounding white matter edema, mass effect, and cortical signal changes can be seen. DWI can be used to confirm that the extra-axial collection represents an empyema and typically demonstrates restricted diffusion. Subdural hygromas or effusions without enhancement may be seen in some cases. These usually resolve spontaneously without specific therapeutic intervention, but must be differentiated from subdural empyemas that demand more aggressive management. Attention should be paid to the bone adjacent to subdural empyemas to detect early osteomyelitis, as this often necessitates a longer course of antibiotic therapy.

Vascular Complications of Bacterial Meningitis

Focal arterial or venous infarcts may be seen on cross-sectional studies in patients with meningitis. Contrast-enhanced CT venography, which will show a filling defect within the affected sinus and may show hemorrhagic infarcts, is a useful modality to diagnose dural venous sinus thrombosis. MR venography and MRA can also be added to conventional MRI sequences to detect dural venous sinus thrombosis, cortical vein thrombus, or arterial thrombus.

Other Complications

In cases of pneumococcal meningitis, high-resolution postcontrast imaging of the temporal bones can help detect labyrinthitis, and in the subacute stage, CT and MRI can detect early labyrinthitis ossificans.

Viral Meningoencephalitis

Herpes simplex virus (HSV) type 1 remains the most common cause of viral encephalitis.[53] In recent years, however, other viruses such as Epstein-Barr virus (EBV), influenza viruses, and locale-specific viruses such as West Nile virus and Eastern equine encephalitis have been identified in the pediatric population in the United States. The list of potential agents is even broader in the immunocompromised child.

MRI can detect changes in viral encephalitis early in the course of disease. In neonates with herpes simplex encephalitis (HSE), the medial temporal and inferior frontal lobes are typically spared and the condition is usually nonhemorrhagic. Patchy periventricular white matter, low attenuation on CT, and corresponding T2 hyperintensity is seen on MRI. Mild meningeal enhancement may be seen in a small number of cases.[57]

Although some older children and young adults with HSE can have normal MRI scans, the vast majority show signal abnormality in the inferomedial temporal lobes. The imaging findings in HSE are the result of edema, hemorrhage, and necrosis seen on pathology. The distribution of disease in the inferomedial temporal lobes and insular cortex is supportive of route of entry into the brain along small branches of the trigeminal nerve. When findings are bilateral, they are usually asymmetric.[57] Signal changes may also be seen in the limbic system and insular cortex, and less frequently in the cingulate gyrus, basal ganglia, and parietooccipital cortex.[58] Petechial hemorrhage is typical in HSE in older children and young adults, seen as T1 hyperintensity or low signal intensity blooming on T2* or SWI sequences. Cortical hemorrhage may be seen in the acute stage, characterized by gyriform, linear T1 hyperintensities. DWI is shown to be more sensitive than either T2-weighted or FLAIR imaging in early detection of the cytotoxic edema. Although the foci of T2 prolongation persist, the DWI changes disappear over the following 10 to 14 days. In some cases, atrophy of the white matter or progressive ventricular enlargement may be evident on follow-up studies.

Eastern equine encephalitis (EEE) can resemble HSV encephalitis clinically and on electroencephalography, but early and predominant basal ganglia and thalamic involvement in EEE may be helpful in differentiating the 2 conditions (Fig. 6).[59]

Fungal Infections

Fungal CNS infection is rare in the immunocompetent child. In children undergoing chemotherapy for hematological or oncologic malignancy, fungal meningitis or meningoencephalitis must be considered especially, in the presence of systemic infection by a particular agent (eg, Candida).

Cerebellitis

Acute cerebellitis is a rare inflammatory syndrome, usually in early childhood, characterized by cerebellar dysfunction that presents following an infection or vaccination. Presentation may include truncal ataxia, dysmetria, and headache. Although most cases of acute cerebellitis are benign without significant sequelae, in some cases it can result in severe cerebellar atrophy, and on rare occasion, it can be fulminant and result in sudden death. Early on in the acute phase, CT is useful in detecting acute hydrocephalus, cerebellar edema, or brainstem compression. MRI, however, is the modality of choice to assess the posterior fossa. The most common findings on MRI are bilateral diffuse cerebellar hemispheric T2 and FLAIR hyperintensities (Fig. 7).[60] Involvement of a single hemisphere is

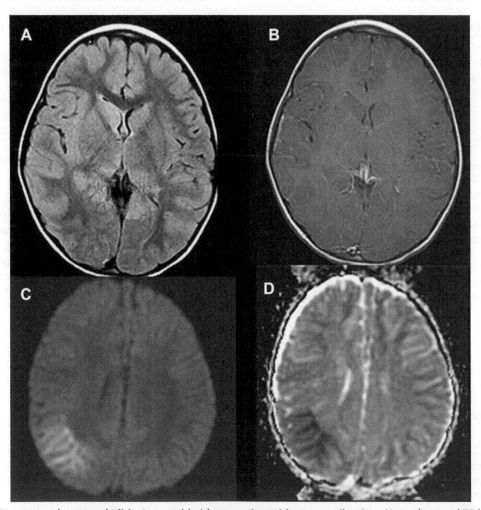

Fig. 6. **Eastern equine encephalitis.** 3-year-old girl presenting with status epilepticus. Note abnormal T2 hyperintensity in the basal ganglia and thalamus on FLAIR imaging (*A*). Postcontrast T1-weighted images show subtle leptomeningeal enhancement (*B*). Diffusion imaging demonstrates an area of decreased diffusion (*C, D*) indicating an infarct, which is an unusual complication in this condition.

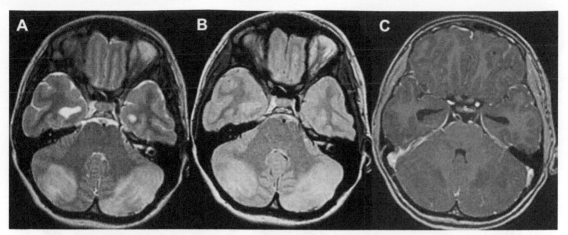

Fig. 7. Acute cerebellitis. 12-year-old girl presenting with headache, vomiting, and diplopia. T2 and FLAIR images (A, B) reveal abnormal bilateral hyperintensity in the cerebellar hemispheres. There is enlargement of the cerebellum and effacement of the fourth ventricle with resultant hydrocephalus. Note the lack of contrast enhancement on the postcontrast T1-weighted image (C).

rarely seen. Leptomeningeal enhancement is seen in the vast majority of patients following contrast administration. DWI in cerebellitis may be helpful in detecting early changes when conventional MRI is normal.[61] The differential diagnosis of acute cerebellitis includes acute disseminated encephalomyelitis (ADEM), Lhermitte-Duclos disease (LDD), diffusely infiltrating glioma or lymphoma, vasculitis, and posterior reversible encephalopathy syndrome (PRES).

Acute Disseminated Encephalomyelitis, Clinically Isolated Syndrome, and Neuromyelitis Optica

Definitions and clinical features
ADEM is defined as the first episode of inflammatory demyelination associated with multifocal neurologic deficits with involvement of multiple sites in the CNS and accompanied by encephalopathy (defined as altered behavior or consciousness). Use of this precise definition is aimed at avoiding the tendency to apply the term ADEM to any child with acute demyelination accompanied by multifocal MRI lesions.[62] ADEM is more common in children younger than 10 years old. It may be preceded by infectious symptoms or history of immunization, although a specific pathogen is rarely implicated. It is classically considered to be an acute, monophasic illness, although not all symptoms and deficits occur contemporaneously. New deficits within 3 months of onset are considered to be part of the same acute episode.

Clinically isolated syndrome (CIS) refers to the first neurologic episode that lasts at least 24 hours, and is caused by inflammation/demyelination at one or more sites in the CNS, but without associated encephalopathy. It can be monofocal, ie, affecting a localized part of the CNS (eg, optic neuritis, transverse myelitis) or multifocal.

Neuromyelitis optica (NMO) is characterized by sequential or concomitant optic neuritis and transverse myelitis, although the spectrum of disease has been expanded to include patients with encephalopathy, seizures, intractable vomiting, and brainstem-mediated hiccups. NMO is more common in nonwhite children and may be associated with systemic autoimmune disease. The presence in serum of antibodies directed against aquaporin 4 (NMO-IgG) appears to be moderately sensitive and very specific to pediatric NMO, particularly relapsing NMO.[62]

Imaging features of ADEM, CIS, and NMO
Imaging findings of ADEM are not specific and typically do not allow differentiation of ADEM from multiple sclerosis (MS) or encephalitis. CT is usually nondiagnostic, although faint hypodensities may be seen if the lesions are large. Characteristic MRI findings include multiple, asymmetrically distributed, poorly defined, foci of hyperintensity on T2 and FLAIR sequences (Fig. 8). Lesions are usually not conspicuous on unenhanced T1-weighted images, except in cases of large lesions, which may be T1 hypointense. Contrast enhancement is variable, although most lesions of ADEM do not enhance. If contrast enhancement is

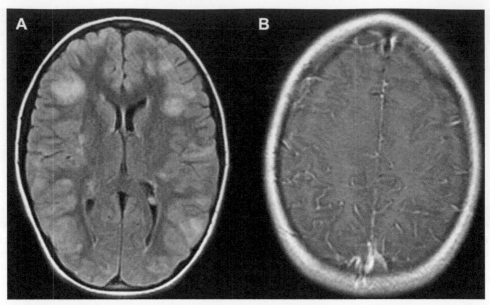

Fig. 8. **Acute disseminated encephalomyelitis (ADEM).** 9-year-old girl presenting with acute ataxia and diplopia 1 week after presumed viral meningitis. Axial FLAIR imaging demonstrates multiple hyperintense foci in the subcortical and deep white matter (A). Subtle leptomeningeal enhancement is present on the postcontrast T1-weighted image (B).

present, it is seen in most of the lesions simultaneously. Multiple lesions involving the white matter and the deep gray matter nuclei (ie, thalamus and basal ganglia) may also be seen. The cerebral cortex may be involved in up to 30% patients.[63] The brainstem, middle cerebellar, peduncle, and cerebellum may also be involved.

Because the imaging features of CIS and NMO overlap with ADEM, the distinction must be based on clinical assessment.

ADEM versus Multiple Sclerosis

Additional ADEM episodes occur rarely and tend to happen in 2 contexts: recurrent ADEM and multiphasic ADEM. Meningismus, fever, and seizures are more commonly seen in ADEM. The outcome after ADEM is favorable, with a complete recovery expected in approximately 70% of cases. An ADEM-like, first demyelinating event can also be the first attack of MS.

The diagnosis of MS in children is based on clinical evidence of a second demyelinating event involving new areas of the CNS. Thus, to diagnose pediatric MS, international consensus definitions require an initial ADEM event followed by 2 subsequent non-ADEM demyelinating events. Another distinction between ADEM and MS is that there is complete, or near-complete, resolution of lesions in ADEM on repeat MRI, whereas follow

up imaging of MS usually demonstrates new, often asymptomatic, lesions.[62]

Presence of well-defined lesions perpendicular to corpus callosum (Dawson's fingers) have been found 100% specific for MS during the first episode of demyelination.[64] More recently, studies have defined new MRI criteria for pediatric MS that warrant further validation. These studies suggest fewer total T2 lesions (≥ 5 vs ≥ 9) are required to identify children with MS with a high sensitivity (94%).[65] Modification of the McDonald criteria to 2 or more lesions in the periventricular region is also considered more sensitive for pediatric MS, while maintaining high specificity. Brainstem lesions are also considered as a more specific criterion for diagnosis of MS in children than the broad category of infratentorial lesions.[66] The value of contrast administration in distinguishing MS from ADEM in children is not yet clear. Further, many features of MS in children are similar to those that characterize MS in adults, although important distinctions may also be noted. Currently, there are no absolute clinical features or radiological, serum, or CSF biomarkers that can distinguish ADEM from pediatric MS.[62]

When demyelinating disease manifests as a single large, or "tumefactive," demyelinating lesion within a cerebral hemisphere in the absence of history of MS, the correct diagnosis is often not made until after surgical biopsy or resection (Fig. 9).

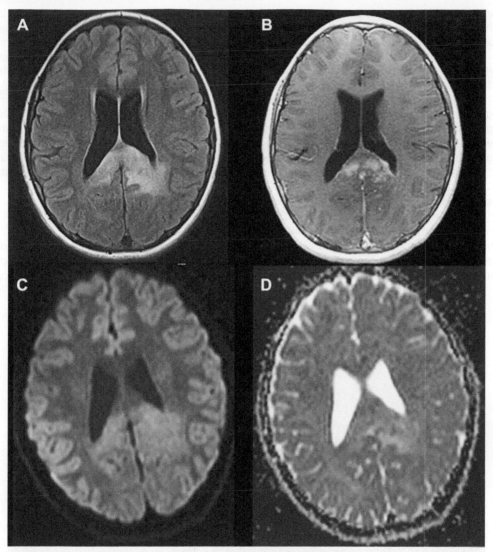

Fig. 9. **Tumefactive demyelination (biopsy-proven).** 12-year-old boy presenting with first-time seizure and right-sided weakness. There is increased T2/FLAIR signal in a thickened splenium of the corpus callosum (A) and patchy enhancement on postcontrast T1-weighted images (B). The trace diffusion (C) and ADC map images (D) demonstrate mild restricted diffusion in the lesion.

ACUTE PRESENTATION OF NEUROMETABOLIC DISEASE

The clues that an acute encephalopathy is the result of an inborn error of metabolism include the following:

1. Acute onset without forewarning in a previously healthy child
2. Progressive and rapid worsening of neurologic symptoms
3. No association, usually, with focal neurologic deficit

4. Initial behavioral disturbance followed by deterioration.

Infants with acute encephalopathy are usually healthy at birth and become ill in the first few days to weeks after birth. Feeding problems, lethargy, irritability, and vomiting usually precede onset of encephalopathy, characterized by decreasing consciousness and/or seizures. Acidosis, hyperammonemia, and tachypnea may also be present. This presentation can be confused, however, with acute infection, hypoxic-ischemic injury, and the sequel of congenital cardiac anomalies. For example, early-onset mitochondrial disease can closely mimic hypoxic-ischemic encephalopathy both clinically and on imaging studies. In such cases, laboratory studies often help in identifying the inborn error of metabolism. In addition, neuroimaging can provide corroborative evidence in making a firm diagnosis, aid in narrowing the list of differential diagnoses, and furnish information leading to the selection of the most appropriate test or tests for follow-up and treatment.

The concept of regional selective vulnerability to toxins and ischemia and the specific cell type injured by the accumulation or deficiency of a metabolite accounts for some of characteristic imaging patterns of damage in these disorders. Patterns of damage from hypoxia or metabolic decompensation can vary with the degree of brain maturation.

DWI and MRS are often useful in narrowing the list of differential diagnoses in acutely ill patients with suspected neurometabolic disorders, and therefore, must be performed in all cases where there is a possibility of a neurometabolic disease. MRS is useful in identifying neonates and children with certain inborn errors of metabolism. For example, N-acetylaspartic acid (NAA) is elevated in children with Canavan disease (Fig. 10), whereas elevated lactate may be a marker for mitochondrial disorders. Many excellent reviews address neurometabolic disorders in children in further detail.[67]

ACUTE PRESENTATION OF NEOPLASTIC LESIONS IN CHILDREN

Intracranial neoplasms usually have a subacute and progressive onset, or may present with episodic seizures. On occasion, however, they may present

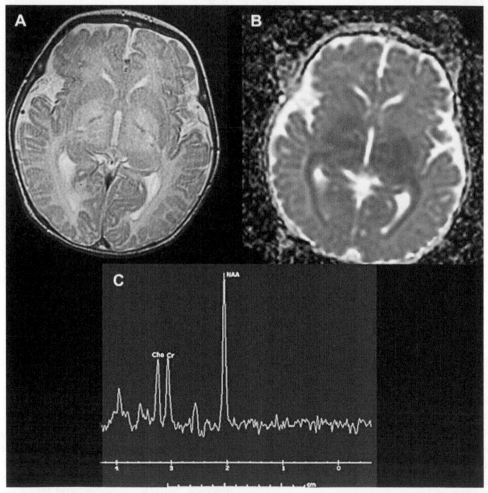

Fig. 10. **Canavan disease.** 5-week-old boy presenting with seizures. Note the T2 prolongation (A) and restricted diffusion on the axial ADC map (B) in the white matter and deep gray nuclei. MR spectroscopy demonstrates a markedly increased NAA peak (C).

acutely with obstructive hydrocephalus, and as previously mentioned, with raised intracranial pressure, seizures, or focal neurologic deficits.

Perilesional edema, intralesional hemorrhage or necrosis into a tumor, or hydrocephalus may be a precipitating event (Fig. 11). In children with pre-existing lesions, changes in tumor characteristics related to radiation or chemotherapy can result in sudden changes in tumor volume and internal architecture. In the acute setting, a noncontrast CT scan may be performed as the initial investigation to achieve rapid screening. If there are signs of acute obstructive hydrocephalus on the CT, emergent, neurosurgical management is imperative as sudden death as a result of cerebral herniation can result in these cases. Obstructive hydrocephalus that is attributable to tumors has been discussed earlier in this article.

After necessary neurosurgical management has been performed, MRI helps delineate the exact size and extent of tumor to aid in tumor diagnosis and surgical planning. Postcontrast imaging of the spine must be considered to identify drop metastases and leptomeningeal seeding, which can have an adverse effect on CSF flow dynamics, and in turn, cause obstructive hydrocephalus.

NEUROLOGIC EMERGENCIES IN CHILDREN WITH ONCOLOGIC DISEASE

Children with systemic cancer are at risk for neurologic disorders that affect normal children, but they are also susceptible to CNS metastases, treatment-related complications of medical and surgical therapy, and paraneoplastic disorders. Unlike adults, headaches and seizures are common presentations of these disorders.[68]

Posterior Reversible Encephalopathy

Posterior reversible leukoencephalopathy (PRES) is an uncommon, but serious, complication of treatment in children with cancer, seen predominantly in patients with leukemia and non-Hodgkin lymphoma. These patients typically have risk factors such as hypertension, and in the setting of prolonged exposure to remission-induction chemotherapy and/or tacrolimus, children may be predisposed to PRES.[69] In addition, PRES may be seen with cyclosporine A therapy after transplantation. These children present with acute neurologic symptoms such as headache, visual disturbance, seizure, or loss of consciousness. Neuroimaging holds the key to accurate and rapid diagnosis in these cases. MRI findings include vasogenic edema, seen predominantly in the white matter of the cerebral hemispheres, especially involving the bilateral parietooccipital regions. Signal abnormalities in the frontal and inferior temporo-occipital junction, brainstem, and cerebellum may be variably involved (Fig. 12). The areas involved are characterized by hyperintensity on T2-weighted and FLAIR images and hypointensity on T1-weighted images. There is *increased*

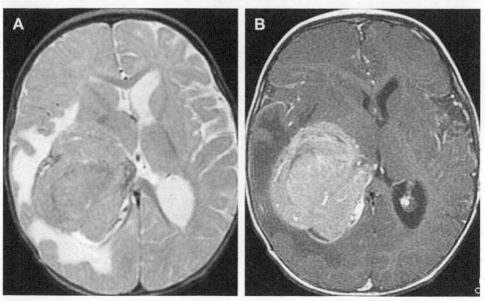

Fig. 11. **Choroid plexus papilloma.** 7-month-old boy presenting with left hemiparesis. There is a large, predominantly T2 intermediate signal intensity mass in the right cerebral hemisphere arising from the choroid plexus with surrounding white matter edema in the region of the right lateral ventricle (*A*). Heterogeneous enhancement within the lesion is noted on the postcontrast T1-weighted image (*B*).

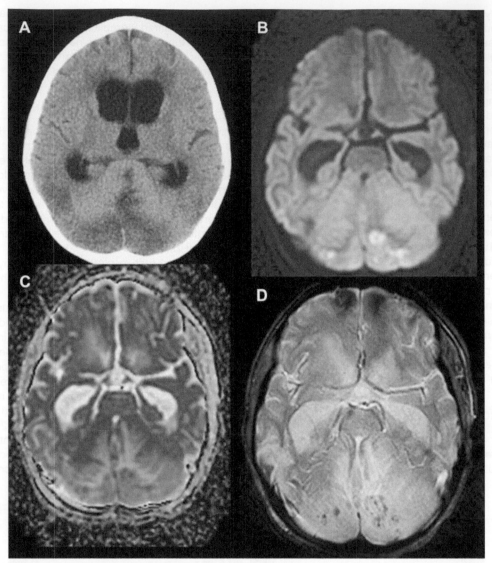

Fig. 12. **Posterior reversible encephalopathy syndrome.** 10-year-old girl status-post bone marrow transplantation for acute lymphocytic leukemia presenting with loss of consciousness and asymmetric pupils. Parietooccipital low density and marked mass effect in the cerebellum and compression of the fourth ventricle is seen on the noncontrast CT (*A*). There is a combination of increased and restricted foci of diffusion in the cerebellum on the trace diffusion and ADC maps (*B, C*), with the foci of decreased diffusion corresponding to multiple small foci of hemorrhage in the cerebellum on the axial gradient-echo sequence (*D*).

diffusion in affected regions in the vast majority of cases, suggesting presence of vasogenic edema. Focal decreased diffusion may be seen in some areas in a small proportion of patients (11% to 26% in adult studies) and there may be hemorrhage in up to 17% of lesions.[70–72] Small pediatric studies suggest a greater prevalence of "atypical" features of PRES in children including chronic clinical sequelae, residual abnormalities seen on MRI, localization-related epilepsy, and persistent abnormal EEG results without further seizure activity.[69,73]

Intracranial vasospasm has been postulated as a pathophysiologic mechanism for the findings and this may be seen on conventional and MR angiography.[71] Sequelae include permanent neurologic deficits, cerebral infarcts, hemorrhage, and even death in untreated cases.

Imaging Goals in Pediatric Patients with Neurologic Emergencies

This article addresses some of the clinical and imaging issues specific to imaging the pediatric patient presenting with a potential neurologic emergency. The challenge faced by the radiologist and emergency medicine specialist lies chiefly in optimizing the use of advanced imaging techniques in the acutely ill pediatric patient to ensure appropriate management. Imaging also must be aimed at obtaining a baseline for follow-up and correlating findings at presentation with structural and functional imaging studies performed in the months and years following the acute presentation.

REFERENCES

1. Brenner DJ, Hall EJ. Computed tomography—an increasing source of radiation exposure. N Engl J Med 2007;357(22):2277–84.

2. Baker C, Kadish H, Schunk JE. Evaluation of pediatric cervical spine injuries. Am J Emerg Med 1999;17(3):230–4.

3. Blahd WH Jr, Iserson KV, Bjelland JC. Efficacy of the posttraumatic cross table lateral view of the cervical spine. J Emerg Med 1985;2(4):243–9.

4. Yngve DA, Harris WP, Herndon WA, et al. Spinal cord injury without osseous spine fracture. J Pediatr Orthop 1988;8(2):153–9.

5. Swischuk LE, John SD, Hendrick EP. Is the open-mouth odontoid view necessary in children under 5 years? Pediatr Radiol 2000;30(3):186–9.

6. Hutchings L, Atijosan O, Burgess C, et al. Developing a spinal clearance protocol for unconscious pediatric trauma patients. J Trauma 2009;67(4):681–6.

7. Proctor MR. Spinal cord injury. Crit Care Med 2002;30(Suppl 11):S489–99.

8. Visocchi M, Chiaretti A, Genovese O, et al. Haemodynamic patterns in children with posttraumatic diffuse brain swelling. A preliminary study in 6 cases with neuroradiological features consistent with diffuse axonal injury. Acta Neurochir (Wien) 2007;149(4):347–56.

9. Kuppermann N. Pediatric head trauma: the evidence regarding indications for emergent neuroimaging. Pediatr Radiol. 2008;38(Suppl 4):S670–4.

10. Lum C, Chakraborty S, Schlossmacher M, et al. Vertebral artery dissection with a normal-appearing lumen at multisection CT angiography: the importance of identifying wall hematoma. AJNR Am J Neuroradiol 2009;30(4):787–92.

11. Vertinsky AT, Schwartz NE, Fischbein NJ, et al. Comparison of multidetector CT angiography and MR imaging of cervical artery dissection. AJNR Am J Neuroradiol 2008;29(9):1753–60.

12. Frush DP, Frush KS. The ALARA concept in pediatric imaging: building bridges between radiology and emergency medicine: consensus conference on imaging safety and quality for children in the emergency setting, Feb. 23-24, 2008, Orlando, FL—Executive Summary. Pediatr Radiol. 2008;38 (Suppl 4):S629–32.

13. Zimmerman RA, Bilaniuk LT, Pollock AN, et al. 3.0 T versus 1.5 T pediatric brain imaging. Neuroimaging Clin N Am 2006;16(2):229–39, ix.

14. Haacke EM, Mittal S, Wu Z, et al. Susceptibility-weighted imaging: technical aspects and clinical applications, part 1. AJNR Am J Neuroradiol 2009; 30(1):19–30.

15. Ashwal S, Babikian T, Gardner-Nichols J, et al. Susceptibility-weighted imaging and proton magnetic resonance spectroscopy in assessment of outcome after pediatric traumatic brain injury. Arch Phys Med Rehabil. 2006;87(12 Suppl 2): S50–8.

16. Du YP, Jin Z, Hu Y, et al. Multi-echo acquisition of MR angiography and venography of the brain at 3 Tesla. J Magn Reson Imaging 2009;30(2):449–54.

17. Barnes SR, Haacke EM. Susceptibility-weighted imaging: clinical angiographic applications. Magn Reson Imaging Clin N Am 2009;17(1):47–61.

18. Galloway NR, Tong KA, Ashwal S, et al. Diffusion-weighted imaging improves outcome prediction in pediatric traumatic brain injury. J Neurotrauma 2008;25(10):1153–62.

19. Le Bihan D, Mangin JF, Poupon C, et al. Diffusion tensor imaging: concepts and applications. J Magn Reson Imaging 2001;13(4):534–46.

20. Hagmann P, Jonasson L, Maeder P, et al. Understanding diffusion MR imaging techniques: from scalar diffusion-weighted imaging to diffusion tensor imaging and beyond. Radiographics. 2006;26 (Suppl 1):S205–23.

21. Kumar R, Husain M, Gupta RK, et al. Serial changes in the white matter diffusion tensor imaging metrics in moderate traumatic brain injury and correlation with neuro-cognitive function. J Neurotrauma 2009; 26(4):481–95.

22. Levin HS, Wilde EA, Chu Z, et al. Diffusion tensor imaging in relation to cognitive and functional outcome of traumatic brain injury in children. J Head Trauma Rehabil 2008;23(4):197–208.

23. Tollard E, Galanaud D, Perlbarg V, et al. Experience of diffusion tensor imaging and 1H spectroscopy for outcome prediction in severe traumatic brain injury: preliminary results. Crit Care Med 2009;37(4): 1448–55.

24. Yuan W, Holland SK, Schmithorst VJ, et al. Diffusion tensor MR imaging reveals persistent white matter alteration after traumatic brain injury experienced during early childhood. AJNR Am J Neuroradiol 2007;28(10):1919–25.

25. Chen J, Licht DJ, Smith SE, et al. Arterial spin labeling perfusion MRI in pediatric arterial ischemic stroke: initial experiences. J Magn Reson Imaging 2009;29(2):282–90.

26. Wintermark P, Moessinger AC, Gudinchet F, et al. Temporal evolution of MR perfusion in neonatal hypoxic-ischemic encephalopathy. J Magn Reson Imaging 2008;27(6):1229–34.

27. Wintermark P, Moessinger AC, Gudinchet F, et al. Perfusion-weighted magnetic resonance imaging patterns of hypoxic-ischemic encephalopathy in term neonates. J Magn Reson Imaging 2008;28(4): 1019–25.

28. Cianfoni A, Niku S, Imbesi SG. Metabolite findings in tumefactive demyelinating lesions utilizing short echo time proton magnetic resonance spectroscopy. AJNR Am J Neuroradiol 2007;28(2): 272–7.

29. Greer DM. Multimodal magnetic resonance imaging for determining prognosis in patients with traumatic brain injury—promising but not ready for primetime. Crit Care Med 2009;37(4):1523–4.

30. Tan MA, DeVeber G, Kirton A, et al. Low detection rate of craniocervical arterial dissection in children using time-of-flight magnetic resonance angiography: causes and strategies to improve diagnosis. J Child Neurol 2009;24(10):1250–7.

31. Teksam M, Moharir M, Deveber G, et al. Frequency and topographic distribution of brain lesions in pediatric cerebral venous thrombosis. AJNR Am J Neuroradiol 2008;29(10):1961–5.

32. Widjaja E, Shroff M, Blaser S, et al. 2D time-of-flight MR venography in neonates: anatomy and pitfalls. AJNR Am J Neuroradiol 2006;27(9): 1913–8.

33. Rekate HL. A contemporary definition and classification of hydrocephalus. Semin Pediatr Neurol 2009; 16(1):9–15.

34. Udayasankar UK, Braithwaite K, Arvaniti M, et al. Low-dose nonenhanced head CT protocol for follow-up evaluation of children with ventriculoperitoneal shunt: reduction of radiation and effect on image quality. AJNR Am J Neuroradiol 2008;29(4): 802–6.

35. Rybka K, Staniszewska AM, Bieganski T. Low-dose protocol for head CT in monitoring hydrocephalus in children. Med Sci Monit. 2007;13(Suppl 1): 147–51.

36. Browd SR, Ragel BT, Gottfried ON, et al. Failure of cerebrospinal fluid shunts: part I: obstruction and mechanical failure. Pediatr Neurol 2006;34(2): 83–92.

37. Desai KR, Babb JS, Amodio JB. The utility of the plain radiograph "shunt series" in the evaluation of suspected ventriculoperitoneal shunt failure in pediatric patients. Pediatr Radiol 2007;37(5): 452–6.

38. Mater A, Shroff M, Al-Farsi S, et al. Test characteristics of neuroimaging in the emergency department evaluation of children for cerebrospinal fluid shunt malfunction. CJEM 2008;10(2):131–5.

39. Barkovich AJ. Pediatric neuroimaging. 4th edition. Philadelphia; London: Lippincott Williams & Wilkins; 2005.

40. Kemp AM, Rajaram S, Mann M, et al. What neuroimaging should be performed in children in whom inflicted brain injury (iBI) is suspected? A systematic review. Clin Radiol 2009;64(5):473–83.

41. Kleinman PK, Barnes PD. Diagnostic imaging of child abuse. 2nd edition. St. Louis (MO); London: Mosby; 1998.

42. Foerster BR, Petrou M, Lin D, et al. Neuroimaging evaluation of non-accidental head trauma with correlation to clinical outcomes: a review of 57 cases. J Pediatr 2009;154(4):573–7.

43. Tong KA, Ashwal S, Obenaus A, et al. Susceptibility-weighted MR imaging: a review of clinical applications in children. AJNR Am J Neuroradiol 2008;29(1): 9–17.

44. Suh DY, Davis PC, Hopkins KL, et al. Nonaccidental pediatric head injury: diffusion-weighted imaging findings. Neurosurgery 2001;49(2):309–18 [discussion: 318–20].

45. McKinney AM, Thompson LR, Truwit CL, et al. Unilateral hypoxic-ischemic injury in young children from abusive head trauma, lacking craniocervical vascular dissection or cord injury. Pediatr Radiol 2008;38(2):164–74.

46. Makoroff KL, Cecil KM, Care M, et al. Elevated lactate as an early marker of brain injury in inflicted traumatic brain injury. Pediatr Radiol 2005;35(7): 668–76.

47. Gaillard WD, Chiron C, Cross JH, et al. Guidelines for imaging infants and children with recent-onset epilepsy. Epilepsia 2009;50(9):2147–53.

48. Garvey MA, Gaillard WD, Rusin JA, et al. Emergency brain computed tomography in children with seizures: who is most likely to benefit? J Pediatr 1998;133(5):664–9.

49. Maytal J, Krauss JM, Novak G, et al. The role of brain computed tomography in evaluating children with new onset of seizures in the emergency department. Epilepsia 2000;41(8):950–4.

50. McAbee GN, Barasch ES, Kurfist LA. Results of computed tomography in "neurologically normal" children after initial onset of seizures. Pediatr Neurol 1989;5(2):102–6.

51. Sharma S, Riviello JJ, Harper MB, et al. The role of emergent neuroimaging in children with new-onset afebrile seizures. Pediatrics 2003;111(1):1–5.

52. Warden CR, Brownstein DR, Del Beccaro MA. Predictors of abnormal findings of computed tomography of the head in pediatric patients presenting with seizures. Ann Emerg Med 1997;29(4): 518–23.

53. Kastrup O, Wanke I, Maschke M. Neuroimaging of infections of the central nervous system. Semin Neurol 2008;28(4):511–22.

54. Jan W, Zimmerman RA, Bilaniuk LT, et al. Diffusion-weighted imaging in acute bacterial meningitis in infancy. Neuroradiology 2003;45(9):634–9.

55. Luthra G, Parihar A, Nath K, et al. Comparative evaluation of fungal, tubercular, and pyogenic brain abscesses with conventional and diffusion MR imaging and proton MR spectroscopy. AJNR Am J Neuroradiol 2007;28(7):1332–8.

56. Garg M, Gupta RK, Husain M, et al. Brain abscesses: etiologic categorization with in vivo proton MR spectroscopy. Radiology 2004;230(2):519–27.

57. Baskin HJ, Hedlund G. Neuroimaging of herpesvirus infections in children. Pediatr Radiol 2007;37(10): 949–63.

58. Wasay M, Mekan SF, Khelaeni B, et al. Extra temporal involvement in herpes simplex encephalitis. Eur J Neurol 2005;12(6):475–9.

59. Deresiewicz RL, Thaler SJ, Hsu L, et al. Clinical and neuroradiographic manifestations of eastern equine encephalitis. N Engl J Med 1997;336(26):1867–74.

60. De Bruecker Y, Claus F, Demaerel P, et al. MRI findings in acute cerebellitis. Eur Radiol 2004;14(8): 1478–83.

61. Matsukuma E, Kato Z, Orii K, et al. Acute mumps cerebellitis with abnormal findings in MRI diffusion-weighted images. Eur J Pediatr 2008;167(7):829–30.

62. Dale RC, Brilot F, Banwell B. Pediatric central nervous system inflammatory demyelination: acute disseminated encephalomyelitis, clinically isolated syndromes, neuromyelitis optica, and multiple sclerosis. Curr Opin Neurol 2009;22(3):233–40.

63. Dale RC, de Sousa C, Chong WK, et al. Acute disseminated encephalomyelitis, multiphasic disseminated encephalomyelitis and multiple sclerosis in children. Brain. 2000;123(Pt 12):2407–22.

64. Mikaeloff Y, Adamsbaum C, Husson B, et al. MRI prognostic factors for relapse after acute CNS inflammatory demyelination in childhood. Brain 2004;127(Pt 9):1942–7.

65. Banwell B, Shroff M, Ness JM, et al. MRI features of pediatric multiple sclerosis. Neurology 2007;68(16 Suppl 2):S46–53.

66. Callen DJA, Shroff MM, Branson HM, et al. MRI in the diagnosis of pediatric multiple sclerosis. Neurology 2009;72:961–7.

67. Blaser S, Feigenbaum A. A neuroimaging approach to inborn errors of metabolism. Neuroimaging Clin N Am 2004;14(2):307–29, ix.

68. Antunes NL, De Angelis LM. Neurologic consultations in children with systemic cancer. Pediatr Neurol 1999;20(2):121–4.

69. Morris EB, Laningham FH, Sandlund JT, et al. Posterior reversible encephalopathy syndrome in children with cancer. Pediatr Blood Cancer 2007;48(2): 152–9.

70. Covarrubias DJ, Luetmer PH, Campeau NG. Posterior reversible encephalopathy syndrome: prognostic utility of quantitative diffusion-weighted MR images. AJNR Am J Neuroradiol 2002;23(6): 1038–48.

71. Bartynski WS. Posterior reversible encephalopathy syndrome, part 2: controversies surrounding pathophysiology of vasogenic edema. AJNR Am J Neuroradiol 2008;29(6):1043–9.

72. McKinney AM, Short J, Truwit CL, et al. Posterior reversible encephalopathy syndrome: incidence of atypical regions of involvement and imaging findings. AJR Am J Roentgenol 2007;189(4): 904–12.

73. Lucchini G, Grioni D, Colombini A, et al. Encephalopathy syndrome in children with hemato-oncological disorders is not always posterior and reversible. Pediatr Blood Cancer 2008;51(5): 629–33.

Index

Note: Page numbers of article titles are in **boldface** type.

neuroimaging.theclinics.com

United States Postal Service

Statement of Ownership, Management, and Circulation
(All Periodicals Publications Except Requester Publications)

1. Publication Title	2. Publication Number	3. Filing Date
Neuroimaging Clinics of North America	0 1 0 - 5 4 8	9/15/10

4. Issue Frequency	5. Number of Issues Published Annually	6. Annual Subscription Price
Feb, May, Aug, Nov	4	$293.00

7. Complete Mailing Address of Known Office of Publication (Not printer) (Street, city, county, state, and ZIP+4®)

Elsevier Inc.
360 Park Avenue South
New York, NY 10010-1710

Contact Person
Stephen Bushing
Telephone (Include area code)
215-239-3688

8. Complete Mailing Address of Headquarters or General Business Office of Publisher (Not printer)

Elsevier Inc., 360 Park Avenue South, New York, NY 10010-1710

9. Full Names and Complete Mailing Addresses of Publisher, Editor, and Managing Editor (Do not leave blank)

Publisher (Name and complete mailing address)

Kim Murphy, Elsevier, Inc., 1600 John F. Kennedy Blvd. Suite 1800, Philadelphia, PA 19103-2899

Editor (Name and complete mailing address)

Joanne Husovski, Elsevier, Inc., 1600 John F. Kennedy Blvd. Suite 1800, Philadelphia, PA 19103-2899

Managing Editor (Name and complete mailing address)

Catherine Bewick, Elsevier, Inc., 1600 John F. Kennedy Blvd. Suite 1800, Philadelphia, PA 19103-2899

10. Owner (Do not leave blank. If the publication is owned by a corporation, give the name and address of the corporation immediately followed by the names and addresses of all stockholders owning or holding 1 percent or more of the total amount of stock. If not owned by a corporation, give the names and addresses of the individual owners. If owned by a partnership or other unincorporated firm, give its name and address as well as those of each individual owner. If the publication is published by a nonprofit organization, give its name and address.)

Full Name	Complete Mailing Address
Wholly owned subsidiary of	4520 East-West Highway
Reed/Elsevier, US holdings	Bethesda, MD 20814

11. Known Bondholders, Mortgagees, and Other Security Holders Owning or Holding 1 Percent or More of Total Amount of Bonds, Mortgages, or Other Securities. If none, check box. → ☐ None

Full Name	Complete Mailing Address
N/A	

12. Tax Status (For completion by nonprofit organizations authorized to mail at nonprofit rates) (Check one)
The purpose, function, and nonprofit status of this organization and the exempt status for federal income tax purposes:
☐ Has Not Changed During Preceding 12 Months
☐ Has Changed During Preceding 12 Months (Publisher must submit explanation of change with this statement)

PS Form 3526, September 2007 (Page 1 of 3 (Instructions Page 3)) PSN 7530-01-000-9931 PRIVACY NOTICE: See our Privacy policy in www.usps.com

---

13. Publication Title	14. Issue Date for Circulation Data Below
Neuroimaging Clinics of North America	August 2010

15. Extent and Nature of Circulation		Average No. Copies Each Issue During Preceding 12 Months	No. Copies of Single Issue Published Nearest to Filing Date
a. Total Number of Copies (Net press run)		2266	2166
b. Paid Circulation (By Mail and Outside the Mail)	(1) Mailed Outside-County Paid Subscriptions Stated on PS Form 3541. (Include paid distribution above nominal rate, advertiser's proof copies, and exchange copies)	1135	1064
	(2) Mailed In-County Paid Subscriptions Stated on PS Form 3541 (Include paid distribution above nominal rate, advertiser's proof copies, and exchange copies)		
	(3) Paid Distribution Outside the Mails Including Sales Through Dealers and Carriers, Street Vendors, Counter Sales, and Other Paid Distribution Outside USPS®	348	346
	(4) Paid Distribution by Other Classes Mailed Through the USPS (e.g. First-Class Mail®)		
c. Total Paid Distribution (Sum of 15b (1), (2), (3), and (4))	→	1483	1410
d. Free or Nominal Rate Distribution (By Mail and Outside the Mail)	(1) Free or Nominal Rate Outside-County Copies Included on PS Form 3541	96	72
	(2) Free or Nominal Rate In-County Copies Included on PS Form 3541		
	(3) Free or Nominal Rate Copies Mailed at Other Classes Through the USPS (e.g. First-Class Mail)		
	(4) Free or Nominal Rate Distribution Outside the Mail (Carriers or other means)		
e. Total Free or Nominal Rate Distribution (Sum of 15d (1), (2), (3) and (4))	→	96	72
f. Total Distribution (Sum of 15c and 15e)	→	1579	1482
g. Copies not Distributed (See instructions to publishers #4 (page #3))	→	687	684
h. Total (Sum of 15f and g)	→	2266	2166
i. Percent Paid (15c divided by 15f times 100)	→	93.92%	95.14%

16. Publication of Statement of Ownership

If the publication is a general publication, publication of this statement is required. Will be printed in the November 2010 issue of this publication. ☐ Publication not required

17. Signature and Title of Editor, Publisher, Business Manager, or Owner	Date
Stephen R Bushing Stephen R. Bushing – Fulfillment/Inventory Specialist	September 15, 2010

I certify that all information furnished on this form is true and complete. I understand that anyone who furnishes false or misleading information on this form or who omits material or information requested on the form may be subject to criminal sanctions (including fines and imprisonment) and/or civil sanctions (including civil penalties).

PS Form 3526, September 2007 (Page 2 of 3)

Moving?

Make sure your subscription moves with you!

To notify us of your new address, find your **Clinics Account Number** (located on your mailing label above your name), and contact customer service at:

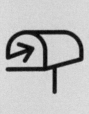

Email: journalscustomerservice-usa@elsevier.com

800-654-2452 (subscribers in the U.S. & Canada)
314-447-8871 (subscribers outside of the U.S. & Canada)

Fax number: 314-447-8029

Elsevier Health Sciences Division
Subscription Customer Service
3251 Riverport Lane
Maryland Heights, MO 63043

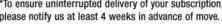

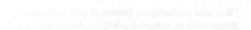

Printed and bound by CPI Group (UK) Ltd, Croydon, CR0 4YY

03/10/2024

01040351-0013